MEDITERRANEAN
COOKBOOK

800 Recipes to Discover the Famous European Diet for Healthy Eating and Staying in Shape

MARCO SALEMI

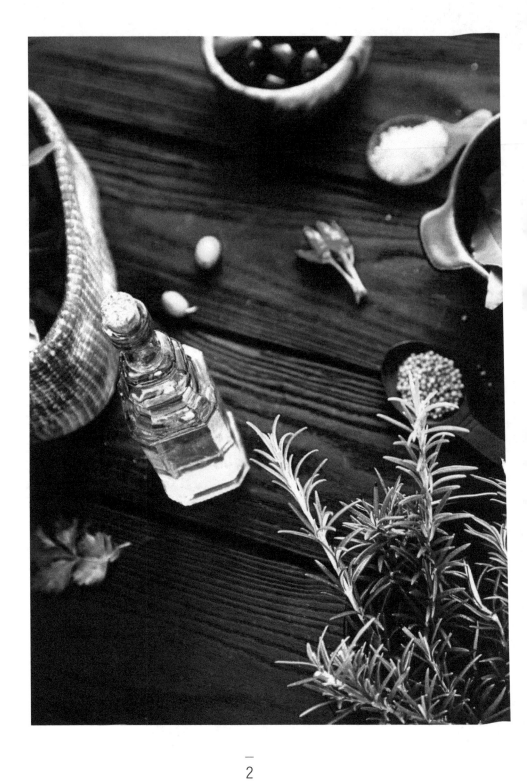

Table of Contents

Sommario

—

—

Introduction

The " Mediterranean diet " can be a generic term that supports the normal eating habits within the countries bordering the Mediterranean. There is no standard Mediterranean diet. A minimum of 16 countries borders the Mediterranean. Eating styles vary between these countries and also between regions within each country due to differences in culture, ethnicity, religion, economy, geography, and agricultural production. However, there are some common factors.

A Mediterranean-style diet typically includes:

lots of fruits, vegetables, bread and other grains, potatoes, beans, nuts, and seeds;
olive oil as the primary source of fat; and
dairy products, eggs, fish, and poultry in low to moderate amounts.
Fish and poultry are used more than meat during this diet. It also focuses on minimally processed plant foods. Wine could also be consumed in low to moderate amounts, usually with meals. Fruit could be a common dessert rather than a sweet treat.

Is the Mediterranean diet a healthy diet to eat?

Year after year, the Mediterranean diet comes out on top of U.S. News and World Report's annual ranking of best diets. A panel of experts judges various popular food plans and diets on criteria including how healthy they are, how well they work, and how easy they are to follow.

The Mediterranean diet is also considered one of the healthiest by many health organizations and dietitians.

So, does it live up to its good reputation?

Does the AHA recommend a Mediterranean-style diet?

Yes. A Mediterranean-style diet can help you achieve the American Heart Association's recommendations for a healthy dietary pattern that:

- emphasizes vegetables, fruits, whole grains, beans, and legumes;

- includes low-fat or fat-free dairy products, fish, poultry, non-tropical vegetable oils and nuts; and

- limits added sugars, sugary drinks, sodium, highly processed foods, refined carbohydrates, saturated fats, and fatty or processed meats.

This type of diet can play a huge role in preventing heart conditions and stroke and reducing risk factors such as obesity, diabetes, high cholesterol, and high vital sign. There is some evidence that a Mediterranean diet rich in virgin vegetable oil can help the body remove excess cholesterol from the arteries and keep blood vessels clear.

What about other popular diets?

You may have heard of popular diets such as paleo, ketogenic (or keto), Atkins, interval, zone, and Whole30. Not all fad diets meet the AHA's science-based criteria for a healthy eating pattern. Some show dramatic results but in the short term and are not heart-healthy.

DASH, or Dietary Methods to Prevent Hypertension, is another eating plan that aligns with AHA recommendations and has been shown to improve health. The DASH diet allows more dairy and meat, while the Mediterranean diet includes regular use of vegetable oil.

A plant-based, vegetarian, or vegan diet can also be a healthy diet to follow.

The most important thing is to focus on the overall quality of your diet, instead of individual nutrients or foods. Try to incorporate more nutrient-dense foods such as vegetables, fruits, legumes, and lean proteins. Limit foods that provide a lot of calories but little nutritional value.

What are the other benefits of a healthy diet?

What you eat affects many aspects of your overall health, including brain health. A healthy diet can improve your ability to think, remember and process information as you age.

In one study, the healthiest consumers at age 50 had a nearly 90 percent lower risk of dementia than those who had the least amount of healthy diets. The Mediterranean and DASH diets have been shown to improve brain health and heart health.

This cookbook offers you a variety of recipes for your Mediterranean diet to follow a healthier and more balanced diet and to improve your energy efficiency and quality of life. Enjoy!

Breakfast

Spinach and Egg Breakfast Wraps

Prep time: 10 minutes | Cook time: 7 minutes | Serves 2

Ingredients:
1 tablespoon olive oil
¼ cup minced onion
3 to 4 tablespoons minced sun-dried tomatoes in olive oil and herbs
3 large eggs, whisked
1½ cups packed baby spinach
ounce (28 g) crumbled feta cheese
Salt, to taste
(8-inch) whole-wheat tortillas

Directions:
Heat the olive oil in a large skillet over medium-high heat.
Sauté the onion and tomatoes for about 3 minutes, stirring
occasionally, until softened.
Reduce the heat to medium. Add the whisked eggs and stir-fry for 1 to
2 minutes.
Stir in the baby spinach and scatter with the crumbled feta cheese.
Season as needed with salt.
Remove the egg mixture from the heat to a plate. Set aside.
Working in batches, place 2 tortillas on a microwave-safe dish and
microwave for about 20 seconds to make them warm.
Spoon half of the egg mixture into each tortilla. Fold them in half and
roll up, then serve.

Per Serving:
calories: 434 | fat: 28.1g | protein: 17.2g | carbs: 30.8g | fiber: 6.0g |
sodium:
551mg

Pumpkin Pie Parfait

Prep time: 5 minutes | Cook time: 0 minutes | Serves 4

Ingredients:
1 (15-ounce / 425-g) can pure pumpkin purée
4 teaspoons honey
teaspoon pumpkin pie spice
¼ teaspoon ground cinnamon
cups plain Greek yogurt
1 cup honey granola

Directions:
Combine the pumpkin purée, honey, pumpkin pie spice, and cinnamon in a large bowl and stir to mix well.
Cover the bowl with plastic wrap and chill in the refrigerator for at least 2 hours.
Make the parfaits: Layer each parfait glass with ¼ cup pumpkin mixture in the bottom. Top with ¼ cup of yogurt and scatter each top with ¼ cup of honey granola. Repeat the layers until the glasses are full. Serve immediately.

Per Serving:
calories: 263 | fat: 8.9g | protein: 15.3g | carbs: 34.6g | fiber: 6.0g | sodium:
91mg

Banana-Blueberry Breakfast Cookies

Prep time: 10 minutes | Cook time: 13 minutes | Serves 4

Ingredients:
2 medium bananas, sliced
4 tablespoons almond butter
4 large eggs, lightly beaten
½ cup unsweetened applesauce
1 teaspoon vanilla extract
⅔ cup coconut flour
¼ teaspoon salt
1 cup fresh or frozen blueberries

Directions:
Preheat the oven to 375°F (190°C). Line a baking sheet with parchment paper.
Stir together the bananas and almond butter in a medium bowl until well incorporated.
Fold in the beaten eggs, applesauce, and vanilla and blend well.
Add the coconut flour and salt and mix well. Add the blueberries and stir to just incorporate.
Drop about 2 tablespoons of dough onto the parchment paper-lined baking sheet for each cookie. Using your clean hand, flatten each into a rounded biscuit shape, until it is 1 inch thick.
Bake in the preheated oven for about 13 minutes, or until the top is golden brown and a toothpick inserted in the center comes out clean. Let the cookies cool for 5 to 10 minutes before serving.

Per Serving:
(3 cookies) calories: 264 | fat: 13.9g | protein: 7.3g | carbs: 27.6g | fiber: 5.2g | sodium:
219mg

Blackberry-Yogurt Green Smoothie

Prep time: 5 minutes | Cook time: 0 minutes | Serves 2

Ingredients:
1 cup plain Greek yogurt
1 cup baby spinach
½ cup frozen blackberries
½ cup unsweetened almond milk
½ teaspoon peeled and grated fresh ginger
¼ cup chopped pecans

Directions:
Process the yogurt, baby spinach, blackberries, almond milk, and ginger in a food processor until smoothly blended.
Divide the mixture into two bowls and serve topped with the chopped pecans.

Per Serving:
calories: 201 | fat: 14.5g | protein: 7.1g | carbs: 14.9g | fiber: 4.3g | sodium: 103mg

Parmesan Oatmeal with Greens

Prep time: 10 minutes | Cook time: 18 minutes | Serves 2

Ingredients:
tablespoon olive oil
¼ cup minced onion
cups greens (arugula, baby spinach, chopped kale, or Swiss chard)
¾ cup gluten-free old-fashioned oats
1½ cups water, or low-sodium chicken stock
2 tablespoons Parmesan cheese
Salt, to taste
Pinch freshly ground black pepper

Directions:
Heat the olive oil in a saucepan over medium-high heat. Add the minced onion and sauté for 2 minutes, or until softened.
Add the greens and stir until they begin to wilt. Transfer this mixture to a bowl and set aside.
Add the oats to the pan and let them toast for about 2 minutes. Add the water and bring the oats to a boil.
Reduce the heat to low, cover, and let the oats cook for 10 minutes, or until the liquid is absorbed and the oats are tender.
Stir the Parmesan cheese into the oats, and add the onion and greens back to the pan. Add additional water if needed, so the oats are creamy and not dry.
Stir well and season with salt and black pepper to taste. Serve warm.

Per Serving:
calories: 257 | fat: 14.0g | protein: 12.2g | carbs: 30.2g | fiber: 6.1g | sodium: 262mg

Cinnamon Pistachio Smoothie

Prep time: 5 minutes | Cook time: 0 minutes | Serves 1

Ingredients:
½ cup unsweetened almond milk, plus more as needed
½ cup plain Greek yogurt
Zest and juice of ½ orange
1 tablespoon extra-virgin olive oil
1 tablespoon shelled pistachios, coarsely chopped
¼ to ½ teaspoon ground allspice
¼ teaspoon vanilla extract
¼ teaspoon ground cinnamon

Directions:
In a blender, combine ½ cup almond milk, yogurt, orange zest and juice, olive oil, pistachios, allspice, vanilla, and cinnamon. Blend until smooth and creamy, adding more almond milk to achieve your desired consistency.
Serve chilled.

Per Serving:
calories: 264 | fat: 22.0g | protein: 6.0g | carbs: 12.0g | fiber: 2.0g | sodium: 127mg

Baked Eggs in Avocado

Prep time: 5 minutes | Cook time: 10 to 15 minutes | Serves 2

Ingredients:
ripe large avocado
large eggs
Salt and freshly ground black pepper, to taste
4 tablespoons jarred pesto, for serving
2 tablespoons chopped tomato, for serving
2 tablespoons crumbled feta cheese, for serving (optional)

Directions:
Preheat the oven to 425°F (220°C).
Slice the avocado in half, remove the pit and scoop out a generous tablespoon of flesh from each half to create a hole big enough to fit an egg.
Transfer the avocado halves (cut-side up) to a baking sheet.
Crack 1 egg into each avocado half and sprinkle with salt and pepper.
Bake in the preheated oven for 10 to 15 minutes, or until the eggs are cooked to your preferred doneness.
Remove the avocado halves from the oven. Scatter each avocado half evenly with the jarred pesto, chopped tomato, and crumbled feta cheese (if desired). Serve immediately.

Per Serving:
calories: 301 | fat: 25.9g | protein: 8.1g | carbs: 9.8g | fiber: 5.0g | sodium: 435mg

Crustless Tiropita (Greek Cheese Pie)

Prep time: 10 minutes | Cook time: 35 to 40 minutes | Serves 6

Ingredients:

4 tablespoons extra-virgin olive oil, divided
½ cup whole-milk ricotta cheese
1¼ cups crumbled feta cheese
tablespoon chopped fresh dill
tablespoons chopped fresh mint
½ teaspoon lemon zest
¼ teaspoon freshly ground black pepper
2 large eggs
½ teaspoon baking powder

Directions:

Preheat the oven to 350°F (180°C). Coat the bottom and sides of a baking dish with 2 tablespoons of olive oil. Set aside.

Mix together the ricotta and feta cheese in a medium bowl and stir with a fork until well combined. Add the dill, mint, lemon zest, and black pepper and mix well.

In a separate bowl, whisk together the eggs and baking powder. Pour the whisked eggs into the bowl of cheese mixture. Blend well.

Slowly pour the mixture into the coated baking dish and drizzle with the remaining 2 tablespoons of olive oil.

Bake in the preheated oven for about 35 to 40 minutes, or until the pie is browned around the edges and cooked through.

Cool for 5 minutes before slicing into wedges.

Per Serving:

calories: 181 | fat: 16.6g | protein: 7.0g | carbs: 1.8g | fiber: 0g | sodium: 321mg

Buckwheat Porridge

Prep time: 5 minutes | Cook time: 40 minutes | Serves 4

Ingredients:
3 cups water
2 cups raw buckwheat groats
Pinch sea salt
1 cup unsweetened almond milk

Directions:
In a medium saucepan, add the water, buckwheat groats, and sea salt
and bring to a boil over medium-high heat.
Once it starts to boil, reduce the heat to low. Cook for about 20
minutes, stirring occasionally, or until most of the water is absorbed.
Fold in the almond milk and whisk well. Continue cooking for about
15 minutes, or until the buckwheat groats are very softened.
Ladle the porridge into bowls and serve warm.

Per Serving:
calories: 121 | fat: 1.0g | protein: 6.3g | carbs: 21.5g | fiber: 3.0g |
sodium: 47mg

Healthy Chia Pudding

Prep time: 5 minutes | Cook time: 0 minutes | Serves 4

Ingredients:
4 cups unsweetened almond milk
¾ cup chia seeds
1 teaspoon ground cinnamon
Pinch sea salt

Directions:
In a medium bowl, whisk together the almond milk, chia seeds,
cinnamon, and sea salt until well incorporated.
Cover and transfer to the refrigerator to thicken for about 1 hour, or
until a pudding-like texture is achieved.
Serve chilled.

Per Serving:
calories: 236 | fat: 9.8g | protein: 13.1g | carbs: 24.8g | fiber: 11.0g |
sodium: 133mg

Savory Breakfast Oatmeal

Prep time: 5 minutes | Cook time: 15 minutes | Serves 2

Ingredients:
½ cup steel-cut oats
1 cup water
1 medium cucumber, chopped
1 large tomato, chopped
1 tablespoon olive oil
Pinch freshly grated Parmesan cheese
Sea salt and freshly ground pepper, to taste
Flat-leaf parsley or mint, chopped, for garnish

Directions:
Combine the oats and water in a medium saucepan and bring to a boil over high heat, stirring continuously, or until the water is absorbed, about 15 minutes.
Divide the oatmeal between 2 bowls and scatter the tomato and cucumber on top. Drizzle with the olive oil and sprinkle with the Parmesan cheese.
Season with salt and pepper to taste. Serve garnished with the parsley.

Per Serving:
calories: 197| fat: 8.9g | protein: 6.3g | carbs: 23.1g | fiber: 6.4g | sodium: 27mg

Feta and Olive Scrambled Eggs

Prep time: 5 minutes | Cook time: 5 minutes | Serves 2

Ingredients:

4 large eggs
1 tablespoon unsweetened almond milk
Sea salt and freshly ground pepper, to taste
1 tablespoon olive oil
¼ cup crumbled feta cheese
10 Kalamata olives, pitted and sliced
Small bunch fresh mint, chopped, for garnish

Directions:

Beat the eggs in a bowl until just combined. Add the milk and a pinch of sea salt and whisk well.

Heat a medium nonstick skillet over medium-high heat and add the olive oil.

Pour in the egg mixture and stir constantly, or until they just begin to curd and firm up, about 2 minutes. Add the feta cheese and olive slices, and stir until evenly combined. Season to taste with salt and pepper. Divide the mixture between 2 plates and serve garnished with the fresh chopped mint.

Per Serving:

calories: 244 | fat: 21.9g | protein: 8.4g | carbs:3.5g | fiber: 0.6g | sodium: 339mg

Creamy Peach Smoothie

Prep time: 15 minutes | Cook time: 0 minutes | Serves 2

Ingredients:
2 cups packed frozen peaches, partially thawed
½ ripe avocado
½ cup plain or vanilla Greek yogurt
2 tablespoons flax meal
1 tablespoon honey
1 teaspoon orange extract 1 teaspoon vanilla extract

Directions:
Place all the ingredients in a blender and blend until completely mixed and smooth.
Divide the mixture into two bowls and serve immediately.

Per Serving:
calories: 212 | fat: 13.1g | protein: 6.0g | carbs: 22.5g | fiber: 7.2g | sodium: 40mg

Blueberry Smoothie

Prep time: 5 minutes | Cook time: 0 minutes | Serves 1

Ingredients:
cup unsweetened almond milk, plus additional as needed
¼ cup frozen blueberries
tablespoons unsweetened almond butter
1 tablespoon extra-virgin olive oil
1 tablespoon ground flaxseed or chia seeds
1 to 2 teaspoons maple syrup
½ teaspoon vanilla extract
¼ teaspoon ground cinnamon

Directions:
Blend all the ingredients in a blender until smooth and creamy.
You can add additional almond milk to reach your preferred
consistency as needed. Serve immediately.

Per Serving:
calories: 459 | fat: 40.1g | protein: 8.9g | carbs: 20.0g | fiber: 10.1g |
sodium: 147mg

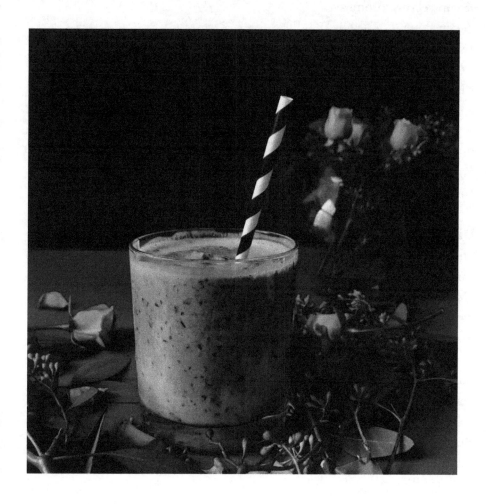

Banana Corn Fritters

Prep time: 5 minutes | Cook time: 10 minutes | Serves 2

Ingredients:
½ cup yellow cornmeal
¼ cup flour
2 small ripe bananas, peeled and mashed
2 tablespoons unsweetened almond milk
1 large egg, beaten
½ teaspoon baking powder
¼ to ½ teaspoon ground chipotle chili
¼ teaspoon ground cinnamon
¼ teaspoon sea salt
1 tablespoon olive oil

Directions:
Stir together all ingredients except for the olive oil in a large bowl until smooth.
Heat a nonstick skillet over medium-high heat. Add the olive oil and drop about 2 tablespoons of batter for each fritter. Cook for 2 to 3 minutes until the bottoms are golden brown, then flip. Continue cooking for 1 to 2 minutes more, until cooked through. Repeat with the remaining batter.
Serve warm.

Per Serving:
calories: 396 | fat: 10.6g | protein: 7.3g | carbs: 68.0g | fiber: 4.8g | sodium: 307mg

Apple-Tahini Toast

Prep time: 5 minutes | Cook time: 0 minutes | Serves 1

Ingredients:
2 slices whole-wheat bread, toasted
2 tablespoons tahini
1 small apple of your choice, cored and thinly sliced
1 teaspoon honey

Directions:
Spread the tahini on the toasted bread.
Place the apple slices on the bread and drizzle with the honey. Serve immediately.

Per Serving:
calories: 458 | fat: 17.8g | protein: 11.0g | carbs: 63.5g | fiber: 10.5g | sodium: 285mg

Kale and Apple Smoothie

Prep time: 5 minutes | Cook time: 0 minutes | Serves 2

Ingredients:
2 cups shredded kale
1 cup unsweetened almond milk
¼ cup 2 percent plain Greek yogurt
½ Granny Smith apple, unpeeled, cored and chopped
½ avocado, diced
3 ice cubes

Directions:
Put all ingredients in a blender and blend until smooth and thick.
Pour into two glasses and serve immediately.

Per Serving:
calories: 177 | fat: 6.8g | protein: 8.2g | carbs: 22.0g | fiber: 4.1g |
sodium: 112mg

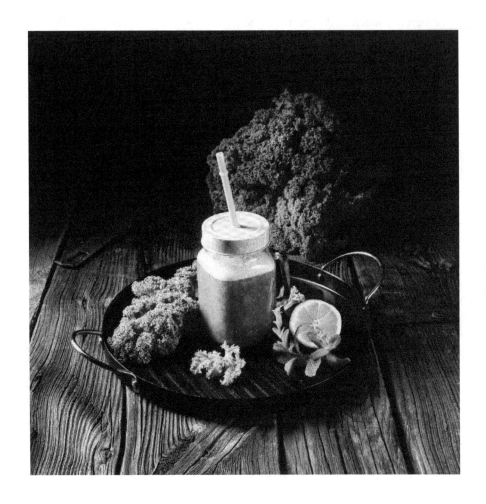

Cauliflower Breakfast Porridge

Prep time: 5 minutes | Cook time: 5 minutes | Serves 2

Ingredients:
2 cups riced cauliflower

¾ cup unsweetened almond milk

4 tablespoons extra-virgin olive oil, divided

2 teaspoons grated fresh orange peel (from ½ orange)

½ teaspoon almond extract or vanilla extract

½ teaspoon ground cinnamon

⅛ teaspoon salt

4 tablespoons chopped walnuts, divided

1 to 2 teaspoons maple syrup (optional)

Directions:
Place the riced cauliflower, almond milk, 2 tablespoons of olive oil, orange peel, almond extract, cinnamon, and salt in a medium saucepan. Stir to incorporate and bring the mixture to a boil over medium-high heat, stirring often.

Remove from the heat and add 2 tablespoons of chopped walnuts and maple syrup (if desired).

Stir again and divide the porridge into bowls. To serve, sprinkle each bowl evenly with remaining 2 tablespoons of walnuts and olive oil.

Per Serving:
calories: 381 | fat: 37.8g | protein: 5.2g | carbs: 10.9g | fiber: 4.0g | sodium: 228mg

Mediterranean Eggs (Shakshuka)

Prep time: 5 minutes | Cook time: 20 minutes | Serves 4

Ingredients:
2 tablespoons extra-virgin olive oil
1 cup chopped shallots
1 teaspoon garlic powder
1 cup finely diced potato
1 cup chopped red bell peppers
1 (14.5-ounce/ 411-g) can diced tomatoes, drained
¼ teaspoon ground cardamom
¼ teaspoon paprika
¼ teaspoon turmeric
4 large eggs
¼ cup chopped fresh cilantro

Directions:
Preheat the oven to 350°F (180°C).
Heat the olive oil in an ovenproof skillet over medium-high heat until it shimmers.
Add the shallots and sauté for about 3 minutes, stirring occasionally, until fragrant.
Fold in the garlic powder, potato, and bell peppers and stir to combine. Cover and cook for 10 minutes, stirring frequently.
Add the tomatoes, cardamon, paprika, and turmeric and mix well.
When the mixture begins to bubble, remove from the heat and crack the eggs into the skillet.
Transfer the skillet to the preheated oven and bake for 5 to 10 minutes, or until the egg whites are set and the yolks are cooked to your liking.
Remove from the oven and garnish with the cilantro before serving.

Per Serving:
calories: 223 | fat: 11.8g | protein: 9.1g | carbs: 19.5g | fiber: 3.0g | sodium: 277mg

Breakfast Yogurt Sundae

Prep time: 5 minutes | Cook time: 0 minutes | Serves 1

Ingredients:
¾ cup plain Greek yogurt
¼ cup fresh mixed berries (blueberries, strawberries, blackberries)
2 tablespoons walnut pieces
tablespoon ground flaxseed
fresh mint leaves, shredded

Directions:
Pour the yogurt into a tall parfait glass and sprinkle with the mixed berries, walnut pieces, and flaxseed.
Garnish with the shredded mint leaves and serve immediately.

Per Serving:
calories: 236 | fat: 10.8g | protein: 21.1g | carbs: 15.9g | fiber: 4.1g | sodium: 63mg

Avocado Toast with Goat Cheese

Prep time: 5 minutes | Cook time: 2 to 3 minutes | Serves 2

Ingredients:
2 slices whole-wheat thin-sliced bread
½ avocado
2 tablespoons crumbled goat cheese
Salt, to taste

Directions:
Toast the bread slices in a toaster for 2 to 3 minutes on each side until browned.

Scoop out the flesh from the avocado into a medium bowl and mash it with a fork to desired consistency. Spread the mash onto each piece of toast.

Scatter the crumbled goat cheese on top and season as needed with salt.

Serve immediately.

Per Serving:
calories: 136 | fat: 5.9g | protein: 5.0g | carbs: 17.5g | fiber: 5.1g | sodium: 194mg

Breakfast Pancakes with Berry Sauce

Prep time: 5 minutes | Cook time: 10 minutes | Serves 4

Ingredients:
1 cup almond flour
1 teaspoon baking powder
¼ teaspoon salt
6 tablespoon extra-virgin olive oil, divided
2 large eggs, beaten
Zest and juice of 1 lemon ½ teaspoon vanilla extract Berry Sauce:
1 cup frozen mixed berries
1 tablespoon water, plus more as needed
½ teaspoon vanilla extract

Directions:
In a large bowl, combine the almond flour, baking powder, and salt and stir to break up any clumps. Add 4 tablespoons olive oil, beaten eggs, lemon zest and juice, and vanilla extract and stir until well mixed.
Heat 1 tablespoon of olive oil in a large skillet. Spoon about 2 tablespoons of batter for each pancake. Cook until bubbles begin to form, 4 to 5 minutes. Flip and cook for another 2 to 3 minutes. Repeat with the remaining 1 tablespoon of olive oil and batter. Make the Berry Sauce Combine the frozen berries, water, and vanilla extract in a small saucepan and heat over medium-high heat for 3 to 4 minutes until bubbly, adding more water as needed. Using the back of a spoon or fork, mash the berries and whisk until smooth.
Serve the pancakes with the berry sauce.

Per Serving:
calories: 275 | fat: 26.0g | protein: 4.0g | carbs: 8.0g | fiber: 2.0g | sodium: 271mg

Avocado Smoothie

Prep time: 2 minutes | Cook time: 0 minutes | Serves 2

Ingredients:
large avocado
1½ cups unsweetened coconut milk
tablespoons honey

Directions:
Place all ingredients in a blender and blend until smooth and creamy.
Serve immediately.

Per Serving:
calories: 686 | fat: 57.6g | protein: 6.2g | carbs: 35.8g | fiber: 10.7g |
sodium: 35mg

Morning Overnight Oats with Raspberries

Prep time: 5 minutes | Cook time: 0 minutes | Serves 2

Ingredients:
⅔ cup unsweetened almond milk
¼ cup raspberries
⅓ cup rolled oats
1 teaspoon honey
¼ teaspoon turmeric
⅛ teaspoon ground cinnamon
Pinch ground cloves

Directions:
Place the almond milk, raspberries, rolled oats, honey, turmeric, cinnamon, and cloves in a mason jar. Cover and shake to combine. Transfer to the refrigerator for at least 8 hours, preferably 24 hours. Serve chilled.

Per Serving:
calories: 81 | fat: 1.9g | protein: 2.1g | carbs: 13.8g | fiber: 3.0g | sodium: 97mg

Tomato and Egg Scramble

Prep time: 10 minutes | Cook time: 20 minutes | Serves 4

Ingredients:
2 tablespoons extra-virgin olive oil
¼ cup finely minced red onion
1½ cups chopped fresh tomatoes
2 garlic cloves, minced
½ teaspoon dried thyme
½ teaspoon dried oregano
8 large eggs
½ teaspoon salt
¼ teaspoon freshly ground black pepper
¾ cup crumbled feta cheese
¼ cup chopped fresh mint leaves

Directions:
Heat the olive oil in a large skillet over medium heat.
Sauté the red onion and tomatoes in the hot skillet for 10 to 12 minutes, or until the tomatoes are softened.
Stir in the garlic, thyme, and oregano and sauté for 2 to 4 minutes, or until the garlic is fragrant.
Meanwhile, beat the eggs with the salt and pepper in a medium bowl until frothy.
Pour the beaten eggs into the skillet and reduce the heat to low.
Scramble for 3 to 4 minutes, stirring constantly, or until the eggs are set.
Remove from the heat and scatter with the feta cheese and mint. Serve warm.

Per Serving:
calories: 260 | fat: 21.9g | protein: 10.2g | carbs: 5.8g | fiber: 1.0g | sodium: 571mg

Feta and Spinach Frittata

Prep time: 10 minutes | Cook time: 15 minutes | Serves 2

Ingredients:

4 large eggs, beaten

2 tablespoons fresh chopped herbs, such as rosemary, thyme, oregano, basil or 1 teaspoon dried herbs

¼ teaspoon salt

Freshly ground black pepper, to taste

4 tablespoons extra-virgin olive oil, divided

1 cup fresh spinach, arugula, kale, or other leafy greens

4 ounces (113 g) quartered artichoke hearts, rinsed, drained, and thoroughly dried

8 cherry tomatoes, halved

½ cup crumbled soft goat cheese

Directions:

Preheat the broiler to Low.

In a small bowl, combine the beaten eggs, herbs, salt, and pepper and whisk well with a fork. Set aside. In an ovenproof skillet, heat 2 tablespoons of olive oil over medium heat. Add the spinach, artichoke hearts, and cherry tomatoes and sauté until just wilted, 1 to 2 minutes. Pour in the egg mixture and let it cook undisturbed over medium heat for 3 to 4 minutes, until the eggs begin to set on the bottom.

Sprinkle the goat cheese across the top of the egg mixture and transfer the skillet to the oven. Broil for 4 to 5 minutes, or until the frittata is firm in the center and golden brown on top. Remove from the oven and run a rubber spatula around the edge to loosen the sides. Slice the frittata in half and serve drizzled with the remaining 2 tablespoons of olive oil.

Per Serving:

calories: 529 | fat: 46.5g | protein: 21.4g | carbs: 7.1g | fiber: 3.1g | sodium: 762mg

Avocado and Egg Toast

Prep time: 5 minutes | Cook time: 8 minutes | Serves 2

Ingredients:

2 tablespoons ground flaxseed
½ teaspoon baking powder
2 large eggs, beaten
1 teaspoon salt, plus additional for serving
½ teaspoon freshly ground black pepper, plus additional for serving
½ teaspoon garlic powder, sesame seed, caraway seed, or other dried
herbs (optional)
3 tablespoons extra-virgin olive oil, divided
medium ripe avocado, peeled, pitted, and sliced
tablespoons chopped ripe tomato

Directions:

In a small bowl, combine the flaxseed and baking powder, breaking up
any lumps in the baking powder. Add the beaten eggs, salt, pepper, and
garlic powder (if desired) and whisk well. Let sit for 2 minutes.
In a small nonstick skillet, heat 1 tablespoon of olive oil over medium
heat. Pour the egg mixture into the skillet and let cook undisturbed
until the egg begins to set on bottom, 2 to 3 minutes. Using a rubber
spatula, scrape down the sides to allow uncooked egg to reach the
bottom. Cook for an additional 2 to 3 minutes. Once almost set, flip
like a pancake and allow the top to fully cook, another 1 to 2 minutes.
Remove from the skillet and allow to cool slightly, then slice into 2
pieces. Top each piece with avocado slices, additional salt and pepper,
chopped tomato, and drizzle with the remaining 2 tablespoons of olive
oil. Serve immediately.

Per Serving:

calories: 297 | fat: 26.1g | protein: 8.9g | carbs: 12.0g | fiber: 7.1g |
sodium: 1132mg

Berry and Nut Parfait

Prep time: 10 minutes | Cook time: 0 minutes | Serves 2

Ingredients:
2 cups plain Greek yogurt
2 tablespoons honey
1 cup fresh raspberries
1 cup fresh blueberries
½ cup walnut pieces

Directions:
In a medium bowl, whisk the yogurt and honey. Spoon into 2 serving bowls.

Top each with ½ cup blueberries, ½ cup raspberries, and ¼ cup walnut pieces. Serve immediately.

Per Serving:
calories: 507 | fat: 23.0g | protein: 24.1g | carbs: 57.0g | fiber: 8.2g | sodium: 172mg

Creamy Breakfast Bulgur with Berries

Prep time: 2 minutes | Cook time: 10 minutes | Serves 2

Ingredients:
½ cup medium-grain bulgur wheat
1 cup water
Pinch sea salt
¼ cup unsweetened almond milk
1 teaspoon pure vanilla extract
¼ teaspoon ground cinnamon
1 cup fresh berries of your choice

Directions:
Put the bulgur in a medium saucepan with the water and sea salt, and bring to a boil.
Cover, remove from heat, and let stand for 10 minutes until water is absorbed.
Stir in the milk, vanilla, and cinnamon until fully incorporated. Divide between 2 bowls and top with the fresh berries to serve.

Per Serving:
calories: 173 | fat: 1.6g | protein: 5.7g | carbs: 34.0g | fiber: 6.0g | sodium: 197mg

Fluffy Almond Flour Pancakes with Strawberries

Prep time: 5 minutes | Cook time: 15 minutes | Serves 4

Ingredients:
1 cup plus 2 tablespoons unsweetened almond milk
cup almond flour
large eggs, whisked
⅓ cup honey
teaspoon baking soda
¼ teaspoon salt
tablespoons extra-virgin olive oil
1 cup sliced strawberries

Directions:
Combine the almond milk, almond flour, whisked eggs, honey, baking soda, and salt in a large bowl and whisk to incorporate.
Heat the olive oil in a large skillet over medium-high heat.
Make the pancakes: Pour ⅓ cup of batter into the hot skillet and swirl the pan so the batter covers the bottom evenly. Cook for 2 to 3 minutes until the pancake turns golden brown around the edges.
Gently flip the pancake with a spatula and cook for 2 to 3 minutes until cooked through. Repeat with the remaining batter.
Serve the pancakes with the sliced strawberries on top.

Per Serving:
calories: 298 | fat: 11.7g | protein: 11.8g | carbs: 34.8g | fiber: 3.9g | sodium: 195mg

Creamy Vanilla Oatmeal

Prep time: 5 minutes | Cook time: 40 minutes | Serves 4

Ingredients:
4 cups water
Pinch sea salt
cup steel-cut oats
¾ cup unsweetened almond milk
teaspoons pure vanilla extract

Directions:
Add the water and salt to a large saucepan over high heat and bring to a boil.
Once boiling, reduce the heat to low and add the oats. Mix well and cook for 30 minutes, stirring occasionally.
Fold in the almond milk and vanilla and whisk to combine. Continue cooking for about 10 minutes, or until the oats are thick and creamy.
Ladle the oatmeal into bowls and serve warm.

Per Serving:
calories: 117 | fat: 2.2g | protein: 4.3g | carbs: 20.0g | fiber: 3.8g | sodium: 38mg

Tomato and Egg Breakfast Pizza

Prep time: 5 minutes | Cook time: 15 minutes | Serves 2

Ingredeients:
2 (6- to 8-inch-long) slices of whole-wheat naan bread
2 tablespoons prepared pesto
medium tomato, sliced
large eggs

Directions:
Heat a large nonstick skillet over medium-high heat. Place the naan bread in the skillet and let warm for about 2 minutes on each side, or until softened.

Spread 1 tablespoon of the pesto on one side of each slice and top with tomato slices.

Remove from the skillet and place each one on its own plate.

Crack the eggs into the skillet, keeping them separated, and cook until the whites are no longer translucent and the yolk is cooked to desired doneness.

Using a spatula, spoon one egg onto each bread slice. Serve warm.

Per Serving:
calories: 429 | fat: 16.8g | protein: 18.1g | carbs: 12.0g | fiber: 4.8g | sodium: 682mg

Classic Shakshuka

Prep time: 15 minutes | Cook time: 30 minutes | Serves 2

Ingredients:

tablespoon olive oil
½ red pepper, diced
½ medium onion, diced
small garlic cloves, minced
½ teaspoon smoked paprika
½ teaspoon cumin
Pinch red pepper flakes
1 (14.5-ounce / 411-g) can fire-roasted tomatoes
¼ teaspoon salt
Pinch freshly ground black pepper
1 ounce (28 g) crumbled feta cheese (about ¼ cup)
3 large eggs
3 tablespoons minced fresh parsley

Directions:

Heat the olive oil in a skillet over medium-high heat and add the pepper, onion, and garlic. Sauté until the vegetables start to turn golden. Add the paprika, cumin, and red pepper flakes and stir to toast the spices for about 30 seconds. Add the tomatoes with their juices. Reduce the heat and let the sauce simmer for 10 minutes, or until it starts to thicken. Add the salt and pepper. Taste the sauce and adjust seasonings as necessary. Scatter the feta cheese on top. Make 3 wells in the sauce and crack one egg into each well. Cover and let the eggs cook for about 7 minutes. Remove the lid and continue cooking for 5 minutes more, or until the yolks are cooked to desired doneness. Garnish with fresh parsley and serve.

Per Serving:

calories: 289 | fat: 18.2g | protein: 15.1g | carbs: 18.5g | fiber: 4.9g | sodium: 432

Basil Scrambled Eggs

Prep time: 5 minutes | Cook time: 8 minutes | Serves 2

Ingredients:
4 large eggs
2 tablespoons grated Gruyère cheese
2 tablespoons finely chopped fresh basil
1 tablespoon plain Greek yogurt
tablespoon olive oil
cloves garlic, minced
Sea salt and freshly ground pepper, to taste

Directions:
In a large bowl, beat together the eggs, cheese, basil, and yogurt with a whisk until just combined.
Heat the oil in a large, heavy nonstick skillet over medium-low heat. Add the garlic and cook until golden, about 1 minute.
Pour the egg mixture into the skillet over the garlic. Work the eggs continuously and cook until fluffy and soft.
Season with sea salt and freshly ground pepper to taste. Divide between 2 plates and serve immediately.

Per Serving:
calories: 243 | fat: 19.7g | protein: 15.6g | carbs: 3.4g | fiber: 0.1g | sodium: 568mg

Cinnamon Oatmeal with Dried Cranberries

Prep time: 5 minutes | Cook time: 8 minutes | Serves 2

Ingredients:
1 cup almond milk
1 cup water
Pinch sea salt
1 cup old-fashioned oats
½ cup dried cranberries
1 teaspoon ground cinnamon

Directions:
In a medium saucepan over high heat, bring the almond milk, water, and salt to a boil.

Stir in the oats, cranberries, and cinnamon. Reduce the heat to medium and cook for 5 minutes, stirring occasionally.

Remove the oatmeal from the heat. Cover and let it stand for 3 minutes. Stir before serving.

Per Serving:
calories: 107 | fat: 2.1g | protein: 3.2g | carbs: 18.2g | fiber: 4.1g | sodium: 122mg

Ricotta Toast with Strawberries

Prep time: 10 minutes | Cook time: 0 minutes | Serves 2

Ingredients:
½ cup crumbled ricotta cheese
1 tablespoon honey, plus additional as needed
Pinch of sea salt, plus additional as needed
4 slices of whole-grain bread, toasted
1 cup sliced fresh strawberries
4 large fresh basil leaves, sliced into thin shreds

Directions:
Mix together the cheese, honey, and salt in a small bowl until well incorporated.
Taste and add additional salt and honey as needed.
Spoon 2 tablespoons of the cheese mixture onto each slice of bread and spread it all over.
Sprinkle the sliced strawberry and basil leaves on top before serving.

Per Serving:
calories: 274 | fat: 7.9g | protein: 15.1g | carbs: 39.8g | fiber: 5.0g | sodium: 322mg

Egg Bake

Prep time: 10 minutes | Cook time: 30 minutes | Serves 2

Ingredients:
1 tablespoon olive oil
1 slice whole-grain bread
4 large eggs
3 tablespoons unsweetened almond milk
½ teaspoon onion powder ¼ teaspoon garlic powder
¾ cup chopped cherry tomatoes
¼ teaspoon salt
Pinch freshly ground black pepper

Directions:
Preheat the oven to 375°F (190°C).
Coat two ramekins with the olive oil and transfer to a baking sheet.
Line the bottom of each ramekin with ½ of bread slice.
In a medium bowl, whisk together the eggs, almond milk, onion powder, garlic powder, tomatoes, salt, and pepper until well combined.
Pour the mixture evenly into two ramekins. Bake in the preheated oven for 30 minutes, or until the eggs are completely set.
Cool for 5 minutes before serving.

Per Serving:
calories: 240 | fat: 17.4g | protein: 9.0g | carbs: 12.2g | fiber: 2.8g | sodium: 396mg

Cheesy Broccoli and Mushroom Egg Casserole

Prep time: 10 minutes | Cook time: 40 minutes | Serves 4

Ingredients:
2 tablespoons extra-virgin olive oil
½ sweet onion, chopped
1 teaspoon minced garlic
1 cup sliced button mushrooms
1 cup chopped broccoli
8 large eggs
¼ cup unsweetened almond milk
1 tablespoon chopped fresh basil
1 cup shredded Cheddar cheese
Sea salt and freshly ground black pepper, to taste

Directions:
Preheat the oven to 375°F (190°C).

Heat the olive oil in a large ovenproof skillet over medium-high heat. Add the onion, garlic, and mushrooms to the skillet and sauté for about 5 minutes, stirring occasionally. Stir in the broccoli and sauté for 5 minutes until the vegetables start to soften. Meanwhile, beat the eggs with the almond milk and basil in a small bowl until well mixed. Remove the skillet from the heat and pour the egg mixture over the top. Scatter the Cheddar cheese all over. Bake uncovered in the preheated oven for about 30 minutes, or until the top of the casserole is golden brown and a fork inserted in the center comes out clean. Remove from the oven and sprinkle with the sea salt and pepper. Serve hot.

Per Serving:
calories: 326 | fat: 27.2g | protein: 14.1g | carbs: 6.7g | fiber: 0.7g | sodium: 246mg

Quinoa Breakfast Bowls

Prep time: 5 minutes | Cook time: 17 minutes | Serves 1

Ingredients:
¼ cup quinoa, rinsed
¾ cup water, plus additional as needed
1 carrot, grated
½ small broccoli head, finely chopped
¼ teaspoon salt
1 tablespoon chopped fresh dill

Directions:
Add the quinoa and water to a small pot over high heat and bring to a boil.

Once boiling, reduce the heat to low. Cover and cook for 5 minutes, stirring occasionally.

Stir in the carrot, broccoli, and salt and continue cooking for 1o to 12 minutes, or until the quinoa is cooked though and the vegetables are forktender. If the mixture gets too thick, you can add additional water as needed.

Add the dill and serve warm.

Per Serving:
calories: 219 | fat: 2.9g | protein: 10.0g | carbs: 40.8g | fiber: 7.1g | sodium: 666mg

Warm Bulgur Breakfast Bowls with Fruits

Prep time: 5 minutes | Cook time: 15 minutes | Serves 6

Ingredients:
2 cups unsweetened almond milk
1½ cups uncooked bulgur
cup water
½ teaspoon ground cinnamon
cups frozen (or fresh, pitted) dark sweet cherries
8 dried (or fresh) figs, chopped
½ cup chopped almonds
¼ cup loosely packed fresh mint, chopped

Directions:
Combine the milk, bulgur, water, and cinnamon in a medium saucepan, stirring, and bring just to a boil.
Cover, reduce the heat to medium-low, and allow to simmer for 10 minutes, or until the liquid is absorbed.
Turn off the heat, but keep the pan on the stove, and stir in the frozen cherries (no need to thaw), figs, and almonds. Cover and let the hot bulgur thaw the cherries and partially hydrate the figs, about 1 minute. Fold in the mint and stir to combine, then serve.

Per Serving: calories: 207 | fat: 6.0g | protein: 8.0g | carbs: 32.0g | fiber: 4.0g | sodium: 82mg

Marinara Poached Eggs

Prep time: 5 minutes | Cook time: 15 minutes | Serves 6

Ingredients:
1 tablespoon extra-virgin olive oil
cup chopped onion
garlic cloves, minced
2 (14.5-ounce / 411-g) cans no-salt-added Italian diced tomatoes,
undrained
6 large eggs
½ cup chopped fresh flat-leaf parsley

Directions:
Heat the olive oil in a large skillet over medium-high heat.
Add the onion and sauté for 5 minutes, stirring occasionally. Add the
garlic and cook for 1 minute more.
Pour the tomatoes with their juices over the onion mixture and cook
for 2 to 3 minutes until bubbling.
Reduce the heat to medium and use a large spoon to make six
indentations in the tomato mixture. Crack the eggs, one at a time, into
each indentation.
Cover and simmer for 6 to 7 minutes, or until the eggs are cooked to
your preference.
Serve with the parsley sprinkled on top.

Per Serving:
calories: 89 | fat: 6.0g | protein: 4.0g | carbs: 4.0g | fiber: 1.0g |
sodium: 77mg

Spinach Cheese Pie

Prep time: 5 minutes | Cook time: 25 minutes | Serves 8

Ingredients:
2 tablespoons extra-virgin olive oil
1 onion, chopped
1 pound (454 g) frozen spinach, thawed
¼ teaspoon ground nutmeg
¼ teaspoon garlic salt
¼ teaspoon freshly ground black pepper
4 large eggs, divided
cup grated Parmesan cheese, divided
puff pastry doughs, at room temperature
4 hard-boiled eggs, halved
Nonstick cooking spray

Directions:

Preheat the oven to 350°F (180°C). Spritz a baking sheet with nonstick cooking spray and set aside.

Heat a large skillet over medium-high heat. Add the olive oil and onion and sauté for about 5 minutes, stirring occasionally, or until translucent. Squeeze the excess water from the spinach, then add to the skillet and cook, uncovered, so that any excess water from the spinach can evaporate.

Season with the nutmeg, garlic salt, and black pepper. Remove from heat and set aside to cool.

Beat 3 eggs in a small bowl. Add the beaten eggs and ½ cup of Parmesan cheese to the spinach mixture, stirring well.

Roll out the pastry dough on the prepared baking sheet. Layer the spinach mixture on top of the dough, leaving 2 inches around each edge.

Once the spinach is spread onto the pastry dough, evenly place the hardboiled egg halves throughout the pie, then cover with the second pastry dough. Pinch the edges closed.

Beat the remaining 1 egg in the bowl. Brush the egg wash over the pastry dough.

Bake in the preheated oven for 15 to 20 minutes until golden brown. Sprinkle with the remaining ½ cup of Parmesan cheese. Cool for 5 minutes before cutting and serving.

Per Serving:

calories: 417 | fat: 28.0g | protein: 17.0g | carbs: 25.0g | fiber: 3.0g | sodium: 490mg

Baked Ricotta with Honey Pears

Prep time: 5 minutes | Cook time: 22 to 25 minutes | Serves 4

Ingredients:
(1-pound / 454-g) container whole-milk ricotta cheese
large eggs
¼ cup whole-wheat pastry flour
1 tablespoon sugar
1 teaspoon vanilla extract
¼ teaspoon ground nutmeg
pear, cored and diced
tablespoons water
1 tablespoon honey
Nonstick cooking spray

Directions:
Preheat the oven to 400°F (205°C). Spray four ramekins with nonstick cooking spray.
Beat together the ricotta, eggs, flour, sugar, vanilla, and nutmeg in a large bowl until combined. Spoon the mixture into the ramekins.
Bake in the preheated oven for 22 to 25 minutes, or until the ricotta is just set.
Meanwhile, in a small saucepan over medium heat, simmer the pear in the water for 10 minutes, or until slightly softened. Remove from the heat, and stir in the honey.
Remove the ramekins from the oven and cool slightly on a wire rack. Top the ricotta ramekins with the pear and serve.

Per Serving:
calories: 329 | fat: 19.0g | protein: 17.0g | carbs: 23.0g | fiber: 3.0g | sodium: 109mg

Mediterranean Omelet

Prep time: 8 minutes | Cook time: 15 minutes | Serves 2

Ingredients:

2 teaspoons extra-virgin olive oil, divided
garlic clove, minced
½ yellow bell pepper, thinly sliced
½ red bell pepper, thinly sliced
¼ cup thinly sliced red onion
tablespoons chopped fresh parsley, plus extra for garnish
2 tablespoons chopped fresh basil
½ teaspoon salt
½ teaspoon freshly ground black pepper
4 large eggs, beaten

Directions:

In a large, heavy skillet, heat 1 teaspoon of the olive oil over medium heat. Add the garlic, peppers, and onion to the skillet and sauté, stirring frequently, for 5 minutes.

Add the parsley, basil, salt, and pepper, increase the heat to medium-high, and sauté for 2 minutes. Slide the vegetable mixture onto a plate and return the skillet to the heat.

Heat the remaining 1 teaspoon of olive oil in the skillet and pour in the beaten eggs, tilting the pan to coat evenly. Cook the eggs just until the edges are bubbly and all but the center is dry, 3 to 5 minutes.

Spoon the vegetable mixture onto one-half of the omelet and use a spatula to fold the empty side over the top. Slide the omelet onto a platter or cutting board.

To serve, cut the omelet in half and garnish with extra fresh parsley.

Per Serving:

calories: 206 | fat: 14.2g | protein: 13.7g | carbs: 7.2g | fiber: 1.2g | sodium: 729mg

Sides, Salads, and Soups

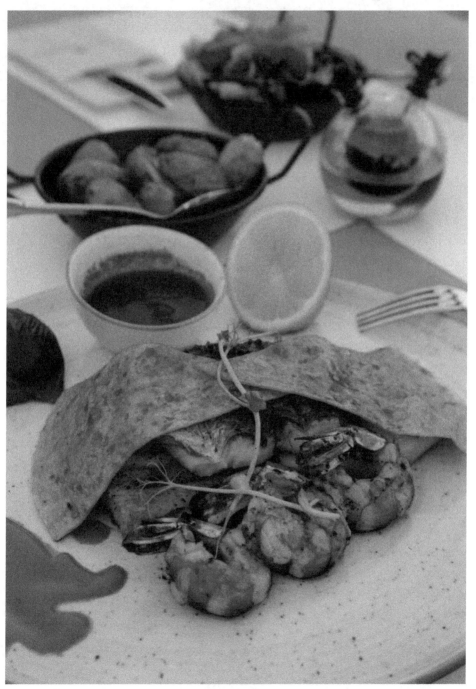

Chicken and Pastina Soup

Prep time: 5 minutes | Cook time: 20 minutes | Serves 6

Ingredients:

tablespoon extra-virgin olive oil

garlic cloves, minced

cups packed chopped kale, center ribs removed

1 cup minced carrots

8 cups no-salt-added chicken or vegetable broth

¼ teaspoon kosher or sea salt

¼ teaspoon freshly ground black pepper

¾ cup uncooked acini de pepe or pastina pasta

cups shredded cooked chicken (about 12 ounces / 340 g)

tablespoons grated Parmesan cheese

Directions:

In a large stockpot over medium heat, heat the oil. Add the garlic and cook for 30 seconds, stirring frequently. Add the kale and carrots and cook for 5 minutes, stirring occasionally.

Add the broth, salt, and pepper, and turn the heat to high. Bring the broth to a boil, and add the pasta. Reduce the heat to medium and cook for 10 minutes, or until the pasta is cooked through, stirring every few minutes so the pasta doesn't stick to the bottom. Add the chicken, and cook for another 2 minutes to warm through.

Ladle the soup into six bowls. Top each with ½ tablespoon of cheese and serve.

Per Serving:

calories: 275 | fat: 19.0g | protein: 16.0g | carbs: 11.0g | fiber: 2.0g | sodium: 298mg

Mushroom Barley Soup

Prep time: 5 minutes | Cook time: 20 to 23 minutes | Serves 6

Ingredients:
2 tablespoons extra-virgin olive oil
1 cup chopped carrots
1 cup chopped onion
5½ cups chopped mushrooms
6 cups no-salt-added vegetable broth
cup uncooked pearled barley
¼ cup red wine
tablespoons tomato paste
4 sprigs fresh thyme or ½ teaspoon dried thyme
1 dried bay leaf
6 tablespoons grated Parmesan cheese

Directions:
In a large stockpot over medium heat, heat the oil. Add the onion and carrots and cook for 5 minutes, stirring frequently. Turn up the heat to medium-high and add the mushrooms. Cook for 3 minutes, stirring frequently.
Add the broth, barley, wine, tomato paste, thyme, and bay leaf. Stir, cover, and bring the soup to a boil. Once it's boiling, stir a few times, reduce the heat to medium-low, cover, and cook for another 12 to 15 minutes, until the barley is cooked through.
Remove the bay leaf and serve the soup in bowls with 1 tablespoon of cheese sprinkled on top of each.

Per Serving:
calories: 195 | fat: 4.0g | protein: 7.0g | carbs: 34.0g | fiber: 6.0g | sodium: 173mg

Garlic Wilted Greens

Prep time: 10 minutes | Cook time: 5 minutes | Serves 2

Ingredients:
tablespoon olive oil
garlic cloves, minced
cups sliced greens (spinach, chard, beet greens, dandelion greens, or acombination)
Pinch salt
Pinch red pepper flakes (or more to taste)

Directions:
Heat the olive oil in a skillet over medium-high heat.
Add garlic and sauté for 30 seconds, or just until fragrant.
Add the greens, salt, and pepper flakes and stir to combine. Let the greens wilt, but do not overcook.
Remove from the skillet and serve on a plate.

Per Serving:
calories: 93 | fat: 6.8g | protein: 1.2g | carbs: 7.3g | fiber: 3.1g | sodium: 112mg

Arugula and Fig Salad

Prep time: 15 minutes | Cook time: 0 minutes | Serves 2

Ingredients:
cups arugula

fresh, ripe figs (or 4 to 6 dried figs), stemmed and sliced

2 tablespoons olive oil

¼ cup lightly toasted pecan halves

2 tablespoons crumbled blue cheese

1 to 2 tablespoons balsamic glaze

Directions:
Toss the arugula and figs with the olive oil in a large bowl until evenly coated.

Add the pecans and blue cheese to the bowl. Toss the salad lightly.

Drizzle with the balsamic glaze and serve immediately.

Per Serving:
calories: 517 | fat: 36.2g | protein: 18.9g | carbs: 30.2g | fiber: 6.1g | sodium: 481mg

Green Bean and Halloumi Salad

Prep time: 20 minutes | Cook time: 5 minutes | Serves 2

Dressing:
¼ cup unsweetened coconut milk
tablespoon olive oil
teaspoons freshly squeezed lemon juice
¼ teaspoon garlic powder ¼ teaspoon onion powder
Pinch salt
Pinch freshly ground black pepper Salad:
½ pound (227 g) fresh green beans, trimmed
2 ounces (57 g) Halloumi cheese, sliced into 2 (½-inch-thick) slices
½ cup halved cherry or grape tomatoes
¼ cup thinly sliced sweet onion

Make the Dressing:

Combine the coconut milk, olive oil, lemon juice, onion powder, garlic powder, salt, and pepper in a small bowl and whisk well. Set aside.

Make the Salad Fill a medium-size pot with about 1 inch of water and add the green beans.

Cover and steam them for about 3 to 4 minutes, or just until beans are tender.

Do not overcook.

Drain beans, rinse them immediately with cold water, and set them aside to cool.

Heat a nonstick skillet over medium-high heat and place the slices of Halloumi in the hot pan. After about 2 minutes, check to see if the cheese is golden on the bottom.

If it is, flip the slices and cook for another minute or until the second side is golden.

Remove cheese from the pan and cut each piece into cubes (about 1-inch square).

Place the green beans, halloumi slices, tomatoes, and onion in a large bowl and toss to combine.

Drizzle the dressing over the salad and toss well to combine.

Serve immediately.

Per Serving:

calories: 274 | fat: 18.1g | protein: 8.0g | carbs: 16.8g | fiber: 5.1g | sodium: 499mg

Avgolemono (Lemon Chicken Soup)

Prep time: 15 minutes | Cook time: 60 minutes | Serves 2

Ingredients:
½ large onion
2 medium carrots
1 celery stalk
1 garlic clove
5 cups low-sodium chicken stock
¼ cup brown rice
1½ cups (about 5 ounces / 142 g) shredded rotisserie chicken
3 tablespoons freshly squeezed lemon juice
egg yolk
tablespoons chopped fresh dill
2 tablespoons chopped fresh parsley
Salt, to taste

Directions:

Put the onion, carrots, celery, and garlic in a food processor and pulse until the vegetables are minced.

Add the vegetables and chicken stock to a stockpot and bring it to a boil over high heat.

Reduce the heat to medium-low and add the rice, shredded chicken and lemon juice.

Cover and let the soup simmer for 40 minutes, or until the rice is cooked.

In a small bowl, whisk the egg yolk lightly.

Slowly, while whisking with one hand, pour about ½ of a ladle of the broth into the egg yolk to warm, or temper, the yolk.

Slowly add another ladle of broth and continue to whisk.

Remove the soup from the heat and pour the whisked egg yolk–broth mixture into the pot. Stir well to combine.

Add the fresh dill and parsley. Season with salt to taste and serve.

Per Serving:

calories: 172 | fat: 4.2g | protein: 18.2g | carbs: 16.1g | fiber: 2.1g | sodium: 232mg

Greens, Fennel, and Pear Soup with Cashews

Prep time: 15 minutes | Cook time: 15 minutes | Serves 4 to 6

Ingredients:
2 tablespoons olive oil
fennel bulb, cut into ¼-inch-thick slices
leeks, white part only, sliced
2 pears, peeled, cored, and cut into ½-inch cubes
teaspoon sea salt
¼ teaspoon freshly ground black pepper
½ cup cashews
cups packed blanched spinach
cups low-sodium vegetable soup

Directions:
Heat the olive oil in a stockpot over high heat until shimmering.
Add the fennel and leeks, then sauté for 5 minutes or until tender.
Add the pears and sprinkle with salt and pepper, then sauté for another
3 minutes or until the pears are soft.
Add the cashews, spinach, and vegetable soup. Bring to a boil. Reduce
the heat to low. Cover and simmer for 5 minutes.
Pour the soup in a food processor, then pulse until creamy and
smooth.
Pour the soup back to the pot and heat over low heat until heated
through.
Transfer the soup to a large serving bowl and serve immediately.

Per Serving:
calories: 266 | fat: 15.1g | protein: 5.2g | carbs: 32.9g | fiber: 7.0g |
sodium: 628mg

Moroccan Lentil, Tomato, and Cauliflower Soup

Prep time: 15 minutes | Cook time: 4 hours | Serves 6

Ingredients:

1 cup chopped carrots

1 cup chopped onions

3 cloves garlic, minced

½ teaspoon ground coriander

1 teaspoon ground cumin

1 teaspoon ground turmeric

¼ teaspoon ground cinnamon

¼ teaspoon freshly ground black pepper

1 cup dry lentils

28 ounces (794 g) tomatoes, diced, reserve the juice

1½ cups chopped cauliflower

4 cups low-sodium vegetable soup

1 tablespoon no-salt-added tomato paste

1 teaspoon extra-virgin olive oil

1 cup chopped fresh spinach

¼ cup chopped fresh cilantro

1 tablespoon red wine vinegar (optional)

Directions:

Put the carrots and onions in the slow cooker, then sprinkle with minced garlic, coriander, cumin, turmeric, cinnamon, and black pepper. Stir to combine well. Add the lentils, tomatoes, and cauliflower, then pour in the vegetable soup and tomato paste. Drizzle with olive oil. Stir to combine well. Put the slow cooker lid on and cook on high for 4 hours or until the vegetables are tender. In the last 30 minutes during the cooking time, open the lid and stir the soup, then fold in the spinach. Pour the cooked soup in a large serving bowl, then spread with cilantro and drizzle with vinegar. Serve immediately.

Per Serving: calories: 131 | fat: 2.1g | protein: 5.6g | carbs: 25.0g | fiber: 5.5g | sodium: 364mg

Zesty Spanish Potato Salad

Prep time: 10 minutes | Cook time: 5 to 7 minutes | Serves 6 to 8

Ingredients:
4 russet potatoes, peeled and chopped
3 large hard-boiled eggs, chopped
1 cup frozen mixed vegetables, thawed
½ cup plain, unsweetened, full-fat Greek yogurt
5 tablespoons pitted Spanish olives
½ teaspoon freshly ground black pepper
½ teaspoon dried mustard seed
½ tablespoon freshly squeezed lemon juice
½ teaspoon dried dill
Salt, to taste

Directions:
Place the potatoes in a large pot of water and boil for 5 to 7 minutes, until just fork-tender, checking periodically for doneness. You don't have to overcook them.
Meanwhile, in a large bowl, mix the eggs, vegetables, yogurt, olives, pepper, mustard, lemon juice, and dill. Season with salt to taste. Once the potatoes are cooled somewhat, add them to the large bowl, then toss well and serve.

Per Serving:
calories: 192 | fat: 5.0g | protein: 9.0g | carbs: 30.0g | fiber: 2.0g | sodium: 59mg

Greek Salad with Dressing

Prep time: 10 minutes | Cook time: 0 minutes | Serves 4 to 6

Ingredients:
head iceberg lettuce
cups cherry tomatoes
1 large cucumber
1 medium onion
¼ cup lemon juice
½ cup extra-virgin olive oil
1 teaspoon salt
1 clove garlic, minced
1 cup Kalamata olives, pitted
1 (6-ounce / 170-g) package feta cheese, crumbled

Directions:
Cut the lettuce into 1-inch pieces and put them in a large salad bowl.
Cut the tomatoes in half and add them to the salad bowl.
Slice the cucumber into bite-sized pieces and add them to the salad bowl.
Thinly slice the onion and add it to the salad bowl.
In a separate bowl, whisk together the olive oil, lemon juice, salt, and garlic. Pour the dressing over the salad and gently toss to evenly coat.
Top the salad with the Kalamata olives and feta cheese and serve.

Per Serving:
calories: 539 | fat: 50.0g | protein: 9.0g | carbs: 18.0g | fiber: 4.0g | sodium: 1758mg

Ritzy Summer Fruit Salad

Prep time: 10 minutes | Cook time: 0 minutes | Serves 8

Ingredients:
cup fresh blueberries
cups cubed cantaloupe
2 cups red seedless grapes
cup sliced fresh strawberries
cups cubed honeydew melon
Zest of 1 large lime
½ cup unsweetened toasted coconut flakes Dressing:
¼ cup raw honey
Juice of 1 large lime
¼ teaspoon sea salt
½ cup extra-virgin olive oil

Directions:
Combine the ingredients for the salad in a large salad bowl, then toss to combine well.
Combine the ingredients for the dressing in a small bowl, then stir to mix well.
Dress the salad and serve immediately.

Per Serving:
calories: 242 | fat: 15.5g | protein: 1.3g | carbs: 28.0g | fiber: 2.4g | sodium: 90mg

Roasted Broccoli and Tomato Panzanella

Prep time: 10 minutes | Cook time: 20 minutes | Serves 4

Ingredients:

1 pound (454 g) broccoli (about 3 medium stalks), trimmed, cut into 1inch florets and ½-inch stem slices 2 tablespoons extra-virgin olive oil, divided

1½ cups cherry tomatoes

1½ teaspoons honey, divided

3 cups cubed whole-grain crusty bread

1 tablespoon balsamic vinegar

¼ teaspoon kosher salt

½ teaspoon freshly ground black pepper

¼ cup grated Parmesan cheese, for serving (optional)

¼ cup chopped fresh oregano leaves, for serving (optional)

Directions:

Preheat the oven to 450°F (235°C).

Toss the broccoli with 1 tablespoon of olive oil in a large bowl to coat well. Arrange the broccoli on a baking sheet, then add the tomatoes to the same bowl and toss with the remaining olive oil. Add 1 teaspoon of honey and toss again to coat well. Transfer the tomatoes on the baking sheet beside the broccoli. Place the baking sheet in the preheated oven and roast for 15 minutes, then add the bread cubes and flip the vegetables. Roast for an additional 3 minutes or until the broccoli is lightly charred and the bread cubes are golden brown. Meanwhile, combine the remaining ingredients, except for the Parmesan and oregano, in a small bowl. Stir to mix well. Transfer the roasted vegetables and bread cubes to the large salad bowl, then dress them and spread with Parmesan and oregano leaves. Toss and serve immediately.

Per Serving: calories: 162 | fat: 6.8g | protein: 8.2g | carbs: 18.9g | fiber: 6.0g | sodium: 397mg

Barley, Parsley, and Pea Salad

Prep time: 10 minutes | Cook time: 10 minutes | Serves 4

Ingredients:
2 cups water
1 cup quick-cooking barley
small bunch flat-leaf parsley, chopped (about 1 to 1½ cups)
cups sugar snap pea pods
Juice of 1 lemon
½ small red onion, diced
2 tablespoons extra-virgin olive oil
Sea salt and freshly ground pepper, to taste

Directions:
Pour the water in a saucepan. Bring to a boil. Add the barley to the saucepan, then put the lid on.
Reduce the heat to low. Simmer the barley for 10 minutes or until the liquid is absorbed, then let sit for 5 minutes.
Open the lid, then transfer the barley in a colander and rinse under cold running water.
Pour the barley in a large salad bowl and add the remaining ingredients. Toss to combine well.
Serve immediately.

Per Serving:
calories: 152 | fat: 7.4g | protein: 3.7g | carbs: 19.3g | fiber: 4.7g| sodium: 20mg

Cheesy Peach and Walnut Salad

Prep time: 10 minutes | Cook time: 0 minutes | Serves 1

Ingredients:
1 ripe peach, pitted and sliced
¼ cup chopped walnuts, toasted
¼ cup shredded Parmesan cheese
1 teaspoon raw honey
Zest of 1 lemon
1 tablespoon chopped fresh mint

Directions:
Combine the peach, walnut, and cheese in a medium bowl, then drizzle with honey. Spread the lemon zest and mint on top. Toss to combine everything well.
Serve immediately.

Per Serving:
calories: 373 | fat: 26.4g | protein: 12.9g | carbs: 27.0g | fiber: 4.7g | sodium: 453mg

Cheesy Roasted Broccolini

Prep time: 5 minutes | Cook time: 10 minutes | Serves 2

Ingredients:
1 bunch broccolini (about 5 ounces / 142 g)
tablespoon olive oil
½ teaspoon garlic powder
¼ teaspoon salt
tablespoons grated Romano cheese

Directions:
Preheat the oven to 400°F (205°C). Line a sheet pan with parchment paper.

Slice the tough ends off the broccolini and put in a medium bowl. Add the olive oil, garlic powder, and salt and toss to coat well. Arrange the broccolini on the prepared sheet pan.

Roast in the preheated oven for 7 minutes, flipping halfway through the cooking time.

Remove the pan from the oven and sprinkle the cheese over the broccolini. Using tongs, carefully flip the broccolini over to coat all sides.

Return to the oven and cook for an additional 2 to 3 minutes, or until the cheese melts and starts to turn golden. Serve warm.

Per Serving:
calories: 114 | fat: 9.0g | protein: 4.0g | carbs: 5.0g | fiber: 2.0g | sodium: 400mg

Orange-Honey Glazed Carrots

Prep time: 10 minutes | Cook time: 15 to 20 minutes | Serves 2

Ingredients:
½ pound (227 g) rainbow carrots, peeled
2 tablespoons fresh orange juice
1 tablespoon honey
½ teaspoon coriander
Pinch salt

Directions:
Preheat the oven to 400°F (205°C).
Cut the carrots lengthwise into slices of even thickness and place in a large bowl.
Stir together the orange juice, honey, coriander, and salt in a small bowl. Pour the orange juice mixture over the carrots and toss until well coated.
Spread the carrots in a baking dish in a single layer. Roast for 15 to 20 minutes until fork-tender.
Let cool for 5 minutes before serving.

Per Serving:
calories: 85 | fat: 0g | protein: 1.0g | carbs: 21.0g | fiber: 3.0g | sodium: 156mg

Paella Soup

Prep time: 6 minutes | Cook time: 24 minutes | Serves 6

Ingredients:
2 tablespoons extra-virgin olive oil
cup chopped onion
1½ cups coarsely chopped green bell pepper
1½ cups coarsely chopped red bell pepper
garlic cloves, chopped
1 teaspoon ground turmeric
teaspoon dried thyme
teaspoons smoked paprika
2½ cups uncooked instant brown rice
2 cups low-sodium or no-salt-added chicken broth
2½ cups water
1 cup frozen green peas, thawed
1 (28-ounce / 794-g) can low-sodium or no-salt-added crushed tomatoes
1 pound (454 g) fresh raw medium shrimp, shells and tails removed

Directions:
In a large stockpot over medium-high heat, heat the oil. Add the onion, bell peppers, and garlic. Cook for 8 minutes, stirring occasionally. Add the turmeric, thyme, and smoked paprika, and cook for 2 minutes more, stirring often. Stir in the rice, broth, and water. Bring to a boil over high heat. Cover, reduce the heat to medium-low, and cook for 10 minutes. Stir the peas, tomatoes, and shrimp into the soup. Cook for 4 minutes, until the shrimp is cooked, turning from gray to pink and white. The soup will be very thick, almost like stew, when ready to serve. Ladle the soup into bowls and serve hot.

Per Serving:
calories: 431 | fat: 5.7g | protein: 26.0g | carbs: 69.1g | fiber: 7.4g | sodium: 203mg

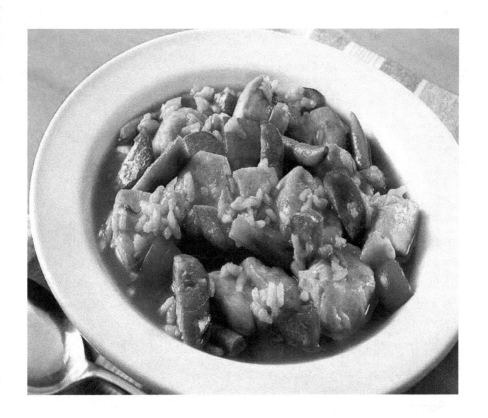

Parmesan Roasted Red Potatoes

Prep time: 10 minutes | Cook time: 55 minutes | Serves 2

Ingredients:

12 ounces (340 g) red potatoes (3 to 4 small potatoes), scrubbed and diced into 1-inch pieces 1 tablespoon olive oil

½ teaspoon garlic powder

¼ teaspoon salt

1 tablespoon grated Parmesan cheese

1 teaspoon minced fresh rosemary (from 1 sprig)

Directions:

Preheat the oven to 425°F (220°C). Line a baking sheet with parchment paper.

In a mixing bowl, combine the potatoes, olive oil, garlic powder, and salt. Toss well to coat.

Lay the potatoes on the parchment paper and roast for 10 minutes.

Flip the potatoes over and roast for another 10 minutes.

Check the potatoes to make sure they are golden brown on the top and bottom. Toss them again, turn the heat down to 350°F (180°C), and roast for 30 minutes more.

When the potatoes are golden brown, scatter the Parmesan cheese over them and toss again. Return to the oven for 3 minutes to melt the cheese.

Remove from the oven and sprinkle with the fresh rosemary before serving.

Per Serving:

calories: 200 | fat: 8.2g | protein: 5.1g | carbs: 30.0g | fiber: 3.2g | sodium: 332mg

Greek Chicken, Tomato, and Olive Salad

Prep time: 10 minutes | Cook time: 0 minutes | Serves 2

Ingredients:

2 grilled boneless, skinless chicken breasts, sliced (about 1 cup)
10 cherry tomatoes, halved
8 pitted Kalamata olives, halved
½ cup thinly sliced red onion Dressing:
¼ cup balsamic vinegar
teaspoon freshly squeezed lemon juice
¼ teaspoon sea salt
¼ teaspoon freshly ground black pepper
teaspoons extra-virgin olive oilFor Serving:
2 cups roughly chopped romaine lettuce
½ cup crumbled feta cheese

Directions:

Combine the ingredients for the salad in a large bowl. Toss to combine well.

Combine the ingredients for the dressing in a small bowl. Stir to mix well.

Pour the dressing the bowl of salad, then toss to coat well. Wrap the bowl in plastic and refrigerate for at least 2 hours.

Remove the bowl from the refrigerator. Spread the lettuce on a large plate, then top with marinated salad. Scatter the salad with feta cheese and serve immediately.

Per Serving:

calories: 328 | fat: 16.9g | protein: 27.6g | carbs: 15.9g | fiber: 3.1g| sodium: 1102mg

Sumptuous Greek Vegetable Salad
Prep time: 20 minutes | Cook time: 0 minutes | Serves 6

Ingredients:
1 (15-ounce / 425-g) can chickpeas, drained and rinsed
1 (14-ounce / 397-g) can artichoke hearts, drained and halved
1 head Bibb lettuce, chopped (about 2½ cups)
1 cucumber, peeled deseeded, and chopped (about 1½ cups)
1½ cups grape tomatoes, halved
¼ cup chopped basil leaves
½ cup sliced black olives
½ cup cubed feta cheese Dressing:
1 tablespoon freshly squeezed lemon juice (from about ½ small lemon)
¼ teaspoon freshly ground black pepper
tablespoon chopped fresh oregano
tablespoons extra-virgin olive oil
1 tablespoon red wine vinegar
1 teaspoon honey

Directions:
Combine the ingredients for the salad in a large salad bowl, then toss to combine well.
Combine the ingredients for the dressing in a small bowl, then stir to mix well.
Dress the salad and serve immediately.

Per Serving:
calories: 165 | fat: 8.1g | protein: 7.2g | carbs: 17.9g | fiber: 7.0g | sodium: 337mg

Sautéed Kale with Olives

Prep time: 10 minutes | Cook time: 10 minutes | Serves 2

Ingredients:
1 bunch kale, leaves chopped and stems minced
½ cup celery leaves, roughly chopped, or additional parsley
½ bunch flat-leaf parsley, stems and leaves roughly chopped
4 garlic cloves, chopped
2 teaspoons olive oil
¼ cup pitted Kalamata olives, chopped
Grated zest and juice of 1 lemon
Salt and pepper, to taste

Directions:
Place the kale, celery leaves, parsley, and garlic in a steamer basket set over a medium saucepan. Steam over medium-high heat, covered, for 15 minutes. Remove from the heat and squeeze out any excess moisture.
Place a large skillet over medium heat. Add the oil, then add the kale mixture to the skillet. Cook, stirring often, for 5 minutes.
Remove from the heat and add the olives and lemon zest and juice. Season with salt and pepper and serve.

Per Serving:
calories: 86 | fat: 6.4g | protein: 1.8g | carbs: 7.5g | fiber: 2.1g | sodium: 276mg

Balsamic Brussels Sprouts and Delicata Squash

Prep time: 10 minutes | Cook time: 30 minutes | Serves 2

Ingredients:
½ pound (227 g) Brussels sprouts, ends trimmed and outer leaves removed
1 medium delicata squash, halved lengthwise, seeded, and cut into 1-inch pieces
cup fresh cranberries
teaspoons olive oil
Salt and freshly ground black pepper, to taste
½ cup balsamic vinegar
2 tablespoons roasted pumpkin seeds
2 tablespoons fresh pomegranate arils (seeds)

Directions:
Preheat oven to 400°F (205°C). Line a sheet pan with parchment paper.
Combine the Brussels sprouts, squash, and cranberries in a large bowl.
Drizzle with olive oil, and season lightly with salt and pepper. Toss well to coat and arrange in a single layer on the sheet pan.
Roast in the preheated oven for 30 minutes, turning vegetables halfway through, or until Brussels sprouts turn brown and crisp in spots.
Meanwhile, make the balsamic glaze by simmering the vinegar for 10 to 12 minutes, or until mixture has reduced to about ¼ cup and turns a syrupy consistency.
Remove the vegetables from the oven, drizzle with balsamic syrup, and sprinkle with pumpkin seeds and pomegranate arils before serving.

Per Serving:
calories: 203 | fat: 6.8g | protein: 6.2g | carbs: 22.0g | fiber: 8.2g | sodium: 32mg

Rich Chicken and Small Pasta Broth

Prep time: 10 minutes | Cook time: 4 hours | Serves 6

Ingredients:
6 boneless, skinless chicken thighs
4 stalks celery, cut into ½-inch pieces
4 carrots, cut into 1-inch pieces
medium yellow onion, halved
garlic cloves, minced
2 bay leaves
Sea salt and freshly ground black pepper, to taste
6 cups low-sodium chicken stock
½ cup stelline pasta
¼ cup chopped fresh flat-leaf parsley

Directions:
Combine the chicken thighs, celery, carrots, onion, and garlic in the slow cooker. Spread with bay leaves and sprinkle with salt and pepper. Toss to mix well.
Pour in the chicken stock. Put the lid on and cook on high for 4 hours or until the internal temperature of chicken reaches at least 165°F (74°C).
In the last 20 minutes of the cooking, remove the chicken from the slow cooker and transfer to a bowl to cool until ready to reserve.
Discard the bay leaves and add the pasta to the slow cooker. Put the lid on and cook for 15 minutes or until al dente.
Meanwhile, slice the chicken, then put the chicken and parsley in the slow cooker and cook for 5 minutes or until well combined.
Pour the soup in a large bowl and serve immediately.

Per Serving:
calories: 285 | fat: 10.8g | protein: 27.4g | carbs: 18.8g | fiber: 2.6g | sodium: 815mg

Baby Potato and Olive Salad

Prep time: 10 minutes | Cook time: 20 minutes | Serves 6

Ingredients:

2 pounds (907 g) baby potatoes, cut into 1-inch cubes
1 tablespoon low-sodium olive brine
3 tablespoons freshly squeezed lemon juice (from about 1 medium lemon)
¼ teaspoon kosher salt
3 tablespoons extra-virgin olive oil
½ cup sliced olives
2 tablespoons torn fresh mint
cup sliced celery (about 2 stalks)
tablespoons chopped fresh oregano

Directions:

Put the tomatoes in a saucepan, then pour in enough water to submerge the tomatoes about 1 inch.
Bring to a boil over high heat, then reduce the heat to medium-low.
Simmer for 14 minutes or until the potatoes are soft.
Meanwhile, combine the olive brine, lemon juice, salt, and olive oil in a small bow. Stir to mix well.
Transfer the cooked tomatoes in a colander, then rinse with running cold water. Pat dry with paper towels.
Transfer the tomatoes in a large salad bowl, then drizzle with olive brine mixture. Spread with remaining ingredients and toss to combine well.
Serve immediately.

Per Serving:

calories: 220 | fat: 6.1g | protein: 4.3g | carbs: 39.2g | fiber: 5.0g | sodium: 231mg

Brussels Sprout and Apple Slaw

Prep time: 15 minutes | Cook time: 0 minutes | Serves 4

Salad:
1 pound (454 g) Brussels sprouts, stem ends removed and sliced thinly
1 apple, cored and sliced thinly
½ red onion, sliced thinly

Dressing:
teaspoon Dijon mustard
teaspoons apple cider vinegar
1 tablespoon raw honey
1 cup plain coconut yogurt
1 teaspoon sea salt
For Garnish:
½ cup pomegranate seeds
½ cup chopped toasted hazelnuts

Directions:
Combine the ingredients for the salad in a large salad bowl, then toss to combine well.
Combine the ingredients for the dressing in a small bowl, then stir to mix well.
Dress the salad let sit for 10 minutes. Serve with pomegranate seeds and toasted hazelnuts on top.

Per Serving:
calories: 248 | fat: 11.2g | protein: 12.7g | carbs: 29.9g | fiber: 8.0g | sodium: 645mg

Pumpkin Soup with Crispy Sage Leaves

Prep time: 15 minutes | Cook time: 10 minutes | Serves 4

Ingredients:
tablespoon olive oil
garlic cloves, cut into ⅛-inch-thick slices
onion, chopped
cups freshly puréed pumpkin
4 cups low-sodium vegetable soup
2 teaspoons chipotle powder
1 teaspoon sea salt
½ teaspoon freshly ground black pepper
½ cup vegetable oil
12 sage leaves, stemmed

Dorections:
Heat the olive oil in a stockpot over high heat until shimmering.
Add the garlic and onion, then sauté for 5 minutes or until the onion is translucent.
Pour in the puréed pumpkin and vegetable soup in the pot, then sprinkle with chipotle powder, salt, and ground black pepper. Stir to mix well. 4. Bring to a boil. Reduce the heat to low and simmer for 5 minutes.
Meanwhile, heat the vegetable oil in a nonstick skillet over high heat. Add the sage leaf to the skillet and sauté for a minute or until crispy. Transfer the sage on paper towels to soak the excess oil.
Gently pour the soup in three serving bowls, then divide the crispy sage leaves in bowls for garnish. Serve immediately.

Per Serving:
calories: 380 | fat: 20.1g | protein: 8.9g | carbs: 45.2g | fiber: 18.0g | sodium: 1364mg

Roasted Root Vegetable Soup

Prep time: 10 minutes | Cook time: 35 minutes | Serves 6

Ingredients:
2 parsnips, peeled and sliced
2 carrots, peeled and sliced
2 sweet potatoes, peeled and sliced
1 teaspoon chopped fresh rosemary
1 teaspoon chopped fresh thyme
teaspoon sea salt
½ teaspoon freshly ground black pepper
tablespoons extra-virgin olive oil
4 cups low-sodium vegetable soup
½ cup grated Parmesan cheese, for garnish (optional)

Directions:
Preheat the oven to 400°F (205°C). Line a baking sheet with aluminum foil.

Combine the parsnips, carrots, and sweet potatoes in a large bowl, then sprinkle with rosemary, thyme, salt, and pepper, and drizzle with olive oil. Toss to coat the vegetables well.

Arrange the vegetables on the baking sheet, then roast in the preheated oven for 30 minutes or until lightly browned and soft. Flip the vegetables halfway through the roasting.

Pour the roasted vegetables with vegetable broth in a food processor, then pulse until creamy and smooth.

Pour the puréed vegetables in a saucepan, then warm over low heat until heated through.

Spoon the soup in a large serving bowl, then scatter with Parmesan cheese. Serve immediately.

Per Serving:
calories: 192 | fat: 5.7g | protein: 4.8g | carbs: 31.5g | fiber: 5.7g | sodium: 797mg

Green Beans with Tahini-Lemon Sauce

Prep time: 5 minutes | Cook time: 10 minutes | Serves 2

Ingredients:
pound (454 g) green beans, washed and trimmed
tablespoons tahini
1 garlic clove, minced
Grated zest and juice of 1 lemon
Salt and black pepper, to taste
1 teaspoon toasted black or white sesame seeds (optional)

Directions:
Steam the beans in a medium saucepan fitted with a steamer basket (or by adding ¼ cup water to a covered saucepan) over medium-high heat. Drain, reserving the cooking water.
Mix the tahini, garlic, lemon zest and juice, and salt and pepper to taste. Use the reserved cooking water to thin the sauce as desired.
Toss the green beans with the sauce and garnish with the sesame seeds, if desired. Serve immediately.

Per Serving:
calories: 188 | fat: 8.4g | protein: 7.2g | carbs: 22.2g | fiber: 7.9g | sodium: 200mg

Mixed Salad With Balsamic Honey Dressing

Prep time: 15 minutes | Cook time: 0 minutes | Serves 2

Dressing:
¼ cup balsamic vinegar
¼ cup olive oil
1 tablespoon honey
1 teaspoon Dijon mustard ¼ teaspoon garlic powder
¼ teaspoon salt, or more to taste Pinch freshly ground black pepper

Salad:
4 cups chopped red leaf lettuce
½ cup cherry or grape tomatoes, halved
½ English cucumber, sliced in quarters lengthwise and then cut into bite-size pieces
Any combination fresh, torn herbs (parsley, oregano, basil, or chives)
1 tablespoon roasted sunflower seeds

Directions:
Combine the vinegar, olive oil, honey, mustard, garlic powder, salt, and pepper in a jar with a lid. Shake well. Make the Salad
In a large bowl, combine the lettuce, tomatoes, cucumber, and herbs. Toss well.
Pour all or as much dressing as desired over the tossed salad and toss again to coat the salad with dressing.
Top with the sunflower seeds before serving.

Per Serving:
calories: 337 | fat: 26.1g | protein: 4.2g | carbs: 22.2g | fiber: 3.1g | sodium: 172mg

Cherry, Plum, Artichoke, and Cheese Board

Prep time: 15 minutes | Cook time: 0 minutes | Serves 4

Ingredients:

2 cups rinsed cherries

2 cups rinsed and sliced plums

2 cups rinsed carrots, cut into sticks

1 cup canned low-sodium artichoke hearts, rinsed and drained

1 cup cubed feta cheese

Directions:

Arrange all the ingredients in separated portions on a clean board or a large tray, then serve with spoons, knife, and forks.

Per Serving:

calories: 417 | fat: 13.8g | protein: 20.1g | carbs: 56.2g | fiber: 3.0g | sodium: 715mg

Cucumber Gazpacho

Prep time: 10 minutes | Cook time: 0 minutes | Serves 4

Ingredients:
2 cucumbers, peeled, deseeded, and cut into chunks
½ cup mint, finely chopped
2 cups plain Greek yogurt
2 garlic cloves, minced
2 cups low-sodium vegetable soup
1 tablespoon no-salt-added tomato paste
3 teaspoons fresh dill
Sea salt and freshly ground pepper, to taste

Directions:
Put the cucumber, mint, yogurt, and garlic in a food processor, then pulse until creamy and smooth.
Transfer the puréed mixture in a large serving bowl, then add the vegetable soup, tomato paste, dill, salt, and ground black pepper. Stir to mix well.
Keep the soup in the refrigerator for at least 2 hours, then serve chilled.

Per Serving:
calories: 133 | fat: 1.5g | protein: 14.2g | carbs: 16.5g | fiber: 2.9g | sodium: 331mg

Super Mushroom and Red Wine Soup

Prep time: 40 minutes | Cook time: 35 minutes | Serves 6

Ingredients:
2 ounces (57 g) dried morels
2 ounces (57 g) dried porcini
1 tablespoon extra-virgin olive oil
8 ounces (227 g) button mushrooms, chopped
8 ounces (227 g) portobello mushrooms, chopped
3 shallots, finely chopped
2 cloves garlic, minced
1 teaspoon finely chopped fresh thyme
Sea salt and freshly ground pepper, to taste
⅓ cup dry red wine
4 cups low-sodium chicken broth
½ cup heavy cream
1 small bunch flat-leaf parsley, chopped

Directions:
Put the dried mushrooms in a large bowl and pour in enough water to submerge the mushrooms. Soak for 30 minutes and drain.

Heat the olive oil in a stockpot over medium-high heat until shimmering. Add the mushrooms and shallots to the pot and sauté for 10 minutes or until the mushrooms are tender. Add the garlic and sauté for an additional 1 minute or until fragrant. Sprinkle with thyme, salt, and pepper. Pour in the dry red wine and chicken broth. Bring to a boil over high heat. Reduce the heat to low. Simmer for 20 minutes.

After simmering, pour half of the soup in a food processor, then pulse until creamy and smooth. Pour the puréed soup back to the pot, then mix in the cream and heat over low heat until heated through.

Pour the soup in a large serving bowl and spread with chopped parsley before serving.

Per Serving: calories: 139 | fat: 7.4g | protein: 7.1g | carbs: 14.4g | fiber: 2.8g | sodium: 94mg

Roasted Cauliflower

Prep time: 10 minutes | Cook time: 20 minutes | Serves 2

Ingredients:
½ large head cauliflower, stemmed and broken into florets (about 3 cups)
tablespoon olive oil
tablespoons freshly squeezed lemon juice
2 tablespoons tahini
1 teaspoon harissa paste
Pinch salt

Directions:
Preheat the oven to 400°F (205°C). Line a sheet pan with parchment paper.
Toss the cauliflower florets with the olive oil in a large bowl and transfer to the sheet pan.
Roast in the preheated oven for 15 minutes, flipping the cauliflower once or twice, or until it starts to become golden.
Meanwhile, in a separate bowl, combine the lemon juice, tahini, harissa, and salt and stir to mix well.
Remove the pan from the oven and toss the cauliflower with the lemon tahini sauce. Return to the oven and roast for another 5 minutes. Serve hot.

Per Serving:
calories: 205 | fat: 15.0g | protein: 4.0g | carbs: 15.0g | fiber: 7.0g | sodium: 161mg

Mediterranean Tomato Hummus Soup

Prep time: 10 minutes | Cook time: 10 minutes | Serves 2

Ingredients:
(14.5-ounce / 411-g) can crushed tomatoes with basil
cups low-sodium chicken stock
1 cup roasted red pepper hummus
Salt, to taste
¼ cup thinly sliced fresh basil leaves, for garnish (optional)

Directions:
Combine the canned tomatoes, hummus, and chicken stock in a blender and blend until smooth. Pour the mixture into a saucepan and bring it to a boil. Season with salt to taste.
Serve garnished with the fresh basil, if desired.

Per Serving:
calories: 147 | fat: 6.2g | protein: 5.2g | carbs: 20.1g | fiber: 4.1g | sodium: 682mg

Vegetable Fagioli Soup

Prep time: 30 minutes | Cook time: 60 minutes | Serves 2

Ingredients:
tablespoon olive oil
medium carrots, diced
2 medium celery stalks, diced
½ medium onion, diced
1 large garlic clove, minced
tablespoons tomato paste
cups low-sodium vegetable broth
1 cup packed kale, stemmed and chopped
1 (15-ounce / 425-g) can red kidney beans, drained and rinsed
1 (15-ounce / 425-g) can cannellini beans, drained and rinsed
½ cup chopped fresh basil
Salt and freshly ground black pepper, to taste

Directions:
Heat the olive oil in a stockpot over medium-high heat. Add the carrots, celery, onion, and garlic and sauté for 10 minutes, or until the vegetables start to turn golden.
Stir in the tomato paste and cook for about 30 seconds.
Add the vegetable broth and bring the soup to a boil. Cover and reduce the heat to low. Cook the soup for 45 minutes, or until the carrots are tender.
Using an immersion blender, purée the soup so that it's partly smooth, but with some chunks of vegetables.
Add the kale, beans, and basil. Season with salt and pepper to taste, then serve.

Per Serving:
calories: 217 | fat: 4.2g | protein: 10.0g | carbs: 36.2g | fiber: 10.2g | sodium: 482m

Butternut Squash and Cauliflower Soup

Prep time: 15 minutes | Cook time: 4 hours | Serves 4 to 6

Ingredients:

1 pound (454 g) butternut squash, peeled and cut into 1-inch cubes
1 small head cauliflower, cut into 1-inch pieces
onion, sliced
cups unsweetened coconut milk1 tablespoon curry powder
½ cup no-added-sugar apple juice
4 cups low-sodium vegetable soup
2 tablespoons coconut oil
1 teaspoon sea salt
¼ teaspoon freshly ground white pepper
¼ cup chopped fresh cilantro, divided

Directions:

Combine all the ingredients, except for the cilantro, in the slow cooker.
Stir to mix well.
Cook on high heat for 4 hours or until the vegetables are tender.
Pour the soup in a food processor, then pulse until creamy and
smooth.
Pour the puréed soup in a large serving bowl and garnish with cilantro
before serving.

Per Serving:

calories: 415 | fat: 30.8g | protein: 10.1g | carbs: 29.9g | fiber: 7.0g |
sodium: 1386mg

Veggie Slaw

Prep time: 20 minutes | Cook time: 0 minutes | Serves 4 to 6

Ingredients:

2 large broccoli stems, peeled and shredded
½ celery root bulb, peeled and shredded
¼ cup chopped fresh Italian parsley
large beet, peeled and shredded
carrots, peeled and shredded
small red onion, sliced thin
zucchini, shreddedDressing:
1 teaspoon Dijon mustard
½ cup apple cider vinegar
1 tablespoon raw honey
teaspoon sea salt
¼ teaspoon freshly ground black pepper
tablespoons extra-virgin olive oilTopping:
½ cup crumbled feta cheese

Directions:

Combine the ingredients for the salad in a large salad bowl, then toss to combine well.

Combine the ingredients for the dressing in a small bowl, then stir to mix well.

Dress the salad, then serve with feta cheese on top.

Per Serving:

calories: 387 | fat: 30.2g | protein: 8.1g | carbs: 25.9g | fiber: 6.0g | sodium: 980mg

Lemon-Tahini Hummus

Prep time: 15 minutes | Cook time: 0 minutes | Serves 6

Ingredients:
1 (15-ounce / 425-g) can chickpeas, drained and rinsed
4 tablespoons extra-virgin olive oil, divided
4 to 5 tablespoons tahini (sesame seed paste)
2 lemons, juiced
1 lemon, zested, divided
1 tablespoon minced garlic
Pinch salt

Directions:
In a food processor, combine the chickpeas, 2 tablespoons of olive oil, tahini, lemon juice, half of the lemon zest, and garlic and pulse for up to 1 minute, scraping down the sides of the food processor bowl as necessary.

Taste and add salt as needed. Feel free to add 1 teaspoon of water at a time to thin the hummus to a better consistency.

Transfer the hummus to a serving bowl. Serve drizzled with the remaining 2 tablespoons of olive oil and remaining half of the lemon zest.

Per Serving:
calories: 216 | fat: 15.0g | protein: 5.0g | carbs: 17.0g | fiber: 5.0g | sodium: 12mg

Lemon and Spinach Orzo

Prep time: 5 minutes | Cook time: 10 minutes | Makes 2 cups

Ingredients:
1 cup dry orzo
1 (6-ounce / 170-g) bag baby spinach
cup halved grape tomatoes
tablespoons extra-virgin olive oil
¼ teaspoon salt
Freshly ground black pepper
¾ cup crumbled feta cheese
1 lemon, juiced and zested

Directions:
Bring a medium pot of water to a boil. Stir in the orzo and cook uncovered for 8 minutes. Drain the water, then return the orzo to medium heat.
Add the spinach and tomatoes and cook until the spinach is wilted. Sprinkle with the olive oil, salt, and pepper and mix well. Top with the feta cheese, lemon juice and zest, then toss one or two more times and serve.

Per Serving: (1 cup)
calories: 610 | fat: 27.0g | protein: 21.0g | carbs: 74.0g | fiber: 6.0g | sodium: 990mg

Citrus Salad with Kale and Fennel

Prep time: 15 minutes | Cook time: 0 minutes | Serves 2

Dressing:
3 tablespoons olive oil
2 tablespoons fresh orange juice
1 tablespoon blood orange vinegar, other orange vinegar, or cider vinegar
tablespoon honey
Salt and freshly ground black pepper, to taste Salad:
cups packed baby kale
1 medium navel or blood orange, segmented
½ small fennel bulb, stems and leaves removed, sliced into matchsticks
3 tablespoons toasted pecans, chopped
2 ounces (57 g) goat cheese, crumbled

Make the Dressing:
Mix the olive oil, orange juice, vinegar, and honey in a small bowl and whisk to combine. Season with salt and pepper to taste. Set aside. Make the Salad
Divide the baby kale, orange segments, fennel, pecans, and goat cheese evenly between two plates.
Drizzle half of the dressing over each salad and serve.

Per Serving:
calories: 503 | fat: 39.1g | protein: 13.2g | carbs: 31.2g | fiber: 6.1g | sodium: 156mg

Arugula, Watermelon, and Feta Salad

Prep time: 10 minutes | Cook time: 0 minutes | Serves 2

Ingredients:
3 cups packed arugula

2½ cups watermelon, cut into bite-size cubes

2 ounces (57 g) feta cheese, crumbled

2 tablespoons balsamic glaze

Directions:
Divide the arugula between two plates.

Divide the watermelon cubes between the beds of arugula.

Scatter half of the feta cheese over each salad.

Drizzle about 1 tablespoon of the glaze (or more if desired) over each salad. Serve immediately.

Per Serving:
calories: 157 | fat: 6.9g | protein: 6.1g | carbs: 22.0g | fiber: 1.1g | sodium: 328mg

Artichoke and Arugula Salad

Prep time: 10 minutes | Cook time: 0 minutes | Serves 6

Ingredients:
6 canned oil-packed artichoke hearts, sliced
6 cups baby arugula leaves
6 fresh olives, pitted and chopped 1 cup cherry tomatoes, sliced in half
Dressing:
teaspoon Dijon mustard
tablespoons balsamic vinegar
clove garlic, minced
tablespoons extra-virgin olive oilFor Garnish:
4 fresh basil leaves, thinly sliced

Directions:
Combine the ingredients for the salad in a large salad bowl, then toss to combine well.
Combine the ingredients for the dressing in a small bowl, then stir to mix well.
Dress the salad, then serve with basil leaves on top.

Per Serving:
calories: 134 | fat: 12.1g | protein: 1.6g | carbs: 6.2g | fiber: 3.0g| sodium: 65mg

Grilled Bell Pepper and Anchovy Antipasto

Prep time: 15 minutes | Cook time: 8 minutes | Serves 4

Ingredients:
2 tablespoons extra-virgin olive oil, divided
4 medium red bell peppers, quartered, stem and seeds removed
6 ounces (170 g) anchovies in oil, chopped
2 tablespoons capers, rinsed and drained
1 cup Kalamata olives, pitted
1 small shallot, chopped
Sea salt and freshly ground pepper, to taste

Directions:
Heat the grill to medium-high heat. Grease the grill grates with 1 tablespoon of olive oil.
Arrange the red bell peppers on the preheated grill grates, then grill for 8 minutes or until charred.
Turn off the grill and allow the pepper to cool for 10 minutes.
Transfer the charred pepper in a colander. Rinse and peel the peppers under running cold water, then pat dry with paper towels.
Cut the peppers into chunks and combine with remaining ingredients in a large bowl. Toss to mix well.
Serve immediately.

Per Serving:
calories: 227 | fat: 14.9g | protein: 13.9g | carbs: 9.9g | fiber: 3.8g| sodium: 1913mg

Marinated Mushrooms and Olives

Prep time: 1 hour 10 minutes | Cook time: 0 minutes | Serves 8

Ingredients:
1 pound (454 g) white button mushrooms, rinsed and drained
1 pound (454 g) fresh olives
½ tablespoon crushed fennel seeds
tablespoon white wine vinegar
tablespoons fresh thyme leaves
Pinch chili flakes
Sea salt and freshly ground pepper, to taste
2 tablespoons extra-virgin olive oil

Directions:
Combine all the ingredients in a large bowl. Toss to mix well.
Wrap the bowl in plastic and refrigerate for at least 1 hour to marinate.
Remove the bowl from the refrigerate and let sit under room
temperature for 10 minutes, then serve.

Per Serving:
calories: 111 | fat: 9.7g | protein: 2.4g | carbs: 5.9g | fiber: 2.7g |
sodium: 449mg

Root Vegetable Roast

Prep time: 15 minutes | Cook time: 25 minutes | Serves 4 to 6

Ingredients:

bunch beets, peeled and cut into 1-inch cubes
small sweet potatoes, peeled and cut into 1-inch cubes
parsnips, peeled and cut into 1-inch rounds
carrots, peeled and cut into 1-inch rounds
1 tablespoon raw honey
1 teaspoon sea salt
½ teaspoon freshly ground black pepper
tablespoon extra-virgin olive oil
tablespoons coconut oil, melted

Directions:

Preheat the oven to 400°F (205°C). Line a baking sheet with parchment paper.

Combine all the ingredients in a large bowl. Toss to coat the vegetables well.

Pour the mixture in the baking sheet, then place the sheet in the preheated oven.

Roast for 25 minutes or until the vegetables are lightly browned and soft. Flip the vegetables halfway through the cooking time.

Remove the vegetables from the oven and allow to cool before serving.

Per Serving:

calories: 461 | fat: 18.1g | protein: 5.9g | carbs: 74.2g | fiber: 14.0g | sodium: 759mg

Sardines with Lemony Tomato Sauce

Prep time: 10 minutes | Cook time: 40 minutes | Serves 4

Ingredients:
2 tablespoons olive oil, divided
4 Roma tomatoes, peeled and chopped, reserve the juice
1 small onion, sliced thinly
Zest of 1 orange
Sea salt and freshly ground pepper, to taste
pound (454 g) fresh sardines, rinsed, spine removed, butterflied
½ cup white wine
tablespoons whole-wheat breadcrumbs

Directions:
Preheat the oven to 425°F (220°C). Grease a baking dish with 1 tablespoon of olive oil.
Heath the remaining olive oil in a nonstick skillet over medium-low heat until shimmering.
Add the tomatoes with juice, onion, orange zest, salt, and ground pepper to the skillet and simmer for 20 minutes or until it thickens.
Pour half of the mixture on the bottom of the baking dish, then top with the butterflied sardines. Pour the remaining mixture and white wine over the sardines.
Spread the breadcrumbs on top, then place the baking dish in the preheated oven. Bake for 20 minutes or until the fish is opaque.
Remove the baking sheet from the oven and serve the sardines warm.

Per Serving:
calories: 363 | fat: 20.2g | protein: 29.7g | carbs: 9.7g | fiber: 2.0g| sodium: 381mg

Mushroom and Soba Noodle Soup

Prep time: 15 minutes | Cook time: 10 minutes | Serves 4

Ingredients:
2 tablespoons coconut oil
8 ounces (227 g) shiitake mushrooms, stemmed and sliced thin
1 tablespoon minced fresh ginger
4 scallions, sliced thin 1 garlic clove, minced
1 teaspoon sea salt
4 cups low-sodium vegetable broth
cups water
ounces (113 g) soba noodles
1 bunch spinach, blanched, rinsed and cut into strips
1 tablespoon freshly squeezed lemon juice

Directions:
Heat the coconut oil in a stockpot over medium heat until melted.
Add the mushrooms, ginger, scallions, garlic, and salt. Sauté for 5
minutes or until fragrant and the mushrooms are tender.
Pour in the vegetable broth and water. Bring to a boil, then add the
soba noodles and cook for 5 minutes or until al dente.
Turn off the heat and add the spinach and lemon juice. Stir to mix well.
Pour the soup in a large bowl and serve immediately.

Per Serving:
calories: 254 | fat: 9.2g | protein: 13.1g | carbs: 33.9g | fiber: 4.0g |
sodium: 1773mg

Sautéed White Beans with Rosemary

Prep time: 10 minutes | Cook time: 12 minutes | Serves 2

Ingredients:
tablespoon olive oil
garlic cloves, minced
1 (15-ounce / 425-g) can white cannellini beans, drained and rinsed
1 teaspoon minced fresh rosemary plus 1 whole fresh rosemary sprig
¼ teaspoon dried sage
½ cup low-sodium chicken stock
Salt, to taste

Directions:
Heat the olive oil in a saucepan over medium-high heat.
Add the garlic and sauté for 30 seconds until fragrant.
Add the beans, minced and whole rosemary, sage, and chicken stock and bring the mixture to a boil.
Reduce the heat to medium and allow to simmer for 10 minutes, or until most of the liquid is evaporated. If desired, mash some of the beans with a fork to thicken them.
Season with salt to taste. Remove the rosemary sprig before serving.

Per Serving:
calories: 155 | fat: 7.0g | protein: 6.0g | carbs: 17.0g | fiber: 8.0g | sodium: 153mg

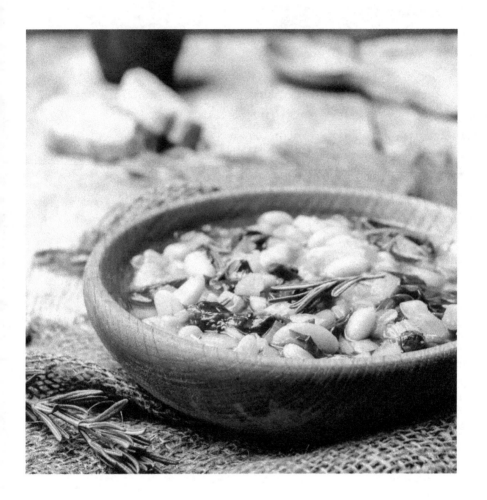

Moroccan Spiced Couscous

Prep time: 10 minutes | Cook time: 8 minutes | Serves 2

Ingredients:
1 tablespoon olive oil
¾ cup couscous
¼ teaspoon cinnamon
¼ teaspoon garlic powder
¼ teaspoon salt, plus more as needed
cup water
tablespoons minced dried apricots
2 tablespoons raisins
2 teaspoons minced fresh parsley

Directions:
Heat the olive oil in a saucepan over medium-high heat until it shimmers.
Add the couscous, cinnamon, garlic powder, and salt. Stir for 1 minute to toast the couscous and spices.
Add the water, apricots, and raisins and bring the mixture to a boil.
Cover and turn off the heat. Allow the couscous to sit for 4 to 5 minutes and then fluff it with a fork. Sprinkle with the fresh parsley. Season with more salt as needed and serve.

Per Serving:
calories: 338 | fat: 8.0g | protein: 9.0g | carbs: 59.0g | fiber: 4.0g | sodium: 299mg

Tricolor Summer Salad

Prep time: 10 minutes | Cook time: 0 minutes | Serves 3 to 4

Ingredients:
¼ cup while balsamic vinegar

2 tablespoons Dijon mustard

1 tablespoon sugar

½ teaspoon garlic salt

½ teaspoon freshly ground black pepper

¼ cup extra-virgin olive oil

1½ cups chopped orange, yellow, and red tomatoes

½ cucumber, peeled and diced

1 small red onion, thinly sliced

¼ cup crumbled feta (optional)

Directions:
In a small bowl, whisk the vinegar, mustard, sugar, pepper, and garlic salt. Then slowly whisk in the olive oil.

In a large bowl, add the tomatoes, cucumber, and red onion. Add the dressing. Toss once or twice, and serve with the feta crumbles (if desired) sprinkled on top.

Per Serving:
calories: 246 | fat: 18.0g | protein: 1.0g | carbs: 19.0g | fiber: 2.0g | sodium: 483mg

Sandwiches, Pizzas, and Wraps

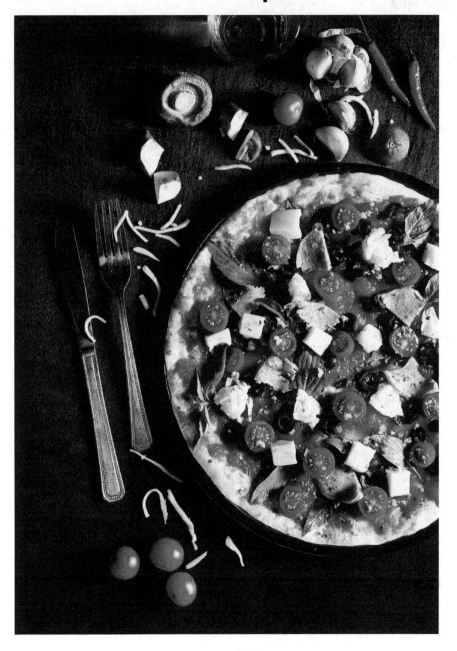

Spicy Black Bean and Poblano Dippers

Prep time: 20 minutes | Cook time: 21 minutes | Serves 8

Ingredients:

2 tablespoons avocado oil, plus more for brushing the dippers

1 (15 ounces / 425 g) can black beans, drained and rinsed

1 poblano, deseeded and quartered

1 jalapeño, halved and deseeded

½ cup fresh cilantro, leaves and tender stems

yellow onion, quartered

garlic cloves

1 teaspoon chili powder

1 teaspoon ground cumin

1 teaspoon sea salt

24 organic corn tortillas

Directions:

Preheat the oven to 400°F (205°C). Line a baking sheet with parchment paper and grease with avocado oil. Combine the remaining ingredients, except for the tortillas, in a food processor, then pulse until chopped finely and the mixture holds together. Make sure not to purée the mixture. Warm the tortillas on the baking sheet in the preheated oven for 1 minute or until softened. Add a tablespoon of the mixture in the middle of each tortilla. Fold one side of the tortillas over the mixture and tuck to roll them up tightly to make the dippers. Arrange the dippers on the baking sheet and brush them with avocado oil. Bake in the oven for 20 minutes or until well browned. Flip the dippers halfway through the cooking time. Serve immediately.

Per Serving:

calories: 388 | fat: 6.5g | protein: 16.2g | carbs: 69.6g | fiber: 13.5g | sodium: 340mg

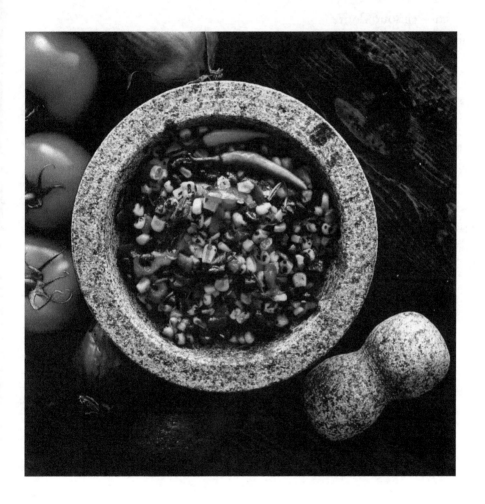

Super Cheeses and Mushroom Tart

Prep time: 30 minutes | Cook time: 1 hour 30 minutes | Serves 4 to 6

Crust:
1¾ cups almond flour
tablespoon raw honey
¾ teaspoon sea salt
¼ cup extra-virgin olive oil
⅓ cup water

Filling:
tablespoons extra-virgin olive oil, divided
1 pound (454 g) white mushrooms, trimmed and sliced thinly
Sea salt, to taste
garlic clove, minced
teaspoons minced fresh thyme
¼ cup shredded Mozzarella cheese
½ cup grated Parmesan cheese
4 ounces (113 g) part-skim ricotta cheese
Ground black pepper, to taste
2 tablespoons ground basil

Make the Crust:

Preheat the oven to 350°F (180°C).

Combine the flour, honey, salt and olive oil in a large bowl. Stir to mix well. Gently mix in the water until a smooth dough forms.

Drop walnut-size clumps from the dough in the single layer on a tart pan. Press the clumps to coat the bottom of the pan.

Bake the crust in the preheated oven for 50 minutes or until firm and browned. Rotate the pan halfway through. Make the Filling

While baking the crust, heat 1 tablespoon of olive oil in a nonstick skillet over medium-high heat until shimmering.

Add the mushrooms and sprinkle with ½ teaspoon of salt. Sauté for 15 minutes or until tender.

Add the garlic and thyme and sauté for 30 seconds or until fragrant. Make the Tart

Meanwhile, combine the cheeses, salt, ground black pepper, and 1 tablespoon of olive oil in a bowl. Stir to mix well.

Spread the cheese mixture over the crust, then top with the mushroom mixture.

Bake in the oven for 20 minutes or until the cheeses are frothy and the tart is heated through. Rotate the pan halfway through the baking time.

Remove the tart from the oven. Allow to cool for at least 10 minutes, then sprinkle with basil. Slice to serve.

Per Serving:

calories: 530 | fat: 26.6g | protein: 11.7g | carbs: 63.5g | fiber: 4.6g | sodium: 785mg

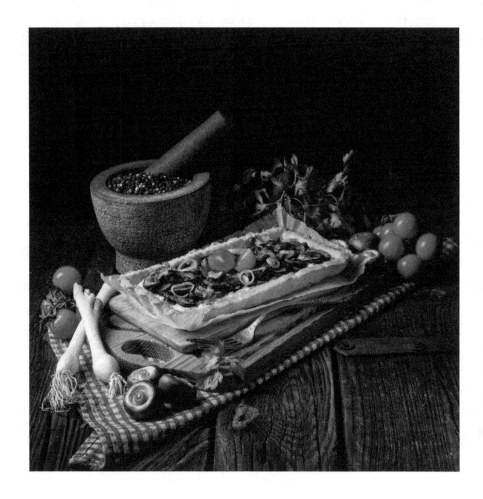

Turkish Eggplant and Tomatoes Pide with Mint

Prep time: 1 day 40 minutes | Cook time: 20 minutes | Makes 6 pides

Dough:
3 cups almond flour
2 teaspoons raw honey
½ teaspoon instant or rapid-rise yeast
1⅓ cups ice water
1 tablespoon extra-virgin olive oil
1½ teaspoons sea salt
Eggplant and Tomato Toppings:
28 ounces (794 g) whole tomatoes, peeled and puréed
5 tablespoons extra-virgin olive oil, divided
1 pound (454 g) eggplant, cut into ½-inch pieces
½ red bell pepper, chopped
Sea salt and ground black pepper, to taste
3 garlic cloves, minced
¼ teaspoon red pepper flakes
½ teaspoon smoked paprika
6 tablespoons minced fresh mint, divided
1½ cups crumbled feta cheese

Make the Dough:
Combine the flour, yeast, and honey in a food processor, pulse to combine well. Gently add water while pulsing. Let the dough sit for 10 minutes.
Mix the olive oil and salt in the dough and knead the dough until smooth. Wrap in plastic and refrigerate for at least 1 day.

Make the Toppings:

Heat 2 tablespoons of olive oil in a nonstick skillet over medium-high heat until shimmering. Add the bell pepper, eggplant, and ½ teaspoon of salt. Sauté for 6 minutes or until the eggplant is lightly browned. Add the red pepper flakes, paprika, and garlic. Sauté for 1 minute or until fragrant. Pour in the puréed tomatoes. Bring to a simmer, then cook for 10 minutes or until the mixture is thickened into about 3½ cups. Turn off the heat and mix in 4 tablespoons of mint, salt, and ground black pepper. Set them aside until ready to use.

Make the Turkish Pide

Preheat the oven to 500°F (260°C). Line three baking sheets with parchment papers. On a clean work surface, divide and shape the dough into six 14 by 5inch ovals. Transfer the dough to the baking sheets. Brush them with 3 tablespoons of olive oil and spread the eggplant mixture and feta cheese on top. Bake in the preheated oven for 12 minutes or until golden brown. Rotate the pide halfway through the baking time.

Remove the pide from the oven and spread with remaining mint and serve immediately.

Per Serving: (1 pide)
calories: 500 | fat: 22.1g | protein: 8.0g | carbs: 69.7g | fiber: 5.8g | sodium: 1001mg

Greek Vegetable Salad Pita

Prep time: 10 minutes | Cook time: 0 minutes | Serves 4

Ingredients:
½ cup baby spinach leaves
½ small red onion, thinly sliced
½ small cucumber, deseeded and chopped
1 tomato, chopped
1 cup chopped romaine lettuce
1 tablespoon extra-virgin olive oil
½ tablespoon red wine vinegar
1 teaspoon Dijon mustard
1 tablespoon crumbled feta cheese
Sea salt and freshly ground pepper, to taste
1 whole-wheat pita

Direction:
Combine all the ingredients, except for the pita, in a large bowl. Toss to mix well.
Stuff the pita with the salad, then serve immediately.

Per Serving:
calories: 137 | fat: 8.1g | protein: 3.1g | carbs: 14.3g | fiber: 2.4g | sodium: 166mg

Artichoke and Cucumber Hoagies

Prep time: 10 minutes | Cook time: 15 minutes | Makes 1

Ingredients:
1 (12-ounce / 340-g) whole grain baguette, sliced in half horizontally
1 cup frozen and thawed artichoke hearts, roughly chopped
cucumber, sliced
tomatoes, sliced
red bell pepper, sliced
⅓ cup Kalamata olives, pitted and chopped
¼ small red onion, thinly sliced
Sea salt and ground black pepper, to taste
tablespoons <u>pesto</u>
Balsamic vinegar, to taste

Directions:
Arrange the baguette halves on a clean work surface, then cut off the top third from each half. Scoop some insides of the bottom half out and reserve as breadcrumbs.
Toast the baguette in a baking pan in the oven for 1 minute to brown lightly.
Put the artichokes, cucumber, tomatoes, bell pepper, olives, and onion in a large bowl. Sprinkle with salt and ground black pepper. Toss to combine well.
Spread the bottom half of the baguette with the vegetable mixture and drizzle with balsamic vinegar, then smear the cut side of the baguette top with pesto. Assemble the two baguette halves.
Wrap the hoagies in parchment paper and let sit for at least an hour before serving.

Per Serving: (1 hoagies)
calories: 1263 | fat: 37.7g | protein: 56.3g | carbs: 180.1g | fiber: 37.8g | sodium: 2137mg

Classic Socca

Prep time: 10 minutes | Cook time: 10 minutes | Serves 4

Ingredients:
1½ cups chickpea flour
½ teaspoon ground turmeric
½ teaspoon sea salt
½ teaspoon ground black pepper
2 tablespoons plus 2 teaspoons extra-virgin olive oil
1½ cups water

Directions:
Combine the chickpea flour, turmeric, salt, and black pepper in a bowl. Stir to mix well, then gently mix in 2 tablespoons of olive oil and water. Stir to mix until smooth.
Heat 2 teaspoons of olive oil in an 8-inch nonstick skillet over mediumhigh heat until shimmering.
Add half cup of the mixture into the skillet and swirl the skillet so the mixture coat the bottom evenly.
Cook for 5 minutes or until lightly browned and crispy. Flip the socca halfway through the cooking time. Repeat with the remaining mixture. Slice and serve warm.

Per Serving:
calories: 207 | fat: 10.2g | protein: 7.9g | carbs: 20.7g | fiber: 3.9g | sodium: 315mg

Alfalfa Sprout and Nut Rolls

Prep time: 40 minutes | Cook time: 0 minutes | Makes 16 bite-size pieces

Ingredients:
cup alfalfa sprouts
tablespoons Brazil nuts
½ cup chopped fresh cilantro 2 tablespoons flaked coconut
garlic clove, minced
tablespoons ground flaxseeds
Zest and juice of 1 lemon
Pinch cayenne pepper
Sea salt and freshly ground black pepper, to taste
tablespoon melted coconut oil
tablespoons water
2 whole-grain wraps

Directions:
Combine all ingredients, except for the wraps, in a food processor, then pulse to combine well until smooth.

Unfold the wraps on a clean work surface, then spread the mixture over the wraps. Roll the wraps up and refrigerate for 30 minutes until set.

Remove the rolls from the refrigerator and slice into 16 bite-sized pieces, if desired, and serve.

Per Serving: (1 piece) calories: 67 | fat: 7.1g | protein: 2.2g | carbs: 2.9g | fiber: 1.0g | sodium: 61mg

Brown Rice and Black Bean Burgers

Prep time: 20 minutes | Cook time: 40 minutes | Makes 8 burgers

Ingredients:
1 cup cooked brown rice
1 (15-ounce / 425-g) can black beans, drained and rinsed
tablespoon olive oil
tablespoons taco or Harissa seasoning
½ yellow onion, finely diced
1 beet, peeled and grated
carrot, peeled and grated
tablespoons no-salt-added tomato paste
tablespoons apple cider vinegar
garlic cloves, minced
¼ teaspoon sea salt
Ground black pepper, to taste 8 whole-wheat hamburger buns

Toppings:
16 lettuce leaves, rinsed well
8 tomato slices, rinsed well
Whole-grain mustard, to taste

Directions:

Line a baking sheet with parchment paper.

Put the brown rice and black beans in a food processor and pulse until mix well. Pour the mixture in a large bowl and set aside.

Heat the olive oil in a nonstick skillet over medium heat until shimmering.

Add the taco seasoning and stir for 1 minute or until fragrant.

Add the onion, beet, and carrot and sauté for 5 minutes or until the onion is translucent and beet and carrot are tender.

Pour in the tomato paste and vinegar, then add the garlic and cook for 3 minutes or until the sauce is thickened. Sprinkle with salt and ground black pepper.

Transfer the vegetable mixture to the bowl of rice mixture, then stir to mix well until smooth.

Divide and shape the mixture into 8 patties, then arrange the patties on the baking sheet and refrigerate for at least 1 hour.

Preheat the oven to 400°F (205°C).

Remove the baking sheet from the refrigerator and allow to sit under room temperature for 10 minutes.

Bake in the preheated oven for 40 minutes or until golden brown on both sides. Flip the patties halfway through the cooking time.

Remove the patties from the oven and allow to cool for 10 minutes. Assemble the buns with patties, lettuce, and tomato slices. Top the filling with mustard and serve immediately.

Per Serving: (1 burger)
calories: 544 | fat: 20.0g | protein: 15.8g | carbs: 76.0g | fiber: 10.6g | sodium: 4

Falafel Balls with Tahini Sauce

Prep time: 2 hours 20 minutes | Cook time: 20 minutes | Serves 4

Ingredients:
Tahini Sauce:
½ cup tahini
2 tablespoons lemon juice
¼ cup finely chopped flat-leaf parsley
2 cloves garlic, minced ½ cup cold water, as needed

Falafel:
1 cup dried chickpeas, soaked overnight, drained
¼ cup chopped flat-leaf parsley
¼ cup chopped cilantro
1 large onion, chopped
1 teaspoon cumin
½ teaspoon chili flakes
4 cloves garlic
1 teaspoon sea salt
5 tablespoons almond flour
1½ teaspoons baking soda, dissolved in 1 teaspoon water
2 cups peanut oil
1 medium bell pepper, chopped
1 medium tomato, chopped
4 whole-wheat pita breads

Directions:

Make the Tahini Sauce

Combine the ingredients for the tahini sauce in a small bowl. Stir to mix well until smooth.

Wrap the bowl in plastic and refrigerate until ready to serve. Make the Falafel

Put the chickpeas, parsley, cilantro, onion, cumin, chili flakes, garlic, and salt in a food processor. Pulse to mix well but not puréed.

Add the flour and baking soda to the food processor, then pulse to form a smooth and tight dough.

Put the dough in a large bowl and wrap in plastic. Refrigerate for at least 2 hours to let it rise.

Divide and shape the dough into walnut-sized small balls.

Pour the peanut oil in a large pot and heat over high heat until the temperature of the oil reaches 375°F (190°C).

Drop 6 balls into the oil each time, and fry for 5 minutes or until golden brown and crispy. Turn the balls with a strainer to make them fried evenly.

Transfer the balls on paper towels with the strainer, then drain the oil from the balls.

Roast the pita breads in the oven for 5 minutes or until golden brown, if needed, then stuff the pitas with falafel balls and top with bell peppers and tomatoes. Drizzle with tahini sauce and serve immediately.

Per Serving:

calories: 574 | fat: 27.1g | protein: 19.8g | carbs: 69.7g | fiber: 13.4g | sodium: 1246mg

Vegetable and Cheese Lavash Pizza

Prep time: 15 minutes | Cook time: 11 minutes | Serves 4

Ingredients:
2 (12 by 9-inch) lavash breads
2 tablespoons extra-virgin olive oil
10 ounces (284 g) frozen spinach, thawed and squeezed dry
1 cup shredded fontina cheese
1 tomato, cored and cut into ½-inch pieces
½ cup pitted large green olives, chopped
¼ teaspoon red pepper flakes
3 garlic cloves, minced
¼ teaspoon sea salt
¼ teaspoon ground black pepper
½ cup grated Parmesan cheese

Directions:
Preheat oven to 475°F (246°C).
Brush the lavash breads with olive oil, then place them on two baking sheet. Heat in the preheated oven for 4 minutes or until lightly browned. Flip the breads halfway through the cooking time.
Meanwhile, combine the spinach, fontina cheese, tomato pieces, olives, red pepper flakes, garlic, salt, and black pepper in a large bowl. Stir to mix well.
Remove the lavash bread from the oven and sit them on two large plates, spread them with the spinach mixture, then scatter with the Parmesan cheese on top.
Bake in the oven for 7 minutes or until the cheese melts and well browned.
Slice and serve warm.

Per Serving:
calories: 431 | fat: 21.5g | protein: 20.0g | carbs: 38.4g | fiber: 2.5g | sodium: 854mg

Dulse, Avocado, and Tomato Pitas

Prep time: 10 minutes | Cook time: 30 minutes | Makes 4 pitas

Ingredients:

2 teaspoons coconut oil

½ cup dulse, picked through and separated

Ground black pepper, to taste

2 avocados, sliced

2 tablespoons lime juice

¼ cup chopped cilantro

2 scallions, white and light green parts, sliced

Sea salt, to taste

4 (8-inch) whole wheat pitas, sliced in half

4 cups chopped romaine

4 plum tomatoes, sliced

Directions:

Heat the coconut oil in a nonstick skillet over medium heat until melted.

Add the dulse and sauté for 5 minutes or until crispy. Sprinkle with ground black pepper and turn off the heat. Set aside.

Put the avocado, lime juice, cilantro, and scallions in a food processor and sprinkle with salt and ground black pepper. Pulse to combine well until smooth.

Toast the pitas in a baking pan in the oven for 1 minute until soft.

Transfer the pitas to a clean work surface and open. Spread the avocado mixture over the pitas, then top with dulse, romaine, and tomato slices.

Serve immediately.

Per Serving: (1 pita)
calories: 412 | fat: 18.7g | protein: 9.1g | carbs: 56.1g | fiber: 12.5g | sodium: 695mg

---

Tuna and Olive Salad Sandwiches

Prep time: 10 minutes | Cook time: 0 minutes | Serves 4

Ingredients:
3 tablespoons freshly squeezed lemon juice
2 tablespoons extra-virgin olive oil
garlic clove, minced
½ teaspoon freshly ground black pepper
(5-ounce / 142-g) cans tuna, drained
1 (2.25-ounce / 64-g) can sliced olives, any green or black variety
½ cup chopped fresh fennel, including fronds
8 slices whole-grain crusty bread

Directions:
In a medium bowl, whisk together the lemon juice, oil, garlic, and pepper. Add the tuna, olives and fennel to the bowl. Using a fork, separate the tuna into chunks and stir to incorporate all the ingredients. Divide the tuna salad equally among 4 slices of bread. Top each with the remaining bread slices.
Let the sandwiches sit for at least 5 minutes so the zesty filling can soak into the bread before serving.

Per Serving:
calories: 952 | fat: 17.0g | protein: 165.0g | carbs: 37.0g | fiber: 7.0g | sodium: 2572mg

Open-Faced Margherita Sandwiches

Prep time: 10 minutes | Cook time: 5 minutes | Serves 4

Ingredients:
2 (6- to 7-inch) whole-wheat submarine or hoagie rolls, sliced open
horizontally
1 tablespoon extra-virgin olive oil
1 garlic clove, halved
1 large ripe tomato, cut into 8 slices
¼ teaspoon dried oregano
1 cup fresh Mozzarella, sliced
¼ cup lightly packed fresh basil leaves, torn into small pieces
¼ teaspoon freshly ground black pepper

Directions:
Preheat the broiler to High with the rack 4 inches under the heating
element.
Put the sliced bread on a large, rimmed baking sheet and broil for 1
minute, or until the bread is just lightly toasted. Remove from the oven.
Brush each piece of the toasted bread with the oil, and rub a garlic half
over each piece.
Put the toasted bread back on the baking sheet. Evenly divide the
tomato slices on each piece. Sprinkle with the oregano and top with the
cheese.
Place the baking sheet under the broiler. Set the timer for 1½ minutes,
but check after 1 minute. When the cheese is melted and the edges are
just starting to get dark brown, remove the sandwiches from the oven.
Top each sandwich with the fresh basil and pepper before serving.

Per Serving:
calories: 93 | fat: 2.0g | protein: 10.0g | carbs: 8.0g | fiber: 2.0g |
sodium: 313mg

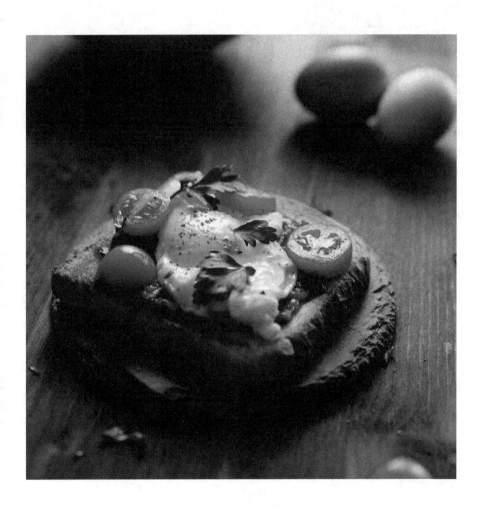

Grilled Caesar Salad Sandwiches

Prep time: 5 minutes | Cook time: 5 minutes | Serves 2

Ingredients:
¾ cup olive oil, divided
romaine lettuce hearts, left intact
to 4 anchovy fillets
Juice of 1 lemon
2 to 3 cloves garlic, peeled
teaspoon Dijon mustard
¼ teaspoon Worcestershire sauce
Sea salt and freshly ground pepper, to taste
slices whole-wheat bread, toasted
Freshly grated Parmesan cheese, for serving

Directions:
Preheat the grill to medium-high heat and oil the grates.
On a cutting board, drizzle the lettuce with 1 to 2 tablespoons of olive oil and place on the grates.
Grill for 5 minutes, turning until lettuce is slightly charred on all sides. Let lettuce cool enough to handle.
In a food processor, combine the remaining olive oil with the anchovies, lemon juice, garlic, mustard, and Worcestershire sauce.
Pulse the ingredients until you have a smooth emulsion. Season with sea salt and freshly ground pepper to taste. Chop the lettuce in half and place on the bread.
Drizzle with the dressing and serve with a sprinkle of Parmesan cheese.

Per Serving:
calories: 949 | fat: 85.6g | protein: 12.9g | carbs: 34.1g | fiber: 13.9g | sodium: 786mg

Green Veggie Sandwiches

Prep time: 20 minutes | Cook time: 0 minutes | Serves 2

Ingredients:

(15-ounce / 425-g) can cannellini beans, drained and rinsed
⅓ cup packed fresh basil leaves
⅓ cup packed fresh parsley
⅓ cup chopped fresh chives
garlic cloves, chopped
Zest and juice of ½ lemon 1 tablespoon apple cider vinegar
Sandwiches:
4 whole-grain bread slices, toasted
8 English cucumber slices
1 large beefsteak tomato, cut into slices
1 large avocado, halved, pitted, and cut into slices
small yellow bell pepper, cut into slices
handfuls broccoli sprouts
2 handfuls fresh spinach

Directions:

In a food processor, combine the cannellini beans, basil, parsley, chives, garlic, lemon zest and juice, and vinegar. Pulse a few times, scrape down the sides, and purée until smooth. You may need to scrape down the sides again to incorporate all the basil and parsley. Refrigerate for at least 1 hour to allow the flavors to blend.
Assemble the Sandwiches Build your sandwiches by spreading several tablespoons of spread on each slice of bread. Layer two slices of bread with the cucumber, tomato, avocado, bell pepper, broccoli sprouts, and spinach. Top with the remaining bread slices and press down lightly. Serve immediately.

Per Serving: calories: 617 | fat: 21.1g | protein: 28.1g | carbs: 86.1g | fiber: 25.6g | sodium: 593mg

Roasted Tomato Panini

Prep time: 15 minutes | Cook time: 3 hours 6 minutes | Serves 2

Ingredients:
2 teaspoons olive oil
4 Roma tomatoes, halved
4 cloves garlic
1 tablespoon Italian seasoning
Sea salt and freshly ground pepper, to taste
4 slices whole-grain bread
4 basil leaves
2 slices fresh Mozzarella cheese

Directions:
Preheat the oven to 250°F (121°C). Grease a baking pan with olive oil.
Place the tomatoes and garlic in the baking pan, then sprinkle with
Italian seasoning, salt, and ground pepper. Toss to coat well.
Roast in the preheated oven for 3 hours or until the tomatoes are
lightly wilted.
Preheat the panini press.
Make the panini: Place two slices of bread on a clean work surface,
then top them with wilted tomatoes. Sprinkle with basil and spread
with Mozzarella cheese. Top them with remaining two slices of bread.
Cook the panini for 6 minutes or until lightly browned and the cheese
melts. Flip the panini halfway through the cooking.
Serve immediately.

Per Serving:
calories: 323 | fat: 12.0g | protein: 17.4g | carbs: 37.5g | fiber: 7.5g |
sodium: 603mg

Samosas in Potatoes

Prep time: 20 minutes | Cook time: 30 minutes | Makes 8

Ingredients:

4 small potatoes
1 teaspoon coconut oil
1 small onion, finely chopped
small piece ginger, minced
garlic cloves, minced
2 to 3 teaspoons curry powder
Sea salt and freshly ground black pepper, to taste
¼ cup frozen peas, thawed
2 carrots, grated
¼ cup chopped fresh cilantro

Directions:

Preheat the oven to 350°F (180°C).
Poke small holes into potatoes with a fork, then wrap with aluminum foil. Bake in the preheated oven for 30 minutes until tender.
Meanwhile, heat the coconut oil in a nonstick skillet over medium-high heat until melted. Add the onion and sauté for 5 minutes or until translucent. Add the ginger and garlic to the skillet and sauté for 3 minutes or until fragrant. Add the curry power, salt, and ground black pepper, then stir to coat the onion. Remove them from the heat.
When the cooking of potatoes is complete, remove the potatoes from the foil and slice in half. Hollow to potato halves with a spoon, then combine the potato fresh with sautéed onion, peas, carrots, and cilantro in a large bowl. Stir to mix well. Spoon the mixture back to the tomato skins and serve immediately.

Per Serving: (1 samosa)
calories: 131 | fat: 13.9g | protein: 3.2g | carbs: 8.8g | fiber: 3.0g | sodium: 111mg

Roasted Vegetable Panini

Prep time: 10 minutes | Cook time: 15 minutes | Serves 4

Ingredients:
2 tablespoons extra-virgin olive oil, divided
1½ cups diced broccoli
1 cup diced zucchini
¼ cup diced onion
¼ teaspoon dried oregano
⅛ teaspoon kosher or sea salt
⅛ teaspoon freshly ground black pepper
(12-ounce / 340-g) jar roasted red peppers, drained and finely chopped
tablespoons grated Parmesan or Asiago cheese
1 cup fresh Mozzarella (about 4 ounces / 113 g), sliced
1 (2-foot-long) whole-grain Italian loaf, cut into 4 equal lengths
Cooking spray

Directions:

Place a large, rimmed baking sheet in the oven. Preheat the oven to 450°F (235°C) with the baking sheet inside.

In a large bowl, stir together 1 tablespoon of the oil, broccoli, zucchini, onion, oregano, salt and pepper.

Remove the baking sheet from the oven and spritz the baking sheet with cooking spray. Spread the vegetable mixture on the baking sheet and roast for 5 minutes, stirring once halfway through cooking.

Remove the baking sheet from the oven. Stir in the red peppers and Parmesan cheese.

In a large skillet over medium-high heat, heat the remaining 1 tablespoon of the oil.

Cut open each section of bread horizontally, but don't cut all the way through. Fill each with the vegetable mix (about ½ cup), and layer 1 ounce (28 g) of sliced Mozzarella cheese on top. Close the sandwiches, and place two of them on the skillet. Place a heavy object on top and grill for 2½ minutes. Flip the sandwiches and grill for another 2½ minutes.

Repeat the grilling process with the remaining two sandwiches.

Serve hot.

Per Serving:

calories: 116 | fat: 4.0g | protein: 12.0g | carbs: 9.0g | fiber: 3.0g | sodium: 569mg

White Pizzas with Arugula and Spinach

Prep time: 10 minutes | Cook time: 20 minutes | Serves 4

Igredients:
pound (454 g) refrigerated fresh pizza dough
tablespoons extra-virgin olive oil, divided
½ cup thinly sliced onion
garlic cloves, minced
cups baby spinach
3 cups arugula
1 tablespoon water
¼ teaspoon freshly ground black pepper
1 tablespoon freshly squeezed lemon juice
½ cup shredded Parmesan cheese
½ cup crumbled goat cheese
Cooking spray

Directions:

Preheat the oven to 500°F (260°C). Spritz a large, rimmed baking sheet with cooking spray.

Take the pizza dough out of the refrigerator.

Heat 1 tablespoon of the oil in a large skillet over medium heat. Add the onion to the skillet and cook for 4 minutes, stirring constantly. Add the garlic and cook for 1 minute, stirring constantly.

Stir in the spinach, arugula, water and pepper. Cook for about 2 minutes, stirring constantly, or until all the greens are coated with oil and they start to cook down. Remove the skillet from the heat and drizzle with the lemon juice.

On a lightly floured work surface, form the pizza dough into a 12-inch circle or a 10-by-12-inch rectangle, using a rolling pin or by stretching with your hands.

Place the dough on the prepared baking sheet. Brush the dough with the remaining 1 tablespoon of the oil. Spread the cooked greens on top of the dough to within ½ inch of the edge. Top with the Parmesan cheese and goat cheese.

Bake in the preheated oven for 10 to 12 minutes, or until the crust starts to brown around the edges.

Remove from the oven and transfer the pizza to a cutting board. Cut into eight pieces before serving.

Per Serving:

calories: 521 | fat: 31.0g | protein: 23.0g | carbs: 38.0g | fiber: 4.0g | sodium: 1073mg

Tuna and Hummus Wraps

Prep time: 10 minutes | Cook time: 0 minutes | Serves 2

Hummus:
cup from 1 (15-ounce / 425-g) can low-sodium chickpeas, drained andrinsed
tablespoons tahini
1 tablespoon extra-virgin olive oil
1 garlic clove
Juice of ½ lemon
¼ teaspoon salt 2 tablespoons water Wraps:
4 large lettuce leaves
1 (5-ounce / 142-g) can chunk light tuna packed in water, drained
1 red bell pepper, seeded and cut into strips
1 cucumber, sliced

Make the Hummus:
In a blender jar, combine the chickpeas, tahini, olive oil, garlic, lemon juice, salt, and water. Process until smooth. Taste and adjust with additional lemon juice or salt, as needed.

Make the Wraps:
On each lettuce leaf, spread 1 tablespoon of hummus, and divide the tuna among the leaves. Top each with several strips of red pepper and cucumber slices.
Roll up the lettuce leaves, folding in the two shorter sides and rolling away from you, like a burrito. Serve immediately.

Per Serving:
calories: 192 | fat: 5.1g | protein: 26.1g | carbs: 15.1g | fiber: 4.1g | sodium: 1065mg

Glazed Mushroom and Vegetable Fajitas

Prep time: 20 minutes | Cook time: 20 minutes | Makes 6

Spicy Glazed Mushrooms:
1 teaspoon olive oil
1 (10- to 12-ounce / 284- to 340-g) package cremini mushrooms, rinsed and drained, cut into thin slices
½ to 1 teaspoon chili powder
Sea salt and freshly ground black pepper, to taste
teaspoon maple syrup

Fajitas:
teaspoons olive oil
1 onion, chopped
Sea salt, to taste
1 bell pepper, any color, deseeded and sliced into long strips
1 zucchini, cut into large matchsticks
6 whole-grain tortilla
carrots, grated
to 4 scallions, sliced
½ cup fresh cilantro, finely chopped

Make the Spicy Glazed Mushrooms:
Heat the olive oil in a nonstick skillet over medium heat until shimmering.
Add the mushrooms and sauté for 10 minutes or until tender.
Sprinkle the mushrooms with chili powder, salt, and ground black pepper. Drizzle with maple syrup. Stir to mix well and cook for 5 to 7 minutes or until the mushrooms are glazed. Set aside until ready to use.

Make the Fajitas:

Heat the olive oil in the same skillet over medium heat until shimmering.

Add the onion and sauté for 5 minutes or until translucent. Sprinkle with salt.

Add the bell pepper and zucchini and sauté for 7 minutes or until tender.

Meanwhile, toast the tortilla in the oven for 5 minutes or until golden brown.

Allow the tortilla to cool for a few minutes until they can be handled, then assemble the tortilla with glazed mushrooms, sautéed vegetables and remaining vegetables to make the fajitas. Serve immediately.

Per Serving:

calories: 403 | fat: 14.8g | protein: 11.2g | carbs: 7.9g | fiber: 7.0g | sodium: 230mg

Mashed Grape Tomato Pizzas

Prep time: 10 minutes | Cook time: 20 minutes | Serves 6

Ingredients:
3 cups grape tomatoes, halved
teaspoon chopped fresh thyme leaves
garlic cloves, minced
¼ teaspoon kosher salt
¼ teaspoon freshly ground black pepper
1 tablespoon extra-virgin olive oil
¾ cup shredded Parmesan cheese
6 whole-wheat pita breads

Directions:
Preheat the oven to 425°F (220°C).
Combine the tomatoes, thyme, garlic, salt, ground black pepper, and olive oil in a baking pan.
Roast in the preheated oven for 20 minutes. Remove the pan from the oven, mash the tomatoes with a spatula and stir to mix well halfway through the cooking time.
Meanwhile, divide and spread the cheese over each pita bread, then place the bread in a separate baking pan and roast in the oven for 5 minutes or until golden brown and the cheese melts.
Transfer the pita bread onto a large plate, then top with the roasted mashed tomatoes. Serve immediately.

Per Serving:
calories: 140 | fat: 5.1g | protein: 6.2g | carbs: 16.9g | fiber: 2.0g | sodium: 466mg

Mini Pork and Cucumber Lettuce Wraps

Prep time: 20 minutes | Cook time: 0 minutes | Makes 12 wraps

Ingredients:
8 ounces (227 g) cooked ground pork
1 cucumber, diced 1 tomato, diced
1 red onion, sliced
1 ounce (28 g) low-fat feta cheese, crumbled
Juice of 1 lemon
1 tablespoon extra-virgin olive oil
Sea salt and freshly ground pepper, to taste
12 small, intact iceberg lettuce leaves

Directions:
Combine the ground pork, cucumber, tomato, and onion in a large
bowl, then scatter with feta cheese. Drizzle with lemon juice and olive
oil, and sprinkle with salt and pepper. Toss to mix well.
Unfold the small lettuce leaves on a large plate or several small plates,
then divide and top with the pork mixture.
Wrap and serve immediately.

Per Serving: (1 warp)
calories: 78 | fat: 5.6g | protein: 5.5g | carbs: 1.4g | fiber: 0.3g |
sodium: 50mg

Za'atar Pizza

Prep time: 10 minutes | Cook time: 1o to 12 minutes | Serves 4 to 6

Ingredients:
1 sheet puff pastry
¼ cup extra-virgin olive oil
⅓ cup za'atar seasoning

Directions:
Preheat the oven to 350°F (180°C). Line a baking sheet with parchment paper.
Place the puff pastry on the prepared baking sheet. Cut the pastry into desired slices.
Brush the pastry with the olive oil. Sprinkle with the za'atar seasoning.
Put the pastry in the oven and bake for 10 to 12 minutes, or until edges are lightly browned and puffed up.
Serve warm.

Per Serving:
calories: 374 | fat: 30.0g | protein: 3.0g | carbs: 20.0g | fiber: 1.0g | sodium: 166mg

Mediterranean Greek Salad Wraps

Prep time: 15 minutes | Cook time: 0 minutes | Serves 4

Ingredients:

1½ cups seedless cucumber, peeled and chopped
1 cup chopped tomato
½ cup finely chopped fresh mint
¼ cup diced red onion
(2.25-ounce / 64-g) can sliced black olives, drained
tablespoons extra-virgin olive oil
1 tablespoon red wine vinegar
¼ teaspoon kosher salt
¼ teaspoon freshly ground black pepper
½ cup crumbled goat cheese
4 whole-wheat flatbread wraps or soft whole-wheat tortillas

Directions:

In a large bowl, stir together the cucumber, tomato, mint, onion and olives.
In a small bowl, whisk together the oil, vinegar, salt, and pepper.
Spread the dressing over the salad. Toss gently to combine.
On a clean work surface, lay the wraps. Divide the goat cheese evenly among the wraps. Scoop a quarter of the salad filling down the center of each wrap.
Fold up each wrap: Start by folding up the bottom, then fold one side over and fold the other side over the top. Repeat with the remaining wraps.
Serve immediately.

Per Serving:

calories: 225 | fat: 12.0g | protein: 12.0g | carbs: 18.0g | fiber: 4.0g | sodium: 349mg

Spicy Tofu Tacos with Cherry Tomato Salsa

Prep time: 20 minutes | Cook time: 11 minutes | Makes 4 tacos

Ingredients:
Cherry Tomato Salsa:
¼ cup sliced cherry tomatoes
½ jalapeño, deseeded and sliced
Juice of 1 lime
garlic clove, minced
Sea salt and freshly ground black pepper, to taste
teaspoons extra-virgin olive oil Spicy Tofu Taco Filling:
4 tablespoons water, divided
½ cup canned black beans, rinsed and drained
2 teaspoons fresh chopped chives, divided
¾ teaspoon ground cumin, divided
¾ teaspoon smoked paprika, divided
Dash cayenne pepper (optional)
¼ teaspoon sea salt
¼ teaspoon freshly ground black pepper
1 teaspoon extra-virgin olive oil
6 ounces (170 g) firm tofu, drained, rinsed, and pressed
4 corn tortillas
¼ avocado, sliced
¼ cup fresh cilantro

Directions:

Make the Cherry Tomato Salsa

Combine the ingredients for the salsa in a small bowl. Stir to mix well. Set aside until ready to use.

Make the Spicy Tofu Taco Filling

Add 2 tablespoons of water into a saucepan, then add the black beans and sprinkle with 1 teaspoon of chives, ½ teaspoon of cumin, ¼ teaspoon of smoked paprika, and cayenne. Stir to mix well.

Cook for 5 minutes over medium heat until heated through, then mash the black beans with the back of a spoon. Turn off the heat and set aside.

Add remaining water into a bowl, then add the remaining chives, cumin, and paprika. Sprinkle with cayenne, salt, and black pepper. Stir to mix well. Set aside.

Heat the olive oil in a nonstick skillet over medium heat until shimmering.

Add the tofu and drizzle with taco sauce, then sauté for 5 minutes or until the seasoning is absorbed. Remove the tofu from the skillet and set aside.

Warm the tortillas in the skillet for 1 minutes or until heated through. Transfer the tortillas onto a large plate and top with tofu, mashed black beans, avocado, cilantro, then drizzle the tomato salsa over. Serve immediately.

Per Serving: (1 taco)
calories: 240 | fat: 9.0g | protein: 11.6g | carbs: 31.6g | fiber: 6.7g | sodium: 195mg

Red Pepper Coques with Pine Nuts

Prep time: 1 day 40 minutes | Cook time: 45 minutes | Makes 4 coques

Dough:
3 cups almond flour
½ teaspoon instant or rapid-rise yeast
teaspoons raw honey
1⅓ cups ice water
tablespoons extra-virgin olive oil
1½ teaspoons sea salt
Red Pepper Topping:
tablespoons extra-virgin olive oil, divided
2 cups jarred roasted red peppers, patted dry and sliced thinly
large onions, halved and sliced thin
garlic cloves, minced
¼ teaspoon red pepper flakes
bay leaves
tablespoons maple syrup
1½ teaspoons sea salt
3 tablespoons red whine vinegar

For Garnish:
¼ cup pine nuts (optional)
1 tablespoon minced fresh parsley

Make the Dough:
Combine the flour, yeast, and honey in a food processor, pulse to combine well. Gently add water while pulsing. Let the dough sit for 10 minutes.
Mix the olive oil and salt in the dough and knead the dough until smooth. Wrap in plastic and refrigerate for at least 1 day.

Make the Topping:

Heat 1 tablespoon of olive oil in a nonstick skillet over medium heat until shimmering.

Add the red peppers, onions, garlic, red pepper flakes, bay leaves, maple syrup, and salt. Sauté for 20 minutes or until the onion is caramelized.

Turn off the heat and discard the bay leaves. Remove the onion from the skillet and baste with wine vinegar. Let them sit until ready to use.

Make the Coques

Preheat the oven to 500°F (260°C). Grease two baking sheets with 1 tablespoon of olive oil. Divide the dough ball into four balls, then press and shape them into equal-sized oval. Arrange the ovals on the baking sheets and pierce each dough about 12 times.

Rub the ovals with 2 tablespoons of olive oil and bake for 7 minutes or until puffed. Flip the ovals halfway through the cooking time.

Spread the ovals with the topping and pine nuts, then bake for an additional 15 minutes or until well browned. Remove the coques from the oven and spread with parsley. Allow to cool for 10 minutes before serving.

Per Serving: (1 coque)
calories: 658 | fat: 23.1g | protein: 3.4g | carbs: 112.0g | fiber: 6.2g | sodium: 1757mg

Ritzy Garden Burgers

Prep time: 1 hour 30 minutes | Cook time: 30 minutes | Serves 6

Ingredients:

1 tablespoon avocado oil

1 yellow onion, diced

½ cup shredded carrots

4 garlic cloves, halved

1 (15 ounces / 425 g) can black beans, rinsed and drained

1 cup gluten-free rolled oats

¼ cup oil-packed sun-dried tomatoes, drained and chopped

½ cup sunflower seeds, toasted

1 teaspoon chili powder

1 teaspoon paprika

1 teaspoon ground cumin

½ cup fresh parsley, stems removed

¼ teaspoon ground red pepper flakes

¾ teaspoon sea salt

¼ teaspoon ground black pepper

¼ cup olive oil For Serving:

6 whole-wheat buns, split in half and toasted

2 ripe avocados, sliced

1 cup kaiware sprouts or mung bean sprouts

1 ripe tomato, sliced

Directions:

Line a baking sheet with parchment paper.

Heat 1 tablespoon of avocado oil in a nonstick skillet over medium heat.

Add the onion and carrots and sauté for 10 minutes or until the onion is caramelized.

Add the garlic and sauté for 30 seconds or until fragrant.

Transfer them into a food processor, then add the remaining ingredients, except for the olive oil. Pulse until chopped fine and the mixture holds together. Make sure not to purée the mixture.

Divide and form the mixture into six 4-inch diameter and ½-inch thick patties.

Arrange the patties on the baking sheet and wrap the sheet in plastic.

Put the baking sheet in the refrigerator and freeze for at least an hour until firm.

Remove the baking sheet from the refrigerator, let them sit under room temperature for 10 minutes.

Heat the olive oil in a nonstick skillet over medium-high heat until shimmering.

Fry the patties in the skillet for 15 minutes or until lightly browned and crispy. Flip the patties halfway through the cooking time. You may need to work in batches to avoid overcrowding.

Assemble the buns with patties, avocados, sprouts, and tomato slices to make the burgers.

Per Serving:

calories: 613 | fat: 23.1g | protein: 26.2g | carbs: 88.3g | fiber: 22.9g | sodium: 456mg

Veg Mix and Blackeye Pea Burritos

Prep time: 15 minutes | Cook time: 40 minutes | Makes 6 burritos

Ingredients:
1 teaspoon olive oil
red onion, diced
garlic cloves, minced
1 zucchini, chopped
1 tomato, diced
1 bell pepper, any color, deseeded and diced
(14-ounce / 397-g) can blackeye peas
teaspoons chili powder
Sea salt, to taste
6 whole-grain tortillas

Directions:
Preheat the oven to 325°F (160°C).
Heat the olive oil in a nonstick skillet over medium heat or until shimmering. Add the onion and sauté for 5 minutes or until translucent. Add the garlic and sauté for 30 seconds or until fragrant. Add the zucchini and sauté for 5 minutes or until tender. Add the tomato and bell pepper and sauté for 2 minutes or until soft. Fold in the black peas and sprinkle them with chili powder and salt. Stir to mix well. Place the tortillas on a clean work surface, then top them with sautéed vegetables mix. Fold one ends of tortillas over the vegetable mix, then tuck and roll them into burritos. Arrange the burritos in a baking dish, seam side down, then pour the juice remains in the skillet over the burritos. Bake in the preheated oven for 25 minutes or until golden brown.
Serve immediately.

Per Serving:calories: 335 | fat: 16.2g | protein: 12.1g | carbs: 8.3g | fiber: 8.0g | sodium: 214mg

Salmon Salad Wraps

Prep time: 10 minutes | Cook time: 0 minutes | Serves 6

Ingredients:
1 pound (454 g) salmon fillets, cooked and flaked
½ cup diced carrots
½ cup diced celery
3 tablespoons diced red onion
3 tablespoons chopped fresh dill
2 tablespoons capers
1½ tablespoons extra-virgin olive oil
1 tablespoon aged balsamic vinegar
¼ teaspoon kosher or sea salt
½ teaspoon freshly ground black pepper
4 whole-wheat flatbread wraps or soft whole-wheat tortillas

Directions:
In a large bowl, stir together all the ingredients, except for the wraps.
On a clean work surface, lay the wraps. Divide the salmon mixture
evenly among the wraps. Fold up the bottom of the wraps, then roll up
the wrap.
Serve immediately.

Per Serving:
calories: 194 | fat: 8.0g | protein: 18.0g | carbs: 13.0g | fiber: 3.0g |
sodium: 536mg

Baked Parmesan Chicken Wraps

Prep time: 10 minutes | Cook time: 18 minutes | Serves 6

Ingredients:
1 pound (454 g) boneless, skinless chicken breasts
1 large egg
¼ cup unsweetened almond milk
⅔ cup whole-wheat bread crumbs
½ cup grated Parmesan cheese
¾ teaspoon garlic powder, divided
1 cup canned low-sodium or no-salt-added crushed tomatoes
1 teaspoon dried oregano
6 (8-inch) whole-wheat tortillas, or whole-grain spinach wraps
1 cup fresh Mozzarella cheese, sliced
1½ cups loosely packed fresh flat-leaf (Italian) parsley, chopped
Cooking spray

Directions:

Preheat the oven to 425°F (220°C). Line a large, rimmed baking sheet with aluminum foil. Place a wire rack on the aluminum foil, and spritz the rack with nonstick cooking spray. Set aside. Place the chicken breasts into a large plastic bag. With a rolling pin, pound the chicken so it is evenly flattened, about ¼ inch thick. Slice the chicken into six portions. In a bowl, whisk together the egg and milk. In another bowl, stir together the bread crumbs, Parmesan cheese and ½ teaspoon of the garlic powder. Dredge each chicken breast portion into the egg mixture, and then into the Parmesan crumb mixture, pressing the crumbs into the chicken so they stick. Arrange the chicken on the prepared wire rack. Bake in the preheated oven for 15 to 18 minutes, or until the internal temperature of the chicken reads 165°F (74°C) on a meat thermometer and any juices run clear. Transfer the chicken to a cutting board, and cut each portion diagonally into ½-inch pieces.

In a small, microwave-safe bowl, stir together the tomatoes, oregano, and the remaining ¼ teaspoon of the garlic powder. Cover the bowl with a paper towel and microwave for about 1 minute on high, until very hot. Set aside. Wrap the tortillas in a damp paper towel and microwave for 30 to 45 seconds on high, or until warmed through. Assemble the wraps: Divide the chicken slices evenly among the six tortillas and top with the sliced Mozzarella cheese. Spread 1 tablespoon of the warm tomato sauce over the cheese on each tortilla, and top each with about ¼ cup of the parsley. Wrap the tortilla: Fold up the bottom of the tortilla, then fold one side over and fold the other side over the top. Serve the wraps warm with the remaining sauce for dipping.

Per Serving:

calories: 358 | fat: 12.0g | protein: 21.0g | carbs: 41.0g | fiber: 7.0g | sodium: 755

Eggplant, Spinach, and Feta Sandwiches

Prep time: 10 minutes | Cook time: 6 to 8 minutes | Serves 2

Ingredients:
medium eggplant, sliced into ½-inch-thick slices
tablespoons olive oil
Sea salt and freshly ground pepper, to taste
5 to 6 tablespoons hummus
4 slices whole-wheat bread, toasted
cup baby spinach leaves
ounces (57 g) feta cheese, softened

Directions:
Preheat the grill to medium-high heat.
Salt both sides of the sliced eggplant, and let sit for 20 minutes to draw out the bitter juices.
Rinse the eggplant and pat dry with a paper towel.
Brush the eggplant slices with olive oil and season with sea salt and freshly ground pepper to taste.
Grill the eggplant until lightly charred on both sides but still slightly firm in the middle, about 3 to 4 minutes per side.
Spread the hummus on the bread slices and top with the spinach leaves, feta cheese, and grilled eggplant. Top with the other slice of bread and serve immediately.

Per Serving:
calories: 493 | fat: 25.3g | protein: 17.1g | carbs: 50.9g | fiber: 14.7g | sodium: 789mg

Pizza Pockets

Prep time: 10 minutes | Cook time: 0 minutes | Serves 2

Ingredients:
½ cup tomato sauce
½ teaspoon oregano
½ teaspoon garlic powder
½ cup chopped black olives
2 canned artichoke hearts, drained and chopped
2 ounces (57 g) pepperoni, chopped
½ cup shredded Mozzarella cheese
1 whole-wheat pita, halved

Directions:
In a medium bowl, stir together the tomato sauce, oregano, and garlic powder.
Add the olives, artichoke hearts, pepperoni, and cheese. Stir to mix.
Spoon the mixture into the pita halves and serve.

Per Serving:
calories: 375 | fat: 23.5g | protein: 17.1g | carbs: 27.1g | fiber: 6.1g | sodium: 1080mg

Mushroom-Pesto Baked Pizza

Prep time: 5 minutes | Cook time: 15 minutes | Serves 2

Ingredients:

teaspoon extra-virgin olive oil
½ cup sliced mushrooms
½ red onion, sliced
Salt and freshly ground black pepper
¼ cup store-bought pesto sauce
whole-wheat flatbreads
¼ cup shredded Mozzarella cheese

Directions:

Preheat the oven to 350°F (180°C).

In a small skillet, heat the oil over medium heat. Add the mushrooms and onion, and season with salt and pepper. Sauté for 3 to 5 minutes until the onion and mushrooms begin to soften.

Spread 2 tablespoons of pesto on each flatbread.

Divide the mushroom-onion mixture between the two flatbreads. Top each with 2 tablespoons of cheese.

Place the flatbreads on a baking sheet and bake for 10 to 12 minutes until the cheese is melted and bubbly. Serve warm.

Per Serving:

calories: 348 | fat: 23.5g | protein: 14.2g | carbs: 28.1g | fiber: 7.1g | sodium: 792mg

Cheesy Fig Pizzas with Garlic Oil

Prep time: 1 day 40 minutes | Cook time: 10 minutes | Makes 2 pizzas

Dough:
cup almond flour
1½ cups whole-wheat flour
¾ teaspoon instant or rapid-rise yeast
teaspoons raw honey
1¼ cups ice water
2 tablespoons extra-virgin olive oil
1¾ teaspoons sea salt

Garlic Oil:
4 tablespoons extra-virgin olive oil, divided
½ teaspoon dried thyme
2 garlic cloves, minced
⅛ teaspoon sea salt
½ teaspoon freshly ground pepper

Topping:
1 cup fresh basil leaves
1 cup crumbled feta cheese
8 ounces (227 g) fresh figs, stemmed and quartered lengthwise
2 tablespoons raw honey

Make the Dough:
Combine the flours, yeast, and honey in a food processor, pulse to combine well. Gently add water while pulsing. Let the dough sit for 10 minutes.

Mix the olive oil and salt in the dough and knead the dough until smooth. Wrap in plastic and refrigerate for at least 1 day.

Make the Garlic Oil:

Heat 2 tablespoons of olive oil in a nonstick skillet over medium-low heat until shimmering.

Add the thyme, garlic, salt, and pepper and sauté for 30 seconds or until fragrant. Set them aside until ready to use.

Make the Pizzas

Preheat the oven to 500°F (260°C). Grease two baking sheets with 2 tablespoons of olive oil. Divide the dough in half and shape into two balls. Press the balls into 13inch rounds. Sprinkle the rounds with a tough of flour if they are sticky.

Top the rounds with the garlic oil and basil leaves, then arrange the rounds on the baking sheets. Scatter with feta cheese and figs.

Put the sheets in the preheated oven and bake for 9 minutes or until lightly browned. Rotate the pizza halfway through.

Remove the pizzas from the oven, then discard the bay leaves. Drizzle with honey. Let sit for 5 minutes and serve immediately.

Per Serving: (1 pizza)
calories: 1350 | fat: 46.5g | protein: 27.5g | carbs: 221.9g | fiber: 23.7g | sodium: 2898mg

Mushroom and Caramelized Onion Musakhan

Prep time: 20 minutes | Cook time: 1 hour 5 minutes | Serves 4

Ingredients:
2 tablespoons sumac, plus more for sprinkling
1 teaspoon ground allspice
½ teaspoon ground cardamom
½ teaspoon ground cumin
3 tablespoons extra-virgin olive oil, divided
pounds (907 g) portobello mushroom caps, gills removed, caps
halvedand sliced ½ inch thick
medium white onions, coarsely chopped
¼ cup water
Kosher salt, to taste
1 whole-wheat Turkish flatbread
¼ cup pine nuts
1 lemon, wedged

Directions:

Preheat the oven to 350°F (180°C).

Combine 2 tablespoons of sumac, allspice, cardamom, and cumin in a small bowl. Stir to mix well.

Heat 2 tablespoons of olive oil in an oven-proof skillet over medium-high heat until shimmering.

Add the mushroom to the skillet and sprinkle with half of sumac mixture. Sauté for 8 minutes or until the mushrooms are tender. You may need to work in batches to avoid overcrowding. Transfer the mushrooms to a plate and set side.

Heat 1 tablespoon of olive oil in the skillet over medium-high heat until shimmering.

Add the onion and sauté for 20 minutes or until caramelized. Sprinkle with remaining sumac mixture, then cook for 1 more minute.

Pour in the water and sprinkle with salt. Bring to a simmer.

Turn off the heat and put the mushroom back to the skillet.

Place the skillet in the preheated oven and bake for 30 minutes.

Remove the skillet from the oven and let the mushroom sit for 10 minutes until cooled down.

Heat the Turkish flatbread in a baking dish in the oven for 5 minutes or until warmed through.

Arrange the bread on a large plate and top with mushrooms, onions, and roasted pine nuts. Squeeze the lemon wedges over and sprinkle with more sumac. Serve immediately.

Per Serving:

calories: 336 | fat: 18.7g | protein: 11.5g | carbs: 34.3g | fiber: 6.9g | sodium: 369mg

Chickpea Lettuce Wraps

Prep time: 15 minutes | Cook time: 0 minutes | Serves 2

Ingredients:
1 (15-ounce / 425-g) can chickpeas, drained and rinsed well
1 celery stalk, diced
½ shallot, minced
1 green apple, cored and diced
3 tablespoons tahini (sesame paste)
2 teaspoons freshly squeezed lemon juice
1 teaspoon raw honey
1 teaspoon Dijon mustard
Dash salt
Filtered water, to thin
4 romaine lettuce leaves

Directions:
In a medium bowl, stir together the chickpeas, celery, shallot, apple, tahini, lemon juice, honey, mustard, and salt. If needed, add some water to thin the mixture.
Place the romaine lettuce leaves on a plate. Fill each with the chickpea filling, using it all. Wrap the leaves around the filling. Serve immediately.

Per Serving:
calories: 397 | fat: 15.1g | protein: 15.1g | carbs: 53.1g | fiber: 15.3g | sodium: 409mg

Zucchini Hummus Wraps

Prep time: 15 minutes | Cook time: 6 minutes | Serves 2

Ingredients:
zucchini, ends removed, thinly sliced lengthwise
½ teaspoon dried oregano
¼ teaspoon freshly ground black pepper
¼ teaspoon garlic powder
¼ cup hummus
whole wheat tortillas
2 Roma tomatoes, cut lengthwise into slices
cup chopped kale
tablespoons chopped red onion
½ teaspoon ground cumin

Directions:
In a skillet over medium heat, add the zucchini slices and cook for 3
minutes per side. Sprinkle with the oregano, pepper, and garlic powder
and remove from the heat.
Spread 2 tablespoons of hummus on each tortilla. Lay half the zucchini
in the center of each tortilla. Top with tomato slices, kale, red onion,
and ¼ teaspoon of cumin. Wrap tightly and serve.

Per Serving:
calories: 248 | fat: 8.1g | protein: 9.1g | carbs: 37.1g | fiber: 8.1g |
sodium: 180mg

Beans, Grains, and Pastas

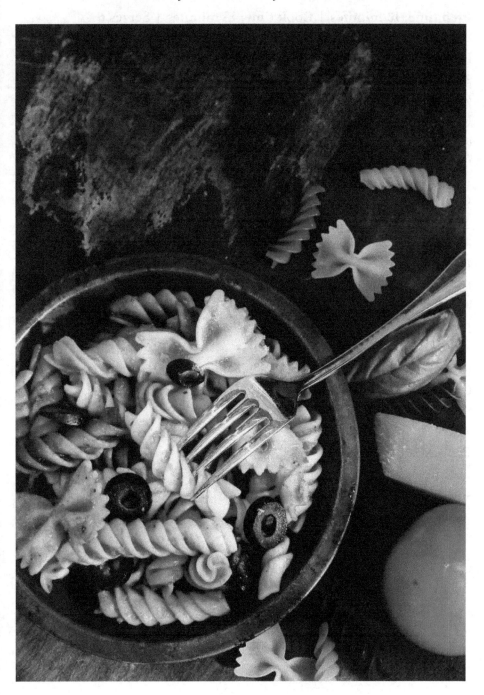

Italian Sautéd Cannellini Beans

Prep time: 10 minutes | Cook time: 15 minutes | Serves 6

Ingredients:
2 teaspoons extra-virgin olive oil
½ cup minced onion
¼ cup red wine vinegar
(12-ounce / 340-g) can no-salt-added tomato paste
tablespoons raw honey
½ cup water
¼ teaspoon ground cinnamon
2 (15-ounce / 425-g) cans cannellini beans

Directions:
Heat the olive oil in a saucepan over medium heat until shimmering.
Add the onion and sauté for 5 minutes or until translucent.
Pour in the red wine vinegar, tomato paste, honey, and water. Sprinkle
with cinnamon. Stir to mix well.
Reduce the heat to low, then pour all the beans into the saucepan.
Cook for 10 more minutes. Stir constantly.
Serve immediately.

Per Serving:
calories: 435 | fat: 2.1g | protein: 26.2g | carbs: 80.3g | fiber: 24.0g |
sodium: 72mg

Lentil and Vegetable Curry Stew

Prep time: 20 minutes | Cook time: 4 hours 7 minutes | Serves 8

Ingredients:

1 tablespoon coconut oil

yellow onion, diced

¼ cup yellow Thai curry paste

cups unsweetened coconut milk

cups dry red lentils, rinsed well and drained

cups bite-sized cauliflower florets

2 golden potatoes, cut into chunks

2 carrots, peeled and diced

8 cups low-sodium vegetable soup, divided

1 bunch kale, stems removed and roughly chopped

Sea salt, to taste

½ cup fresh cilantro, chopped

Pinch crushed red pepper flakes

Directions:

Heat the coconut oil in a nonstick skillet over medium-high heat until melted. Add the onion and sauté for 5 minutes or until translucent. Pour in the curry paste and sauté for another 2 minutes, then fold in the coconut milk and stir to combine well. Bring to a simmer and turn off the heat. Put the lentils, cauliflower, potatoes, and carrot in the slow cooker. Pour in 6 cups of vegetable soup and the curry mixture. Stir to combine well. Cover and cook on high for 4 hours or until the lentils and vegetables are soft. Stir periodically. During the last 30 minutes, fold the kale in the slow cooker and pour in the remaining vegetable soup. Sprinkle with salt. Pour the stew in a large serving bowl and spread the cilantro and red pepper flakes on top before serving hot.

Per Serving:

calories: 530 | fat: 19.2g | protein: 20.3g | carbs: 75.2g | fiber: 15.5g | sodium: 562mg

Butternut Squash and Zucchini with Penne

Prep time: 15 minutes | Cook time: 30 minutes | Serves 6

Ingredients:

1 large zucchini, diced
1 large butternut squash, peeled and diced
large yellow onion, chopped
tablespoons extra-virgin olive oil
1 teaspoon paprika
½ teaspoon garlic powder
½ teaspoon sea salt
½ teaspoon freshly ground black pepper
pound (454 g) whole-grain penne
½ cup dry white wine
tablespoons grated Parmesan cheese

Directions:

Preheat the oven to 400°F (205°C). Line a baking sheet with aluminum foil. Combine the zucchini, butternut squash, and onion in a large bowl. Drizzle with olive oil and sprinkle with paprika, garlic powder, salt, and ground black pepper. Toss to coat well. Spread the vegetables in the single layer on the baking sheet, then roast in the preheated oven for 25 minutes or until the vegetables are tender. Meanwhile, bring a pot of water to a boil, then add the penne and cook for 14 minutes or until al dente. Drain the penne through a colander. Transfer ½ cup of roasted vegetables in a food processor, then pour in the dry white wine. Pulse until smooth. Pour the puréed vegetables in a nonstick skillet and cook with penne over medium-high heat for a few minutes to heat through. Transfer the penne with the purée on a large serving plate, then spread the remaining roasted vegetables and Parmesan on top before serving.

Per Serving:

calories: 340 | fat: 6.2g | protein: 8.0g | carbs: 66.8g | fiber: 9.1g | sodium: 297mg

Small Pasta and Beans Pot

Prep time: 20 minutes | Cook time: 15 minutes | Serves 2 to 4

Ingredients:
1 pound (454 g) small whole wheat pasta
1 (14.5-ounce / 411-g) can diced tomatoes, juice reserved
(15-ounce / 425-g) can cannellini beans, drained and rinsed
tablespoons no-salt-added tomato paste
1 red or yellow bell pepper, chopped
1 yellow onion, chopped
1 tablespoon Italian seasoning mix
3 garlic cloves, minced
¼ teaspoon crushed red pepper flakes, optional
1 tablespoon extra-virgin olive oil
5 cups water
1 bunch kale, stemmed and chopped
½ cup pitted Kalamata olives, chopped
1 cup sliced basil

Directions:
Except for the kale, olives, and basil, combine all the ingredients in a
pot. Stir to mix well. Bring to a boil over high heat. Stir constantly.
Reduce the heat to medium high and add the kale. Cook for 10 minutes
or until the pasta is al dente. Stir constantly.
Transfer all of them on a large plate and serve with olives and basil on
top.

Per Serving:
calories: 357 | fat: 7.6g | protein: 18.2g | carbs: 64.5g | fiber: 10.1g |
sodium: 454mg

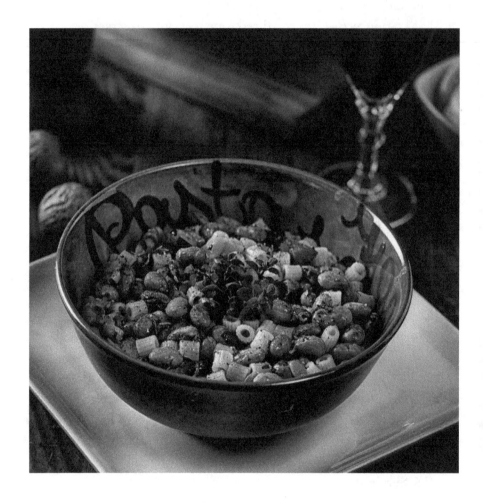

Tomato Basil Pasta

Prep time: 3 minutes | Cook time: 2 minutes | Serves 2

Ingredients:
2 cups dried campanelle or similar pasta
1¾ cups vegetable stock
½ teaspoon salt, plus more as needed
2 tomatoes, cut into large dices
1 or 2 pinches red pepper flakes
½ teaspoon garlic powder ½ teaspoon dried oregano
10 to 12 fresh sweet basil leaves
Freshly ground black pepper, to taste

Directions:
In your Instant Pot, stir together the pasta, stock, and salt. Scatter the tomatoes on top (do not stir).
Secure the lid. Select the Manual mode and set the cooking time for 2 minutes at High Pressure.
Once cooking is complete, do a quick pressure release. Carefully open the lid.
Stir in the red pepper flakes, oregano, and garlic powder. If there's more than a few tablespoons of liquid in the bottom, select Sauté and cook for 2 to 3 minutes until it evaporates.
When ready to serve, chiffonade the basil and stir it in. Taste and season with more salt and pepper, as needed. Serve warm.

Per Serving:
calories: 415 | fat: 2.0g | protein: 15.2g | carbs: 84.2g | fiber: 5.0g | sodium: 485mg

Black Bean Chili with Mangoes

Prep time: 10 minutes | Cook time: 10 minutes | Serves 4

Ingredients:

2 tablespoons coconut oil

onion, chopped

(15-ounce / 425-g) cans black beans, drained and rinsed

1 tablespoon chili powder

1 teaspoon sea salt

¼ teaspoon freshly ground black pepper

cup water

ripe mangoes, sliced thinly

¼ cup chopped fresh cilantro, divided

¼ cup sliced scallions, divided

Directions:

Heat the coconut oil in a pot over high heat until melted.

Put the onion in the pot and sauté for 5 minutes or until translucent.

Add the black beans to the pot. Sprinkle with chili powder, salt, and ground black pepper. Pour in the water. Stir to mix well.

Bring to a boil. Reduce the heat to low, then simmering for 5 minutes or until the beans are tender.

Turn off the heat and mix in the mangoes, then garnish with scallions and cilantro before serving.

Per Serving:

calories: 430 | fat: 9.1g | protein: 20.2g | carbs: 71.9g | fiber: 22.0g | sodium: 608mg

Slow Cooked Turkey and Brown Rice

Prep time: 20 minutes | Cook time: 3 hours 10 minutes | Serves 6

Ingredients:
tablespoon extra-virgin olive oil
1½ pounds (680 g) ground turkey
tablespoons chopped fresh sage, divided
2 tablespoons chopped fresh thyme, divided
teaspoon sea salt
½ teaspoon ground black pepper
cups brown rice
1 (14-ounce / 397-g) can stewed tomatoes, with the juice
¼ cup pitted and sliced Kalamata olives
3 medium zucchini, sliced thinly
¼ cup chopped fresh flat-leaf parsley
1 medium yellow onion, chopped
tablespoon plus 1 teaspoon balsamic vinegar
cups low-sodium chicken stock
2 garlic cloves, minced
½ cup grated Parmesan cheese, for serving

Directions:
Heat the olive oil in a nonstick skillet over medium-high heat until shimmering. Add the ground turkey and sprinkle with 1 tablespoon of sage, 1 tablespoon of thyme, salt and ground black pepper. Sauté for 10 minutes or until the ground turkey is lightly browned. Pour them in the slow cooker, then pour in the remaining ingredients, except for the Parmesan. Stir to mix well. Put the lid on and cook on high for 3 hours or until the rice and vegetables are tender. Pour them in a large serving bowl, then spread with Parmesan cheese before serving.

Per Serving:
calories: 499 | fat: 16.4g | protein: 32.4g | carbs: 56.5g | fiber: 4.7g | sodium: 758mg

Papaya, Jicama, and Peas Rice Bowl
Prep time: 20 minutes | Cook time: 45 minutes | Serves 4

Sauce:
Juice of ¼ lemon
2 teaspoons chopped fresh basil
1 tablespoon raw honey
tablespoon extra-virgin olive oil
Sea salt, to taste

Rice:
1½ cups wild rice
papayas, peeled, seeded, and diced
1 jicama, peeled and shredded
cup snow peas, julienned
cups shredded cabbage
1 scallion, white and green parts, chopped

Directions:
Combine the ingredients for the sauce in a bowl. Stir to mix well. Set aside until ready to use.
Pour the wild rice in a saucepan, then pour in enough water to cover. Bring to a boil.
Reduce the heat to low, then simmer for 45 minutes or until the wild rice is soft and plump. Drain and transfer to a large serving bowl.
Top the rice with papayas, jicama, peas, cabbage, and scallion. Pour the sauce over and stir to mix well before serving.

Per Serving:
calories: 446 | fat: 7.9g | protein: 13.1g | carbs: 85.8g | fiber: 16.0g | sodium: 70mg

Garlic Shrimp Fettuccine

Prep time: 10 minutes | Cook time: 15 minutes | Serves 4 to 6

Ingredients:
8 ounces (227 g) fettuccine pasta
¼ cup extra-virgin olive oil
3 tablespoons garlic, minced
1 pound (454 g) large shrimp, peeled and deveined
⅓ cup lemon juice
1 tablespoon lemon zest
½ teaspoon salt
½ teaspoon freshly ground black pepper

Directions:
Bring a large pot of salted water to a boil. Add the fettuccine and cook for 8 minutes. Reserve ½ cup of the cooking liquid and drain the pasta. In a large saucepan over medium heat, heat the olive oil. Add the garlic and sauté for 1 minute.
Add the shrimp to the saucepan and cook each side for 3 minutes. Remove the shrimp from the pan and set aside.
Add the remaining ingredients to the saucepan. Stir in the cooking liquid. Add the pasta and toss together to evenly coat the pasta.
Transfer the pasta to a serving dish and serve topped with the cooked shrimp.

Per Serving:
calories: 615 | fat: 17.0g | protein: 33.0g | carbs: 89.0g | fiber: 4.0g | sodium: 407mg

Pesto Pasta

Prep time: 10 minutes | Cook time: 8 minutes | Serves 4 to 6

Ingredients:

1 pound (454 g) spaghetti
4 cups fresh basil leaves, stems removed
3 cloves garlic
1 teaspoon salt
½ teaspoon freshly ground black pepper
½ cup toasted pine nuts
¼ cup lemon juice
½ cup grated Parmesan cheese
1 cup extra-virgin olive oil

Directions:

Bring a large pot of salted water to a boil. Add the spaghetti to the pot and cook for 8 minutes.

In a food processor, place the remaining ingredients, except for the olive oil, and pulse.

While the processor is running, slowly drizzle the olive oil through the top opening. Process until all the olive oil has been added.

Reserve ½ cup of the cooking liquid. Drain the pasta and put it into a large bowl. Add the pesto and cooking liquid to the bowl of pasta and toss everything together.

Serve immediately.

Per Serving:

calories: 1067 | fat: 72.0g | protein: 23.0g | carbs: 91..0g | fiber: 6.0g | sodium: 817mg

Cumin Quinoa Pilaf

Prep time: 5 minutes | Cook time: 5 minutes | Serves 2

Ingredients:
2 tablespoons extra virgin olive oil
cloves garlic, minced
cups water
2 cups quinoa, rinsed
2 teaspoons ground cumin
2 teaspoons turmeric
Salt, to taste
1 handful parsley, chopped

Directions:
Press the Sauté button to heat your Instant Pot.
Once hot, add the oil and garlic to the pot, stir and cook for 1 minute.
Add water, quinoa, cumin, turmeric, and salt, stirring well.
Lock the lid. Select the Manual mode and set the cooking time for 1
minute at High Pressure.
When the timer beeps, perform a natural pressure release for 10
minutes, then release any remaining pressure. Carefully remove the lid.
Fluff the quinoa with a fork. Season with more salt, if needed.
Sprinkle the chopped parsley on top and serve.

Per Serving:
calories: 384 | fat: 12.3g | protein: 12.8g | carbs: 57.4g | fiber: 6.9g |
sodium: 448mg

Chickpea, Vegetable, and Fruit Stew

Prep time: 20 minutes | Cook time: 6 hours 4 minutes | Serves 6

Ingredients:

1 large bell pepper, any color, chopped

6 ounces (170 g) green beans, trimmed and cut into bite-size pieces

3 cups canned chickpeas, rinsed and drained

1 (15-ounce / 425-g) can diced tomatoes, with the juice

large carrot, cut into ¼-inch rounds

large potatoes, peeled and cubed

1 large yellow onion, chopped

teaspoon grated fresh ginger

garlic cloves, minced

1¾ cups low-sodium vegetable soup

1 teaspoon ground cumin

1 tablespoon ground coriander

¼ teaspoon ground red pepper flakes

Sea salt and ground black pepper, to taste

8 ounces (227 g) fresh baby spinach

¼ cup diced dried figs

¼ cup diced dried apricots

1 cup plain Greek yogurt

Directions:

Place the bell peppers, green beans, chicken peas, tomatoes and juice, carrot, potatoes, onion, ginger, and garlic in the slow cooker.

Pour in the vegetable soup and sprinkle with cumin, coriander, red pepper flakes, salt, and ground black pepper. Stir to mix well.

Put the slow cooker lid on and cook on high for 6 hours or until the vegetables are soft. Stir periodically.

Open the lid and fold in the spinach, figs, apricots, and yogurt. Stir to mix well.

Cook for 4 minutes or until the spinach is wilted. Pour them in a large serving bowl. Allow to cool for at least 20 minutes, then serve warm.

Per Serving:

calories: 611 | fat: 9.0g | protein: 30.7g | carbs: 107.4g | fiber: 20.8g | sodium: 344mg

Quinoa and Chickpea Vegetable Bowls

Prep time: 20 minutes | Cook time: 15 minutes | Serves 4

Ingredients:

cup red dry quinoa, rinsed and drained
cups low-sodium vegetable soup
2 cups fresh spinach
2 cups finely shredded red cabbage
1 (15-ounce / 425-g) can chickpeas, drained and rinsed
1 ripe avocado, thinly sliced
1 cup shredded carrots
1 red bell pepper, thinly sliced
4 tablespoons Mango Sauce ½ cup fresh cilantro, chopped

Mango Sauce:

1 mango, diced
¼ cup fresh lime juice
½ teaspoon ground turmeric
1 teaspoon finely minced fresh ginger
¼ teaspoon sea salt
Pinch of ground red pepper
teaspoon pure maple syrup
tablespoons extra-virgin olive oil

Directions:

Pour the quinoa and vegetable soup in a saucepan. Bring to a boil. Reduce the heat to low. Cover and cook for 15 minutes or until tender. Fluffy with a fork. Meanwhile, combine the ingredients for the mango sauce in a food processor. Pulse until smooth. Divide the quinoa, spinach, and cabbage into 4 serving bowls, then top with chickpeas, avocado, carrots, and bell pepper. Dress them with the mango sauce and spread with cilantro. Serve immediately.

Per Serving: calories: 366 | fat: 11.1g | protein: 15.5g | carbs: 55.6g | fiber: 17.7g | sodium: 746mg

Tomato Sauce and Basil Pesto Fettuccine

Prep time: 15 minutes | Cook time: 15 minutes | Serves 4

Ingredients:
4 Roma tomatoes, diced
2 teaspoons no-salt-added tomato paste
tablespoon chopped fresh oregano
garlic cloves, minced
1 cup low-sodium vegetable soup
½ teaspoon sea salt
packed cup fresh basil leaves
¼ cup pine nuts
¼ cup grated Parmesan cheese
tablespoons extra-virgin olive oil
1 pound (454 g) cooked whole-grain fettuccine

Directions:
Put the tomatoes, tomato paste, oregano, garlic, vegetable soup, and salt in a skillet. Stir to mix well.
Cook over medium heat for 10 minutes or until lightly thickened.
Put the remaining ingredients, except for the fettuccine, in a food processor and pulse to combine until smooth.
Pour the puréed basil mixture into the tomato mixture, then add the fettuccine. Cook for a few minutes or until heated through and the fettuccine is well coated.
Serve immediately.

Per Serving:
calories: 389 | fat: 22.7g | protein: 9.7g | carbs: 40.2g | fiber: 4.8g | sodium: 616mg

Garlic and Parsley Chickpeas

**Prep time: 10 minutes | Cook time: 18 to 20 minutes |
Serves 4 to 6**

Ingredients:
¼ cup extra-virgin olive oil, divided
4 garlic cloves, sliced thinly
⅛ teaspoon red pepper flakes
onion, chopped finely
¼ teaspoon salt, plus more to taste
Black pepper, to taste
(15-ounce / 425-g) cans chickpeas, rinsed
cup vegetable broth
tablespoons minced fresh parsley
2 teaspoons lemon juice

Directions:
Add 3 tablespoons of the olive oil, garlic, and pepper flakes to a skillet over medium heat. Cook for about 3 minutes, stirring constantly, or until the garlic turns golden but not brown. Stir in the onion and ¼ teaspoon salt and cook for 5 to 7 minutes, or until softened and lightly browned. Add the chickpeas and broth to the skillet and bring to a simmer. Reduce the heat to medium-low, cover, and cook for about 7 minutes, or until the chickpeas are cooked through and flavors meld. Uncover, increase the heat to high and continue to cook for about 3 minutes more, or until nearly all liquid has evaporated. Turn off the heat, stir in the parsley and lemon juice. Season to taste with salt and pepper and drizzle with remaining 1 tablespoon of the olive oil.
Serve warm.

Per Serving:
calories: 220 | fat: 11.4g | protein: 6.5g | carbs: 24.6g | fiber: 6.0g |
sodium: 467mg

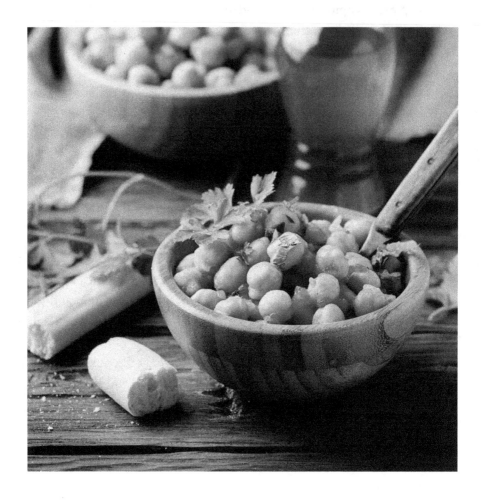

Lentil Risotto

Prep time: 10 minutes | Cook time: 20 minutes | Serves 2

Ingredients:
½ tablespoon olive oil
½ medium onion, chopped
½ cup dry lentils, soaked overnight
½ celery stalk, chopped
1 sprig parsley, chopped
½ cup Arborio (short-grain Italian) rice
garlic clove, lightly mashed
cups vegetable stock

Directions:
Press the Sauté button to heat your Instant Pot.
Add the oil and onion to the Instant Pot and sauté for 5 minutes.
Add the remaining ingredients to the Instant Pot, stirring well.
Secure the lid. Select the Manual mode and set the cooking time for 15 minutes at High Pressure.
Once cooking is complete, do a natural pressure release for 20 minutes, then release any remaining pressure. Carefully open the lid.
Stir and serve hot.

Per Serving:
calories: 261 | fat: 3.6g | protein: 10.6g | carbs: 47.1g | fiber: 8.4g | sodium: 247mg

Ritzy Veggie Chili

Prep time: 15 minutes | Cook time: 5 hours | Serves 4

Ingredients:

1 (28-ounce / 794-g) can chopped tomatoes, with the juice

1 (15-ounce / 425-g) can black beans, drained and rinsed

1 (15-ounce / 425-g) can red beans, drained and rinsed

1 medium green bell pepper, chopped

1 yellow onion, chopped

1 tablespoon onion powder

1 teaspoon paprika

1 teaspoon cayenne pepper

1 teaspoon garlic powder

½ teaspoon sea salt

½ teaspoon ground black pepper

1 tablespoon olive oil

1 large hass avocado, pitted, peeled, and chopped, for garnish

Directions:

Combine all the ingredients, except for the avocado, in the slow cooker. Stir to mix well.

Put the slow cooker lid on and cook on high for 5 hours or until the vegetables are tender and the mixture has a thick consistency.

Pour the chili in a large serving bowl. Allow to cool for 30 minutes, then spread with chopped avocado and serve.

Per Serving:

calories: 633 | fat: 16.3g | protein: 31.7g | carbs: 97.0g | fiber: 28.9g | sodium: 792mg

Spicy Italian Bean Balls with Marinara

Prep time: 20 minutes | Cook time: 30 minutes | Serves 2 to 4

Bean Balls:
1 tablespoon extra-virgin olive oil
½ yellow onion, minced
teaspoon fennel seeds
teaspoons dried oregano
½ teaspoon crushed red pepper flakes
1 teaspoon garlic powder
1 (15-ounce / 425-g) can white beans (cannellini or navy), drained and rinsed
½ cup whole-grain bread crumbs Sea salt and ground black pepper, to taste Marinara:
1 tablespoon extra-virgin olive oil
3 garlic cloves, minced
Handful basil leaves
1 (28-ounce / 794-g) can chopped tomatoes with juice reserved
Sea salt, to taste

Make the Bean Balls:

Preheat the oven to 350°F (180°C). Line a baking sheet with parchment paper.

Heat the olive oil in a nonstick skillet over medium heat until shimmering.

Add the onion and sauté for 5 minutes or until translucent.

Sprinkle with fennel seeds, oregano, red pepper flakes, and garlic powder, then cook for 1 minute or until aromatic.

Pour the sautéed mixture in a food processor and add the beans and bread crumbs. Sprinkle with salt and ground black pepper, then pulse to combine well and the mixture holds together.

Shape the mixture into balls with a 2-ounce (57-g) cookie scoop, then arrange the balls on the baking sheet.

Bake in the preheated oven for 30 minutes or until lightly browned.

Flip the balls halfway through the cooking time.

Make the Marinara

While baking the bean balls, heat the olive oil in a saucepan over medium-high heat until shimmering.

Add the garlic and basil and sauté for 2 minutes or until fragrant.

Fold in the tomatoes and juice. Bring to a boil. Reduce the heat to low.

Put the lid on and simmer for 15 minutes. Sprinkle with salt.

Transfer the bean balls on a large plate and baste with marinara before serving.

Per Serving:

calories: 351 | fat: 16.4g | protein: 11.5g | carbs: 42.9g | fiber: 10.3g | sodium: 377mg

Curry Apple Couscous with Leeks and Pecans

Prep time: 10 minutes | Cook time: 8 minutes | Serves 4

Ingredients:
2 teaspoons extra-virgin olive oil
2 leeks, white parts only, sliced
apple, diced
cups cooked couscous
2 tablespoons curry powder
½ cup chopped pecans

Directions:
Heat the olive oil in a skillet over medium heat until shimmering.
Add the leeks and sauté for 5 minutes or until soft.
Add the diced apple and cook for 3 more minutes until tender.
Add the couscous and curry powder. Stir to combine.
Transfer them in a large serving bowl, then mix in the pecans and
serve.

Per Serving:
calories: 254 | fat: 11.9g | protein: 5.4g | carbs: 34.3g | fiber: 5.9g |
sodium: 15mg

Lebanese Flavor Broken Thin Noodles

Prep time: 10 minutes | Cook time: 25 minutes | Serves 6

Ingredients:

1 tablespoon extra-virgin olive oil
1 (3-ounce / 85-g) cup vermicelli, broken into 1- to 1½-inch pieces
3 cups shredded cabbage
1 cup brown rice
3 cups low-sodium vegetable soup
½ cup water
2 garlic cloves, mashed
¼ teaspoon sea salt
⅛ teaspoon crushed red pepper flakes
½ cup coarsely chopped cilantro
Fresh lemon slices, for serving

Directions:

Heat the olive oil in a saucepan over medium-high heat until shimmering.
Add the vermicelli and sauté for 3 minutes or until toasted.
Add the cabbage and sauté for 4 minutes or until tender.
Pour in the brown rice, vegetable soup, and water. Add the garlic and sprinkle with salt and red pepper flakes.
Bring to a boil over high heat. Reduce the heat to medium low. Put the lid on and simmer for another 10 minutes.
Turn off the heat, then let sit for 5 minutes without opening the lid.
Pour them on a large serving platter and spread with cilantro. Squeeze the lemon slices over and serve warm.

Per Serving:

calories: 127 | fat: 3.1g | protein: 4.2g | carbs: 22.9g | fiber: 3.0g | sodium: 224mg

Cranberry and Almond Quinoa

Prep time: 5 minutes | Cook time: 10 minutes | Serves 2

Ingredients:
2 cups water
1 cup quinoa, rinsed
¼ cup salted sunflower seeds
½ cup slivered almonds
1 cup dried cranberries

Directions:
Combine water and quinoa in the Instant Pot.
Secure the lid. Select the Manual mode and set the cooking time for 10 minutes at High Pressure.
Once cooking is complete, do a quick pressure release. Carefully open the lid.
Add sunflower seeds, almonds, and dried cranberries and gently mix until well combined.
Serve hot.

Per Serving:
calories: 445 | fat: 14.8g | protein: 15.1g | carbs: 64.1g | fiber: 10.2g | sodium: 113mg

Mint Brown Rice

Prep time: 5 minutes | Cook time: 22 minutes | Serves 2

Ingredients:

2 cloves garlic, minced

¼ cup chopped fresh mint, plus more for garnish

1 tablespoon chopped dried chives

1 cup short- or long-grain brown rice

1½ cups water or low-sodium vegetable broth

½ to 1 teaspoon sea salt

Directions:

Place the garlic, mint, chives, rice, and water in the Instant Pot. Stir to combine.

Secure the lid. Select the Manual mode and set the cooking time for 22 minutes at High Pressure.

Once cooking is complete, do a natural pressure release for 10 minutes, then release any remaining pressure. Carefully open the lid.

Add salt to taste and serve garnished with more mint.

Per Serving:

calories: 514 | fat: 6.6g | protein: 20.7g | carbs: 80.4g | fiber: 3.3g | sodium: 786mg

Baked Rolled Oat with Pears and Pecans

Prep time: 15 minutes | Cook time: 30 minutes | Serves 6

Ingredients:
tablespoons coconut oil, melted, plus more for greasing the pan
ripe pears, cored and diced
2 cups unsweetened almond milk
tablespoon pure vanilla extract
¼ cup pure maple syrup
cups gluten-free rolled oats
½ cup raisins
¾ cup chopped pecans
¼ teaspoon ground nutmeg
1 teaspoon ground cinnamon
½ teaspoon ground ginger
¼ teaspoon sea salt

Directions:
Preheat the oven to 350°F (180°C). Grease a baking dish with melted coconut oil, then spread the pears in a single layer on the baking dish evenly.
Combine the almond milk, vanilla extract, maple syrup, and coconut oil in a bowl. Stir to mix well.
Combine the remaining ingredients in a separate large bowl. Stir to mix well. Fold the almond milk mixture in the bowl, then pour the mixture over the pears.
Place the baking dish in the preheated oven and bake for 30 minutes or until lightly browned and set.
Serve immediately.

Per Serving:
calories: 479 | fat: 34.9g | protein: 8.8g | carbs: 50.1g | fiber: 10.8g | sodium: 113mg

Brown Rice Pilaf with Pistachios and Raisins

Prep time: 5 minutes | Cook time: 15 minutes | Serves 6

Ingredients:
1 tablespoon extra-virgin olive oil
1 cup chopped onion
½ cup shredded carrot
½ teaspoon ground cinnamon
teaspoon ground cumin
cups brown rice
1¾ cups pure orange juice
¼ cup water
½ cup shelled pistachios
1 cup golden raisins
½ cup chopped fresh chives

Directions:
Heat the olive oil in a saucepan over medium-high heat until shimmering.
Add the onion and sauté for 5 minutes or until translucent.
Add the carrots, cinnamon, and cumin, then sauté for 1 minutes or until aromatic.
Pour int the brown rice, orange juice, and water. Bring to a boil.
Reduce the heat to medium-low and simmer for 7 minutes or until the liquid is almost absorbed.
Transfer the rice mixture in a large serving bowl, then spread with pistachios, raisins, and chives. Serve immediately.

Per Serving:
calories: 264 | fat: 7.1g | protein: 5.2g | carbs: 48.9g | fiber: 4.0g | sodium: 86mg

Wild Rice, Celery, and Cauliflower Pilaf

Prep time: 10 minutes | Cook time: 45 minutes | Serves 4

Ingredients:

1 tablespoon olive oil, plus more for greasing the baking dish
cup wild rice
cups low-sodium chicken broth
sweet onion, chopped
stalks celery, chopped
teaspoon minced garlic
carrots, peeled, halved lengthwise, and sliced
½ cauliflower head, cut into small florets
1 teaspoon chopped fresh thyme
Sea salt, to taste

Directions:

Preheat the oven to 350°F (180°C). Line a baking sheet with parchment paper and grease with olive oil. Put the wild rice in a saucepan, then pour in the chicken broth. Bring to a boil. Reduce the heat to low and simmer for 30 minutes or until the rice is plump. Meanwhile, heat the remaining olive oil in an oven-proof skillet over medium-high heat until shimmering. Add the onion, celery, and garlic to the skillet and sauté for 3 minutes or until the onion is translucent. Add the carrots and cauliflower to the skillet and sauté for 5 minutes. Turn off the heat and set aside. Pour the cooked rice in the skillet with the vegetables. Sprinkle with thyme and salt. Set the skillet in the preheated oven and bake for 15 minutes or until the vegetables are soft.
Serve immediately.

Per Serving:

calories: 214 | fat: 3.9g | protein: 7.2g | carbs: 37.9g | fiber: 5.0g | sodium: 122mg

Walnut and Ricotta Spaghetti

Prep time: 15 minutes | Cook time: 10 minutes | Serves 6

Ingredients:
pound (454 g) cooked whole-wheat spaghetti
tablespoons extra-virgin olive oil
4 cloves garlic, minced
¾ cup walnuts, toasted and finely chopped
2 tablespoons ricotta cheese
¼ cup flat-leaf parsley, chopped
½ cup grated Parmesan cheese
Sea salt and freshly ground pepper, to taste

Directions:
Reserve a cup of spaghetti water while cooking the spaghetti.
Heat the olive oil in a nonstick skillet over medium-low heat or until shimmering.
Add the garlic and sauté for a minute or until fragrant.
Pour the spaghetti water into the skillet and cook for 8 more minutes.
Turn off the heat and mix in the walnuts and ricotta cheese.
Put the cooked spaghetti on a large serving plate, then pour the walnut sauce over. Spread with parsley and Parmesan, then sprinkle with salt and ground pepper. Toss to serve.

Per Serving:
calories: 264 | fat: 16.8g | protein: 8.6g | carbs: 22.8g | fiber: 4.0g | sodium: 336mg

Caprese Fusilli

Prep time: 15 minutes | Cook time: 7 minutes | Serves 3

Ingredients:
1 tablespoon olive oil
1 onion, thinly chopped
6 garlic cloves, minced
1 teaspoon red pepper flakes
2½ cups dried fusilli
1 (15-ounce / 425-g) can tomato sauce
1 cup tomatoes, halved
1 cup water
¼ cup basil leaves
1 teaspoon salt
cup Ricotta cheese, crumbled
tablespoons chopped fresh basil

Directions:
Warm oil on Sauté. Add red pepper flakes, garlic and onion and cook for 3 minutes until soft.
Mix in fusilli, tomatoes, half of the basil leaves, water, tomato sauce, and salt. Seal the lid, and cook on High Pressure for 4 minutes. Release the pressure quickly.
Transfer the pasta to a serving platter and top with the crumbled ricotta and remaining chopped basil.

Per Serving:
calories: 589 | fat: 17.7g | protein: 19.5g | carbs: 92.8g | fiber: 13.8g | sodium: 879mg

Chicken and Spaghetti Ragù Bolognese

Prep time: 15 minutes | Cook time: 42 minutes | Serves 8

Ingredients:
2 tablespoons olive oil
6 ounces (170 g) bacon, cubed
1 onion, minced
1 carrot, minced
celery stalk, minced
garlic cloves, crushed
¼ cup tomato paste
¼ teaspoon crushed red pepper flakes
1½ pounds (680 g) ground chicken
½ cup white wine
1 cup milk
1 cup chicken broth
Salt, to taste
1 pound (454 g) spaghetti

Directions:
Warm oil on Sauté. Add bacon and fry for 5 minutes until crispy.
Add celery, carrot, garlic and onion and cook for 5 minutes until
fragrant. Mix in red pepper flakes and tomato paste, and cook for 2
minutes. Break chicken into small pieces and place in the pot.
Cook for 10 minutes, as you stir, until browned. Pour in wine and
simmer for 2 minutes. Add chicken broth and milk. Seal the lid and
cook for 15 minutes on High Pressure. Release the pressure quickly.
Add the spaghetti and stir. Seal the lid, and cook on High Pressure for
another 5 minutes.Release the pressure quickly. Check the pasta for
doneness. Taste, adjust the seasoning and serve hot.

Per Serving:
calories: 477 | fat: 20.6g | protein: 28.1g | carbs: 48.5g | fiber: 5.3g |
sodium: 279mg

Lemony Farro and Avocado Bowl
Prep time: 5 minutes | Cook time: 25 minutes | Serves 4

Ingredients:
1 tablespoon plus 2 teaspoons extra-virgin olive oil, divided
½ medium onion, chopped
carrot, shredded
garlic cloves, minced
(6-ounce / 170-g) cup pearled farro
cups low-sodium vegetable soup
2 avocados, peeled, pitted, and sliced
Zest and juice of 1 small lemon
¼ teaspoon sea salt

Directions:
Heat 1 tablespoon of olive oil in a saucepan over medium-high heat until shimmering.
Add the onion and sauté for 5 minutes or until translucent.
Add the carrot and garlic and sauté for 1 minute or until fragrant.
Add the farro and pour in the vegetable soup. Bring to a boil over high heat. Reduce the heat to low. Put the lid on and simmer for 20 minutes or until the farro is al dente.
Transfer the farro in a large serving bowl, then fold in the avocado slices. Sprinkle with lemon zest and salt, then drizzle with lemon juice and 2 teaspoons of olive oil.
Stir to mix well and serve immediately.

Per Serving:
calories: 210 | fat: 11.1g | protein: 4.2g | carbs: 27.9g | fiber: 7.0g | sodium: 152mg

Rice and Blueberry Stuffed Sweet Potatoes

Prep time: 15 minutes | Cook time: 20 minutes | Serves 4

Ingredients:
2 cups cooked wild rice
½ cup dried blueberries
½ cup chopped hazelnuts
½ cup shredded Swiss chard
1 teaspoon chopped fresh thyme
1 scallion, white and green parts, peeled and thinly sliced
Sea salt and freshly ground black pepper, to taste
4 sweet potatoes, baked in the skin until tender

Directions:
Preheat the oven to 400°F (205°C).
Combine all the ingredients, except for the sweet potatoes, in a large bowl. Stir to mix well.
Cut the top third of the sweet potato off length wire, then scoop most of the sweet potato flesh out.
Fill the potato with the wild rice mixture, then set the sweet potato on a greased baking sheet.
Bake in the preheated oven for 20 minutes or until the sweet potato skin is lightly charred.
Serve immediately.

Per Serving:
calories: 393 | fat: 7.1g | protein: 10.2g | carbs: 76.9g | fiber: 10.0g | sodium: 93mg

Creamy Garlic Parmesan Chicken Pasta

Prep time: 5 minutes | Cook time: 15 minutes | Serves 4

Ingredients:

3 tablespoons extra-virgin olive oil

2 boneless, skinless chicken breasts, cut into thin strips

1 large onion, thinly sliced

3 tablespoons garlic, minced

1½ teaspoons salt

1 pound (454 g) fettuccine pasta

1 cup heavy whipping cream

¾ cup freshly grated Parmesan cheese, divided

½ teaspoon freshly ground black pepper

Directions:

In a large skillet over medium heat, heat the olive oil. Add the chicken and cook for 3 minutes.

Add the onion, garlic and salt to the skillet. Cook for 7 minutes, stirring occasionally.

Meanwhile, bring a large pot of salted water to a boil and add the pasta, then cook for 7 minutes.

While the pasta is cooking, add the heavy cream, ½ cup of the Parmesan cheese and black pepper to the chicken. Simmer for 3 minutes.

Reserve ½ cup of the pasta water. Drain the pasta and add it to the chicken cream sauce.

Add the reserved pasta water to the pasta and toss together. Simmer for 2 minutes. Top with the remaining ¼ cup of the Parmesan cheese and serve warm.

Per Serving:

calories: 879 | fat: 42.0g | protein: 35.0g | carbs: 90.0g | fiber: 5.0g | sodium: 1336mg

Bulgur Pilaf with Garbanzo
Prep time: 5 minutes | Cook time: 20 minutes | Serves 4 to 6

Ingredients:
3 tablespoons extra-virgin olive oil
1 large onion, chopped
(1-pound / 454-g) can garbanzo beans, rinsed and drained
cups bulgur wheat, rinsed and drained
1½ teaspoons salt
½ teaspoon cinnamon
4 cups water

Directions:
In a large pot over medium heat, heat the olive oil. Add the onion and cook for 5 minutes.
Add the garbanzo beans and cook for an additional 5 minutes.
Stir in the remaining ingredients.
Reduce the heat to low. Cover and cook for 10 minutes.
When done, fluff the pilaf with a fork. Cover and let sit for another 5 minutes before serving.

Per Serving:
calories: 462 | fat: 13.0g | protein: 15.0g | carbs: 76.0g | fiber: 19.0g | sodium: 890mg

Freekeh Pilaf with Dates and Pistachios

Prep time: 10 minutes | Cook time: 10 minutes | Serves 4 to 6

Ingredients:
2 tablespoons extra-virgin olive oil, plus extra for drizzling
1 shallot, minced
1½ teaspoons grated fresh ginger
¼ teaspoon ground coriander
¼ teaspoon ground cumin
Salt and pepper, to taste
1¾ cups water
1½ cups cracked freekeh, rinsed
3 ounces (85 g) pitted dates, chopped
¼ cup shelled pistachios, toasted and coarsely chopped
1½ tablespoons lemon juice
¼ cup chopped fresh mint

Directions:
Set the Instant Pot to Sauté mode and heat the olive oil until shimmering.
Add the shallot, ginger, coriander, cumin, salt, and pepper to the pot and cook for about 2 minutes, or until the shallot is softened. Stir in the water and freekeh.
Secure the lid. Select the Manual mode and set the cooking time for 4 minutes at High Pressure. Once cooking is complete, do a quick pressure release. Carefully open the lid.
Add the dates, pistachios and lemon juice and gently fluff the freekeh with a fork to combine. Season to taste with salt and pepper.
Transfer to a serving dish and sprinkle with the mint. Serve drizzled with extra olive oil.

Per Serving:
calories: 280 | fat: 8.0g | protein: 8.0g | carbs: 46.0g | fiber: 9.0g | sodium: 200mg

Quinoa with Baby Potatoes and Broccoli

Prep time: 5 minutes | Cook time: 10 minutes | Serves 4

Ingredients:
2 tablespoons olive oil
1 cup baby potatoes, cut in half
cup broccoli florets
cups cooked quinoa
Zest of 1 lemon
Sea salt and freshly ground pepper, to taste

Directions:
Heat the olive oil in a large skillet over medium heat until shimmering.
Add the potatoes and cook for about 6 to 7 minutes, or until softened
and golden brown. Add the broccoli and cook for about 3 minutes, or
until tender.
Remove from the heat and add the quinoa and lemon zest. Season with
salt and pepper to taste, then serve.

Per Serving:
calories: 205 | fat: 8.6g | protein: 5.1g | carbs: 27.3g | fiber: 3.7g |
sodium: 158mg

Pearl Barley Risotto with Parmesan Cheese

Prep time: 5 minutes | Cook time: 20 minutes | Serves 6

Ingredients:

4 cups low-sodium or no-salt-added vegetable broth
1 tablespoon extra-virgin olive oil
cup chopped yellow onion
cups uncooked pearl barley
½ cup dry white wine
1 cup freshly grated Parmesan cheese, divided
¼ teaspoon kosher or sea salt
¼ teaspoon freshly ground black pepper
Fresh chopped chives and lemon wedges, for serving (optional)

Directions:

Pour the broth into a medium saucepan and bring to a simmer.

Heat the olive oil in a large stockpot over medium-high heat. Add the onion and cook for about 4 minutes, stirring occasionally.

Add the barley and cook for 2 minutes, stirring, or until the barley is toasted. Pour in the wine and cook for about 1 minute, or until most of the liquid evaporates. Add 1 cup of the warm broth into the pot and cook, stirring, for about 2 minutes, or until most of the liquid is absorbed.

Add the remaining broth, 1 cup at a time, cooking until each cup is absorbed (about 2 minutes each time) before adding the next. The last addition of broth will take a bit longer to absorb, about 4 minutes.

Remove the pot from the heat, and stir in ½ cup of the cheese, and the salt and pepper.

Serve with the remaining ½ cup of the cheese on the side, along with the chives and lemon wedges (if desired).

Per Serving:

calories: 421 | fat: 11.0g | protein: 15.0g | carbs: 67.0g | fiber: 11.0g | sodium: 641mg

Israeli Couscous with Asparagus

Prep time: 5 minutes | Cook time: 25 minutes | Serves 6

Ingredients:

1½ pounds (680 g) asparagus spears, ends trimmed and stalks chopped into 1-inch pieces
1 garlic clove, minced
1 tablespoon extra-virgin olive oil
¼ teaspoon freshly ground black pepper
1¾ cups water
1 (8-ounce / 227-g) box uncooked whole-wheat or regular Israeli couscous (about 1⅓ cups)
¼ teaspoon kosher salt
1 cup garlic-and-herb goat cheese, at room temperature

Directions:

Preheat the oven to 425°F (220°C).
In a large bowl, stir together the asparagus, garlic, oil, and pepper. Spread the asparagus on a large, rimmed baking sheet and roast for 10 minutes, stirring a few times. Remove the pan from the oven, and spoon the asparagus into a large serving bowl. Set aside.
While the asparagus is roasting, bring the water to a boil in a medium saucepan. Add the couscous and season with salt, stirring well. Reduce the heat to medium-low. Cover and cook for 12 minutes, or until the water is absorbed.
Pour the hot couscous into the bowl with the asparagus. Add the goat cheese and mix thoroughly until completely melted.
Serve immediately.

Per Serving:

calories: 103 | fat: 2.0g | protein: 6.0g | carbs: 18.0g | fiber: 5.0g | sodium: 343mg

Bulgur Pilaf with Kale and Tomatoes

Prep time: 10 minutes | Cook time: 10 minutes | Serves 2

Ingredients:
2 tablespoons olive oil
2 cloves garlic, minced
bunch kale, trimmed and cut into bite-sized pieces
Juice of 1 lemon
cups cooked bulgur wheat
1 pint cherry tomatoes, halved
Sea salt and freshly ground pepper, to taste

Directions:
Heat the olive oil in a large skillet over medium heat. Add the garlic
and sauté for 1 minute.
Add the kale leaves and stir to coat. Cook for 5 minutes until leaves are
cooked through and thoroughly wilted.
Add the lemon juice, bulgur and tomatoes. Season with sea salt and
freshly ground pepper to taste, then serve.

Per Serving:
calories: 300 | fat: 14.0g | protein: 6.2g | carbs: 37.8g | fiber: 8.7g |
sodium: 595mg

Rice and Sweet Potato Pilaf

Prep time: 15 minutes | Cook time: 10 minutes | Serves 4 to 6

Ingredients:
2 tablespoons extra-virgin olive oil
onion, chopped fine
½ teaspoon table salt
garlic cloves, minced
1½ teaspoons ground turmeric
teaspoon ground coriander
⅛ teaspoon cayenne pepper
cups chicken broth
1½ cups long-grain white rice, rinsed
12 ounces (340 g) sweet potato, peeled, quartered lengthwise, and sliced ½ inch thick
½ preserved lemon, pulp and white pith removed, rind rinsed and minced (2 tablespoons)
½ cup shelled pistachios, toasted and chopped
¼ cup fresh cilantro leaves
¼ cup pomegranate seeds

Using highest Sauté function, heat oil in Instant Pot until shimmering. Add onion and salt and cook until onion is softened, about 5 minutes. Stir in garlic, turmeric, coriander, and cayenne and cook until fragrant, about 30 seconds. Stir in broth, rice, and sweet potato.
Lock lid in place and close pressure release valve. Select Manual function and cook for 4 minutes. Turn off Instant Pot and quick release pressure. Carefully remove lid, allowing steam to escape away from you. Add preserved lemon and gently fluff rice with fork to combine. Lay clean dish towel over pot, replace lid, and let sit for 5 minutes. Season with salt and pepper to taste. Transfer to serving dish and sprinkle with pistachios, cilantro, and pomegranate seeds. Serve.
Per Serving: calories: 698 | fat: 22.8g | protein: 36.8g | carbs: 85.5g | fiber: 5.9g | sodium: 802mg

Rice and Bean Stuffed Zucchini

Prep time: 10 minutes | Cook time: 15 minutes | Serves 4

Ingredients:

2 small zucchini, halved lengthwise

½ cup cooked rice

½ cup canned white beans, drained and rinsed

½ cup chopped tomatoes

½ cup chopped toasted cashew nuts

½ cup grated Parmesan cheese

1 tablespoon olive oil

½ teaspoon salt

½ teaspoon freshly ground black pepper

Directions:

Pour 1 cup of water in the instant pot and insert a trivet. Scoop out the pulp of zucchini and chop roughly.

In a bowl, mix the zucchini pulp, rice, tomatoes, cashew nuts, ¼ cup of Parmesan, olive oil, salt, and black pepper. Fill the zucchini boats with the mixture, and arrange the stuffed boats in a single layer on the trivet. Seal the lid and cook for 15 minutes on Steam on High. Do a quick release and serve.

Per Serving:

calories: 239 | fat: 14.7g | protein: 9.4g | carbs: 19.0g | fiber: 2.6g | sodium: 570mg

Chard and Mushroom Risotto

Prep time: 15 minutes | Cook time: 20 minutes | Serves 4

Ingredients:
3 tablespoons olive oil
onion, chopped
Swiss chard, stemmed and chopped
1 cup risotto rice
⅓ cup white wine
cups vegetable stock
½ teaspoon salt
½ cup mushrooms
tablespoons pumpkin seeds, toasted
⅓ cup grated Pecorino Romano cheese

Directions:
Heat oil on Sauté, and cook onion and mushrooms for 5 minutes, stirring, until tender. Add the rice and cook for a minute. Stir in wine and cook for 2 to 3 minutes until almost evaporated.
Pour in stock and season with salt. Seal the lid and cook on High Pressure for 10 minutes. Do a quick release. Stir in chard until wilted, mix in cheese to melt, and serve scattered with pumpkin seeds.

Per Serving:
calories: 420 | fat: 17.7g | protein: 11.8g | carbs: 54.9g | fiber: 4.9g | sodium: 927mg

Chili Halloumi Cheese with Rice

Prep time: 10 minutes | Cook time: 8 minutes | Serves 6

Ingrdeients:

2 cups water

2 tablespoons brown sugar

2 tablespoons rice vinegar

1 tablespoon sweet chili sauce

1 tablespoon olive oil

1 teaspoon fresh minced garlic

20 ounces (567 g) Halloumi cheese, cubed

1 cup rice

¼ cup chopped fresh chives, for garnish

Directions:

Heat the oil on Sauté and fry the halloumi for 5 minutes until golden brown. Set aside.

To the pot, add water, garlic, olive oil, vinegar, sugar, soy sauce, and chili sauce and mix well until smooth. Stir in rice noodles. Seal the lid and cook on High Pressure for 3 minutes. Release the pressure quickly. Split the rice between bowls. Top with fried halloumi and sprinkle with fresh chives before serving.

Per Serving:

calories: 534 | fat: 34.3g | protein: 24.9g | carbs: 30.1g | fiber: 1.0g | sodium: 652mg

Grana Padano Risotto

Prep time: 10 minutes | Cook time: 23 minutes | Serves 6

Ingredients:
1 tablespoon olive oil
white onion, chopped
cups Carnaroli rice, rinsed
¼ cup dry white wine
4 cups chicken stock
teaspoon salt
½ teaspoon ground white pepper
tablespoons Grana padano cheese, grated
¼ tablespoon Grana padano cheese, flakes

Directions:
Warm oil on Sauté. Stir-fry onion for 3 minutes until soft and translucent. Add rice and cook for 5 minutes stirring occasionally. Pour wine into the pot to deglaze, scrape away any browned bits of food from the pan.
Stir in stock, pepper, and salt to the pot. Seal the lid, press Rice and cook on High Pressure for 15 minutes. Release the pressure quickly. Sprinkle with grated Parmesan cheese and stir well. Top with flaked cheese for garnish before serving.

Per Serving:
calories: 307 | fat: 6.0g | protein: 8.2g | carbs: 53.2g | fiber: 2.1g | sodium: 945mg

Turkey and Bell Pepper Tortiglioni

Prep time: 20 minutes | Cook time: 10 minutes | Serves 6

Ingredients:

2 teaspoons chili powder

1 teaspoon salt

1 teaspoon cumin

1 teaspoon onion powder 1 teaspoon garlic powder

½ teaspoon thyme

1½ pounds (680 g) turkey breast, cut into strips

1 tablespoon olive oil

1 red onion, cut into wedges

4 garlic cloves, minced

3 cups chicken broth

1 cup salsa

1 pound (454 g) tortiglioni

1 red bell pepper, chopped diagonally

1 yellow bell pepper, chopped diagonally

1 green bell pepper, chopped diagonally

1 cup shredded Gouda cheese

½ cup sour cream

½ cup chopped parsley

Directions:

In a bowl, mix chili powder, cumin, garlic powder, onion powder, salt, and oregano. Reserve 1 teaspoon of seasoning. Coat turkey with the remaining seasoning.

Warm oil on Sauté. Add turkey strips and sauté for 4 to 5 minutes until browned. Place the turkey in a bowl. Sauté the onion and garlic for 1 minute in the cooker until soft. Press Cancel.

Mix in salsa, broth, and scrape the bottom of any brown bits. Into the broth mixture, stir in tortiglioni pasta and cover with bell peppers and chicken.

Seal the lid and cook for 5 minutes on High Pressure. Do a quick Pressure release.

Open the lid and sprinkle with shredded gouda cheese and reserved seasoning, and stir well. Divide into plates and top with sour cream. Add parsley for garnishing and serve.

Per Serving:

calories: 646 | fat: 21.7g | protein: 41.1g | carbs: 72.9g | fiber: 11.1g | sodium: 201mg

Fava and Garbanzo Bean Ful

Prep time: 10 minutes | Cook time: 10 minutes | Serves 6

Ingredients:

1 (15-ounce / 425-g) can fava beans, rinsed and drained

1 (1-pound / 454-g) can garbanzo beans, rinsed and drained

3 cups water

½ cup lemon juice

3 cloves garlic, peeled and minced

1 teaspoon salt

3 tablespoons extra-virgin olive oil

Directions:

In a pot over medium heat, cook the beans and water for 10 minutes. Drain the beans and transfer to a bowl. Reserve 1 cup of the liquid from the cooked beans.

Add the reserved liquid, lemon juice, minced garlic and salt to the bowl with the beans. Mix to combine well. Using a potato masher, mash up about half the beans in the bowl.

Give the mixture one more stir to make sure the beans are evenly mixed.

Drizzle with the olive oil and serve.

Per Serving:

calories: 199 | fat: 9.0g | protein: 10.0g | carbs: 25.0g | fiber: 9.0g | sodium: 395mg

Triple-Green Pasta with Cheese

Prep time: 5 minutes | Cook time: 14 to 16 minutes | Serves 4

Ingredients:

8 ounces (227 g) uncooked penne

tablespoon extra-virgin olive oil

garlic cloves, minced

¼ teaspoon crushed red pepper

2 cups chopped fresh flat-leaf parsley, including stems

5 cups loosely packed baby spinach

¼ teaspoon ground nutmeg

¼ teaspoon kosher salt

¼ teaspoon freshly ground black pepper

⅓ cup Castelvetrano olives, pitted and sliced

⅓ cup grated Parmesan cheese

Directions:

In a large stockpot of salted water, cook the pasta for about 8 to 10 minutes. Drain the pasta and reserve ¼ cup of the cooking liquid. Meanwhile, heat the olive oil in a large skillet over medium heat. Add the garlic and red pepper and cook for 30 seconds, stirring constantly. Add the parsley and cook for 1 minute, stirring constantly. Add the spinach, nutmeg, salt, and pepper, and cook for 3 minutes, stirring occasionally, or until the spinach is wilted.

Add the cooked pasta and the reserved ¼ cup cooking liquid to the skillet. Stir in the olives and cook for about 2 minutes, or until most of the pasta water has been absorbed.

Remove from the heat and stir in the cheese before serving.

Per Serving:

calories: 262 | fat: 4.0g | protein: 15.0g | carbs: 51.0g | fiber: 13.0g | sodium: 1180mg

Caprese Pasta with Roasted Asparagus

Prep time: 5 minutes | Cook time: 25 minutes | Serves 6

Ingredients:
8 ounces (227 g) uncooked small pasta, like orecchiette (little ears) or farfalle (bow ties)
1½ pounds (680 g) fresh asparagus, ends trimmed and stalks chopped into 1inch pieces
1½ cups grape tomatoes, halved
2 tablespoons extra-virgin olive oil
¼ teaspoon kosher salt
¼ teaspoon freshly ground black pepper
2 cups fresh Mozzarella, drained and cut into bite-size pieces (about 8 ounces / 227 g)
⅓ cup torn fresh basil leaves
2 tablespoons balsamic vinegar

Directions:
Preheat the oven to 400°F (205°C).
In a large stockpot of salted water, cook the pasta for about 8 to 10 minutes. Drain and reserve about ¼ cup of the cooking liquid.
Meanwhile, in a large bowl, toss together the asparagus, tomatoes, oil, salt and pepper. Spread the mixture onto a large, rimmed baking sheet and bake in the oven for 15 minutes, stirring twice during cooking.
Remove the vegetables from the oven and add the cooked pasta to the baking sheet. Mix with a few tablespoons of cooking liquid to help the sauce become smoother and the saucy vegetables stick to the pasta. Gently mix in the Mozzarella and basil. Drizzle with the balsamic vinegar. Serve from the baking sheet or pour the pasta into a large bowl.

Per Serving:
calories: 147 | fat: 3.0g | protein: 16.0g | carbs: 17.0g | fiber: 5.0g | sodium: 420mg

Spaghetti with Pine Nuts and Cheese

Prep time: 10 minutes | Cook time: 11 minutes | Serves 4 to 6

Ingredients:
8 ounces (227 g) spaghetti
4 tablespoons almond butter
1 teaspoon freshly ground black pepper
½ cup pine nuts
1 cup fresh grated Parmesan cheese, divided

Directions:
Bring a large pot of salted water to a boil. Add the pasta and cook for 8 minutes.

In a large saucepan over medium heat, combine the butter, black pepper, and pine nuts. Cook for 2 to 3 minutes, or until the pine nuts are lightly toasted.

Reserve ½ cup of the pasta water. Drain the pasta and place it into the pan with the pine nuts.

Add ¾ cup of the Parmesan cheese and the reserved pasta water to the pasta and toss everything together to evenly coat the pasta.

Transfer the pasta to a serving dish and top with the remaining ¼ cup of the Parmesan cheese. Serve immediately.

Per Serving:
calories: 542 | fat: 32.0g | protein: 20.0g | carbs: 46.0g | fiber: 2.0g | sodium: 552mg

Brown Rice Stuffed Portobello Mushrooms

Prep time: 15 minutes | Cook time: 10 minutes | Serves 4

Ingredients:
4 large portobello mushrooms, stems and gills removed
2 tablespoons olive oil
½ cup brown rice, cooked
1 tomato, seed removed and chopped
¼ cup black olives, pitted and chopped
1 green bell pepper, seeded and diced
½ cup feta cheese, crumbled
Juice of 1 lemon
½ teaspoon salt
½ teaspoon ground black pepper
Minced fresh cilantro, for garnish
1 cup vegetable broth

Directions:
Brush the mushrooms with olive oil. Arrange the mushrooms in a
single layer in an oiled baking pan. In a bowl, mix the rice, tomato,
olives, bell pepper, feta cheese, lemon juice, salt, and black pepper.
Spoon the rice mixture into the mushrooms. Pour in the broth, seal the
lid and cook on High Pressure for 10 minutes. Do a quick release.
Garnish with fresh cilantro and serve immediately.

Per Serving:
calories: 190 | fat: 12.5g | protein: 5.9g | carbs: 15.2g | fiber: 2.6g |
sodium: 682m

Spinach and Ricotta Stuffed Pasta Shells

Prep time: 15 minutes | Cook time: 35 minutes | Serves 6

Ingredients:

2 cups onion, chopped

1 cup carrot, chopped

3 garlic cloves, minced

3½ tablespoons olive oil,

1 (28-ounce / 794-g) canned tomatoes, crushed

12 ounces (340 g) conchiglie pasta

tablespoon olive oil

cups ricotta cheese, crumbled

1½ cups feta cheese, crumbled

2 cups spinach, chopped

¾ cup grated Pecorino Romano cheese

2 tablespoons chopped fresh chives

1 tablespoon chopped fresh dill

Salt and ground black pepper to taste

1 cup shredded Cheddar cheese

Directions:

Warm olive oil on Sauté. Add onion, carrot, and garlic, and cook for 5 minutes until tender. Stir in tomatoes and cook for another 10 minutes. Remove to a bowl and set aside.

Wipe the pot with a damp cloth, add pasta and cover with enough water. Seal the lid and cook for 5 minutes on High Pressure. Do a quick release and drain the pasta. Lightly Grease olive oil to a baking sheet.

In a bowl, combine feta and ricotta cheese. Add spinach, Pecorino Romano cheese, dill, and chives, and stir well. Adjust the seasonings. Using a spoon, fill the shells with the mixture.

Spread 4 cups tomato sauce on the baking sheet. Place the stuffed shells over with seam-sides down and sprinkle Cheddar cheese atop. Use aluminum foil to the cover the baking dish.

Pour 1 cup of water in the pot of the Pressure cooker and insert the trivet. Lower the baking dish onto the trivet. Seal the lid, and cook for 15 minutes on High Pressure. Do a quick pressure release. Take away the foil. Place the stuffed shells to serving plates and top with tomato sauce before serving.

Per Serving:

calories: 730 | fat: 41.5g | protein: 30.0g | carbs: 62.7g | fiber: 10.6g | sodium: 966mg

Carrot Risoni

Prep time: 5 minutes | Cook time: 11 minutes | Serves 6

Ingredients:
cup orzo, rinsed
cups water
2 carrots, cut into sticks
large onion, chopped
tablespoons olive oil
Salt, to taste
Fresh cilantro, chopped, for garnish

Directions:
Heat oil on Sauté. Add onion and carrots and stir-fry for about 10 minutes until tender and crispy. Remove to a plate and set aside. Add water, salt and orzo in the instant pot.
Seal the lid and cook on High Pressure for 1 minute. Do a quick release. Fluff the cooked orzo with a fork. Transfer to a serving plate and top with the carrots and onion. Serve scattered with cilantro.

Per Serving:
calories: 121 | fat: 4.9g | protein: 1.7g | carbs: 18.1g | fiber: 2.9g | sodium: 17mg

Roasted Butternut Squash and Rice

Prep time: 15 minutes | Cook time: 15 minutes | Serves 4

Ingredients:
½ cup water
2 cups vegetable broth
small butternut squash, peeled and sliced
tablespoons olive oil, divided
1 teaspoon salt
1 teaspoon freshly ground black pepper
1 cup feta cheese, cubed
tablespoon coconut aminos
teaspoons arrowroot starch
1 cup jasmine rice, cooked

Directions:
Pour the rice and broth in the pot and stir to combine. In a bowl, toss butternut squash with 1 tablespoon of olive oil and season with salt and black pepper.

In another bowl, mix the remaining olive oil, water and coconut aminos. Toss feta in the mixture, add the arrowroot starch, and toss again to combine well. Transfer to a greased baking dish.

Lay a trivet over the rice and place the baking dish on the trivet. Seal the lid and cook on High for 15 minutes. Do a quick pressure release. Fluff the rice with a fork and serve with squash and feta.

Per Serving:
calories: 258 | fat: 14.9g | protein: 7.8g | carbs: 23.2g | fiber: 1.2g | sodium: 1180mg

Pesto Arborio Rice and Veggie Bowls

Prep time: 10 minutes | Cook time: 1 minute | Serves 2

Ingredients:
cup arborio rice, rinsed and drained
cups vegetable broth
Salt and black pepper to taste
1 potato, peeled, cubed
1 head broccoli, cut into small florets
bunch baby carrots, peeled
¼ cabbage, chopped
eggs
¼ cup pesto sauce
Lemon wedges, for serving

Directions:
In the pot, mix broth, pepper, rice and salt. Set trivet to the inner pot on top of rice and add a steamer basket to the top of the trivet. Mix carrots, potato, eggs and broccoli in the steamer basket. Add pepper and salt for seasoning.
Seal the lid and cook for 1 minute on High Pressure. Quick release the pressure.
Take away the trivet and steamer basket from the pot. Set the eggs in a bowl of ice water. Then peel and halve the eggs. Use a fork to fluff rice. Adjust the seasonings.
In two bowls, equally divide rice, broccoli, eggs, carrots, sweet potatoes, and a dollop of pesto. Serve alongside a lemon wedge.

Per Serving:
calories: 858 | fat: 24.4g | protein: 26.4g | carbs: 136.2g | fiber: 14.1g | sodium: 985mg

Mashed Beans with Cumin

Prep time: 10 minutes | Cook time: 10 to 12 minutes | Serves 4 to 6

Ingredients:

1 tablespoon extra-virgin olive oil, plus extra for serving
4 garlic cloves, minced
teaspoon ground cumin
(15-ounce / 425-g) cans fava beans
tablespoons tahini
2 tablespoons lemon juice, plus lemon wedges for serving
Salt and pepper, to taste
1 tomato, cored and cut into ½-inch pieces
small onion, chopped finely
hard-cooked large eggs, chopped
2 tablespoons minced fresh parsley

Directions:

Add the olive oil, garlic and cumin to a medium saucepan over medium heat. Cook for about 2 minutes, or until fragrant.
Stir in the beans with their liquid and tahini. Bring to a simmer and cook for 8 to 10 minutes, or until the liquid thickens slightly.
Turn off the heat, mash the beans to a coarse consistency with a potato masher. Stir in the lemon juice and 1 teaspoon pepper. Season with salt and pepper.
Transfer the mashed beans to a serving dish. Top with the tomato, onion, eggs and parsley. Drizzle with the extra olive oil.
Serve with the lemon wedges.

Per Serving:

calories: 125 | fat: 8.6g | protein: 4.9g | carbs: 9.1g | fiber: 2.9g | sodium: 131mg

Turkish Canned Pinto Bean Salad

Prep time: 10 minutes | Cook time: 3 minutes | Serves 4 to 6

Ingredients:
¼ cup extra-virgin olive oil, divided
3 garlic cloves, lightly crushed and peeled
2 (15-ounce / 425-g) cans pinto beans, rinsed
cups plus 1 tablespoon water
Salt and pepper, to taste
¼ cup tahini
tablespoons lemon juice
1 tablespoon ground dried Aleppo pepper, plus extra for serving
8 ounces (227 g) cherry tomatoes, halved
¼ red onion, sliced thinly
½ cup fresh parsley leaves
2 hard-cooked large eggs, quartered
1 tablespoon toasted sesame seeds

Directions:
Add 1 tablespoon of the olive oil and garlic to a medium saucepan over medium heat. Cook for about 3 minutes, stirring constantly, or until the garlic turns golden but not brown. Add the beans, 2 cups of the water and 1 teaspoon salt and bring to a simmer. Remove from the heat, cover and let sit for 20 minutes. Drain the beans and discard the garlic. In a large bowl, whisk together the remaining 3 tablespoons of the oil, tahini, lemon juice, Aleppo, the remaining 1 tablespoon of the water and ¼ teaspoon salt. Stir in the beans, tomatoes, onion and parsley. Season with salt and pepper to taste. Transfer to a serving platter and top with the eggs. Sprinkle with the sesame seeds and extra Aleppo before serving.

Per Serving:
calories: 402 | fat: 18.9g | protein: 16.2g | carbs: 44.4g | fiber: 11.2g | sodium: 456mg

Black-Eyed Pea and Vegetable Stew

Prep time: 15 minutes | Cook time: 40 minutes | Serves 2

Ingredients:

½ cup black-eyed peas, soaked in water overnight

3 cups water, plus more as needed

1 large carrot, peeled and cut into ½-inch pieces (about ¾ cup)

1 large beet, peeled and cut into ½-inch pieces (about ¾ cup)

¼ teaspoon turmeric

¼ teaspoon cayenne pepper

¼ teaspoon ground cumin seeds, toasted

¼ cup finely chopped parsley

¼ teaspoon salt (optional)

½ teaspoon fresh lime juice

Directions:

Pour the black-eyed peas and water into a large pot, then cook over medium heat for 25 minutes.

Add the carrot and beet to the pot and cook for 10 minutes more, adding more water as needed.

Add the turmeric, cayenne pepper, cumin, and parsley to the pot and cook for another 6 minutes, or until the vegetables are softened. Stir the mixture periodically. Season with salt, if desired.

Serve drizzled with the fresh lime juice.

Per Serving:

calories: 89 | fat: 0.7g | protein: 4.1g | carbs: 16.6g | fiber: 4.5g | sodium: 367mg

Chickpea Salad with Tomatoes and Basil

Prep time: 5 minutes | Cook time: 45 minutes | Serves 2

Ingredients:
1 cup dried chickpeas, rinsed
1 quart water, or enough to cover the chickpeas by 3 to 4 inches
1½ cups halved grape tomatoes
cup chopped fresh basil leaves
to 3 tablespoons balsamic vinegar
½ teaspoon garlic powder
½ teaspoon salt, or more to taste

Directions:
In your Instant Pot, combine the chickpeas and water.
Secure the lid. Select the Manual mode and set the cooking time for 45 minutes at High Pressure.
Once cooking is complete, do a natural pressure release for 20 minutes, then release any remaining pressure. Carefully open the lid and drain the chickpeas. Refrigerate to cool (unless you want to serve this warm, which is good, too).
While the chickpeas cool, in a large bowl, stir together the basil, tomatoes, vinegar, garlic powder, and salt. Add the beans, stir to combine, and serve.

Per Serving:
calories: 395 | fat: 6.0g | protein: 19.8g | carbs: 67.1g | fiber: 19.0g | sodium: 612mg

Mediterranean-Style Beans and Greens

Prep time: 10 minutes | Cook time: 15 minutes | Serves 2

Ingredients:
1 (14.5-ounce / 411-g) can diced tomatoes with juice
(15-ounce / 425-g) can cannellini beans, drained and rinsed
tablespoons chopped green olives, plus 1 or 2 sliced for garnish
¼ cup vegetable broth, plus more as needed
teaspoon extra-virgin olive oil
cloves garlic, minced
4 cups arugula
¼ cup freshly squeezed lemon juice

Directions:
In a medium saucepan, bring the tomatoes, beans, and chopped olives
to a low boil, adding just enough broth to make the ingredients saucy
(you may need more than ¼ cup if your canned tomatoes don't have a
lot of juice). Reduce heat to low and simmer for about 5 minutes.
Meanwhile, in a large skillet, heat the olive oil over medium-high heat.
When the oil is hot and starts to shimmer, add garlic and sauté just
until it starts to turn slightly tan, about 30 seconds. Add the arugula and
lemon juice, stirring to coat leaves with the olive oil and juice. Cover,
reduce the heat to low, and simmer for 3 to 5 minutes.
Serve the beans over the greens and garnish with olive slices.

Per Serving:
calories: 262 | fat: 5.9g | protein: 13.2g | carbs: 40.4g | fiber: 9.8g |
sodium: 897mg

Broccoli and Carrot Pasta Salad

Prep time: 5 minutes | Cook time: 10 minutes | Serves 2

Ingredients:
8 ounces (227 g) whole-wheat pasta
2 cups broccoli florets
1 cup peeled and shredded carrots
¼ cup plain Greek yogurt
Juice of 1 lemon
1 teaspoon red pepper flakes
Sea salt and freshly ground pepper, to taste

Directions:
Bring a large pot of lightly salted water to a boil. Add the pasta to the boiling water and cook until al dente, about 8 to 10 minutes. Drain the pasta and let rest for a few minutes.

When cooled, combine the pasta with the veggies, yogurt, lemon juice, and red pepper flakes in a large bowl, and stir thoroughly to combine. Taste and season to taste with salt and pepper. Serve immediately.

Per Serving:
calories: 428 | fat: 2.9g | protein: 15.9g | carbs: 84.6g | fiber: 11.7g | sodium: 642mg

Bean and Veggie Pasta

Prep time: 10 minutes | Cook time: 15 minutes | Serves 2

Ingredients:

16 ounces (454 g) small whole wheat pasta, such as penne, farfalle, or macaroni 5 cups water

1 (15-ounce / 425-g) can cannellini beans, drained and rinsed

1 (14.5-ounce / 411-g) can diced (with juice) or crushed tomatoes

1 yellow onion, chopped

red or yellow bell pepper, chopped

tablespoons tomato paste

1 tablespoon olive oil

3 garlic cloves, minced

¼ teaspoon crushed red pepper (optional)

1 bunch kale, stemmed and chopped

1 cup sliced basil

½ cup pitted Kalamata olives, chopped

Directions:

Add the pasta, water, beans, tomatoes (with juice if using diced), onion, bell pepper, tomato paste, oil, garlic, and crushed red pepper (if desired), to a large stockpot. Bring to a boil over high heat, stirring often.

Reduce the heat to medium-high, add the kale, and cook, continuing to stir often, until the pasta is al dente, about 10 minutes.

Remove from the heat and let sit for 5 minutes. Garnish with the basil and olives and serve.

Per Serving:

calories: 565 | fat: 17.7g | protein: 18.0g | carbs: 85.5g | fiber: 16.5g | sodium: 540mg

Cherry, Apricot, and Pecan Brown Rice Bowl

Prep time: 15 minutes | Cook time: 1 hour 1 minutes | Serves 2

Ingredients:
2 tablespoons olive oil
2 green onions, sliced
½ cup brown rice
cup low -sodium chicken stock
tablespoons dried cherries
4 dried apricots, chopped
2 tablespoons pecans, toasted and chopped
Sea salt and freshly ground pepper, to taste

Directions:
Heat the olive oil in a medium saucepan over medium-high heat until shimmering.
Add the green onions and sauté for 1 minutes or until fragrant.
Add the rice. Stir to mix well, then pour in the chicken stock.
Bring to a boil. Reduce the heat to low. Cover and simmer for 50 minutes or until the brown rice is soft.
Add the cherries, apricots, and pecans, and simmer for 10 more minutes or until the fruits are tender.
Pour them in a large serving bowl. Fluff with a fork. Sprinkle with sea salt and freshly ground pepper. Serve immediately.

Per Serving:
calories: 451 | fat: 25.9g | protein: 8.2g | carbs: 50.4g | fiber: 4.6g | sodium: 122mg

Cheesy Tomato Linguine

Prep time: 15 minutes | Cook time: 11 minutes | Serves 4

Ingredients:
2 tablespoons olive oil
small onion, diced
garlic cloves, minced
1 cup cherry tomatoes, halved
1½ cups vegetable stock
¼ cup julienned basil leaves
1 teaspoon salt
½ teaspoon ground black pepper
¼ teaspoon red chili flakes
1 pound (454 g) Linguine noodles, halved
Fresh basil leaves for garnish
½ cup Parmigiano-Reggiano cheese, grated

Directions:
Warm oil on Sauté. Add onion and Sauté for 2 minutes until soft. Mix garlic and tomatoes and sauté for 4 minutes. To the pot, add vegetable stock, salt, julienned basil, red chili flakes and pepper.
Add linguine to the tomato mixture until covered. Seal the lid and cook on High Pressure for 5 minutes.
Naturally release the pressure for 5 minutes. Stir the mixture to ensure it is broken down.
Divide into plates. Top with basil and Parmigiano-Reggiano cheese and serve.

Per Serving:
calories: 311 | fat: 11.3g | protein: 10.3g | carbs: 42.1g | fiber: 1.9g | sodium: 210mg

Beef and Bean Stuffed Pasta Shells

Prep time: 15 minutes | Cook time: 17 minutes | Serves 4

Ingredients:
2 tablespoons olive oil
1 pound (454 g) ground beef
pound (454 g) pasta shells
cups water
15 ounces (425 g) tomato sauce
1 (15-ounce / 425-g) can black beans, drained and rinsed
15 ounces (425 g) canned corn, drained (or 2 cups frozen corn)
10 ounces (283 g) red enchilada sauce
4 ounces (113 g) diced green chiles
1 cup shredded Mozzarella cheese
Salt and ground black pepper to taste
Additional cheese for topping
Finely chopped parsley for garnish

Directions:
Heat oil on Sauté. Add ground beef and cook for 7 minutes until it starts to brown.
Mix in pasta, tomato sauce, enchilada sauce, black beans, water, corn, and green chiles and stir to coat well. Add more water if desired.
Seal the lid and cook on High Pressure for 10 minutes. Do a quick Pressure release. Into the pasta mixture, mix in Mozzarella cheese until melted; add black pepper and salt. Garnish with parsley to serve.

Per Serving:
calories: 1006 | fat: 30.0g | protein: 53.3g | carbs: 138.9g | fiber: 24.4g | sodium: 1139mg

Parmesan Squash Linguine

Prep time: 15 minutes | Cook time: 5 minutes | Serves 4

Ingredients:
cup flour
teaspoons salt
2 eggs
4 cups water
1 cup seasoned breadcrumbs
½ cup grated Parmesan cheese, plus more for garnish
1 yellow squash, peeled and sliced
1 pound (454 g) linguine
24 ounces (680 g) canned seasoned tomato sauce
2 tablespoons olive oil
1 cup shredded Mozzarella cheese
Minced fresh basil, for garnish

Directions:
Break the linguine in half. Put it in the pot and add water and half of
salt. Seal the lid and cook on High Pressure for 5 minutes. Combine
the flour and 1 teaspoon of salt in a bowl. In another bowl, whisk the
eggs and 2 tablespoons of water. In a third bowl, mix the breadcrumbs
and Mozzarella cheese.
Coat each squash slices in the flour. Shake off excess flour, dip in the
egg wash, and dredge in the bread crumbs. Set aside. Quickly release
the pressure. Remove linguine to a serving bowl and mix in the tomato
sauce and sprinkle with fresh basil. Heat oil on Sauté and fry breaded
squash until crispy.
Serve the squash topped Mozzarella cheese with the linguine on side.

Per Serving:
calories: 857 | fat: 17.0g | protein: 33.2g | carbs: 146.7g | fiber: 18.1g
| sodium: 1856mg

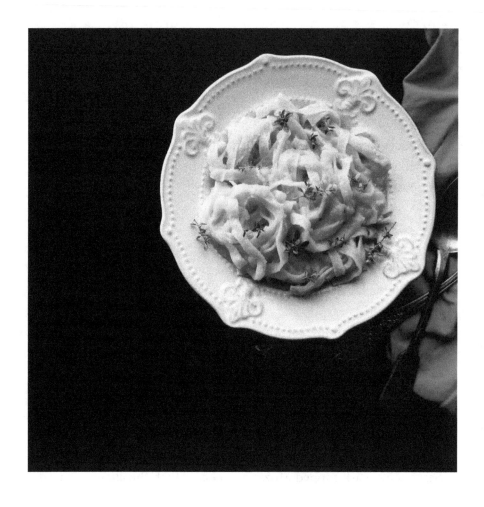

Pork and Spinach Spaghetti

Prep time: 15 minutes | Cook time: 16 minutes | Serves 4

Ingredients:

2 tablespoons olive oil
½ cup onion, chopped 1 garlic clove, minced
pound (454 g) ground pork
cups water
1 (14-ounce / 397-g) can diced tomatoes, drained
½ cup sun-dried tomatoes
1 tablespoon dried oregano
1 teaspoon Italian seasoning
1 fresh jalapeño chile, stemmed, seeded, and minced
1 teaspoon salt
8 ounces (227 g) dried spaghetti, halved
1 cup spinach

Directions:

Warm oil on Sauté. Add onion and garlic and cook for 2 minutes until softened. Stir in pork and cook for 5 minutes. Stir in jalapeño, water, sundried tomatoes, Italian seasoning, oregano, diced tomatoes, and salt with the chicken; mix spaghetti and press to submerge into the sauce. Seal the lid and cook on High Pressure for 9 minutes. Release the pressure quickly. Stir in spinach, close lid again, and simmer on Keep Warm for 5 minutes until spinach is wilted.

Per Serving:

calories: 621 | fat: 32.2g | protein: 29.1g | carbs: 53.9g | fiber: 5.9g | sodium: 738mg

Gouda Beef and Spinach Fettuccine

Prep time: 10 minutes | Cook time: 15 minutes | Serves 6

Ingredients:
10 ounces (283 g) ground beef
1 pound (454 g) fettuccine pasta
1 cup gouda cheese, shredded
1 cup fresh spinach, torn
medium onion, chopped
cups tomatoes, diced
1 tablespoon olive oil
1 teaspoon salt
½ teaspoon ground black pepper

Directions:
Heat the olive oil on Sauté mode in the Instant Pot. Stir-fry the beef and onion for 5 minutes. Add the pasta. Pour water enough to cover and season with salt and pepper. Cook on High Pressure for 5 minutes. Do a quick release. Press Sauté and stir in the tomato and spinach; cook for 5 minutes. Top with Gouda to serve.

Per Serving:
calories: 493 | fat: 17.7g | protein: 20.6g | carbs: 64.3g | fiber: 9.5g | sodium: 561mg

Black-Eyed Peas Salad with Walnuts

Prep time: 10 minutes | Cook time: 0 minutes | Serves 4 to 6

Ingredients:
3 tablespoons extra-virgin olive oil

3 tablespoons dukkah, divided

2 tablespoons lemon juice

2 tablespoons pomegranate molasses

¼ teaspoon salt, or more to taste

⅛ teaspoon pepper, or more to taste

2 (15-ounce / 425-g) cans black-eyed peas, rinsed

½ cup pomegranate seeds

½ cup minced fresh parsley

½ cup walnuts, toasted and chopped 4 scallions, sliced thinly

Directions:
In a large bowl, whisk together the olive oil, 2 tablespoons of the dukkah, lemon juice, pomegranate molasses, salt and pepper.

Stir in the remaining ingredients. Season with salt and pepper.

Sprinkle with the remaining 1 tablespoon of the dukkah before serving.

Per Serving:
calories: 155 | fat: 11.5g | protein: 2.0g | carbs: 12.5g | fiber: 2.1g | sodium: 105mg

Mediterranean Lentils

Prep time: 7 minutes | Cook time: 24 minutes | Serves 2

Ingredients:
1 tablespoon olive oil
1 small sweet or yellow onion, diced
1 garlic clove, diced
1 teaspoon dried oregano
½ teaspoon ground cumin
½ teaspoon dried parsley
½ teaspoon salt, plus more as needed
¼ teaspoon freshly ground black pepper, plus more as needed
1 tomato, diced
1 cup brown or green lentils
2½ cups vegetable stock
1 bay leaf

Directions:
Set your Instant Pot to Sauté and heat the olive oil until it shimmers. Add the onion and cook for 3 to 4 minutes until soft. Turn off the Instant Pot and add the garlic, oregano, cumin, parsley, salt, and pepper. Cook until fragrant, about 1 minute. Stir in the tomato, lentils, stock, and bay leaf. Lock the lid. Select the Manual mode and set the cooking time for 18 minutes at High Pressure. When the timer beeps, perform a natural pressure release for 10 minutes, then release any remaining pressure. Carefully open the lid. Remove and discard the bay leaf. Taste and season with more salt and pepper, as needed. If there's too much liquid remaining, select Sauté and cook until it evaporates. Serve warm.

Per Serving
calories: 426 | fat: 8.1g | protein: 26.2g | carbs: 63.8g | fiber: 31.0g | sodium: 591mg

Roasted Ratatouille Pasta

Prep time: 10 minutes | Cook time: 30 minutes | Serves 2

Ingredients:
1 small eggplant (about 8 ounces / 227 g)
1 small zucchini
1 portobello mushroom
1 Roma tomato, halved
½ medium sweet red pepper, seeded
½ teaspoon salt, plus additional for the pasta water
1 teaspoon Italian herb seasoning
tablespoon olive oil
cups farfalle pasta (about 8 ounces / 227 g)
2 tablespoons minced sun-dried tomatoes in olive oil with herbs
2 tablespoons prepared pesto

Directions:

Slice the ends off the eggplant and zucchini. Cut them lengthwise into ½inch slices.

Place the eggplant, zucchini, mushroom, tomato, and red pepper in a large bowl and sprinkle with ½ teaspoon of salt. Using your hands, toss the vegetables well so that they're covered evenly with the salt. Let them rest for about 10 minutes.

While the vegetables are resting, preheat the oven to 400°F (205°C). Line a baking sheet with parchment paper.

When the oven is hot, drain off any liquid from the vegetables and pat them dry with a paper towel. Add the Italian herb seasoning and olive oil to the vegetables and toss well to coat both sides.

Lay the vegetables out in a single layer on the baking sheet. Roast them for 15 to 20 minutes, flipping them over after about 10 minutes or once they start to brown on the underside. When the vegetables are charred in spots, remove them from the oven.

While the vegetables are roasting, fill a large saucepan with water. Add salt and cook the pasta until al dente, about 8 to 10 minutes. Drain the pasta, reserving ½ cup of the pasta water.

When cool enough to handle, cut the vegetables into large chunks (about 2 inches) and add them to the hot pasta.

Stir in the sun-dried tomatoes and pesto and toss everything well. Serve immediately.

Per Serving:

calories: 613 | fat: 16.0g | protein: 23.1g | carbs: 108.5g | fiber: 23.0g | sodium: 775mg

Lentil and Mushroom Pasta

Prep time: 10 minutes | Cook time: 50 minutes | Serves 2

Ingredients:
2 tablespoons olive oil
large yellow onion, finely diced
portobello mushrooms, trimmed and chopped finely
tablespoons tomato paste
garlic cloves, chopped
1 teaspoon oregano
2½ cups water
1 cup brown lentils
1 (28-ounce / 794-g) can diced tomatoes with basil (with juice if diced)
1 tablespoon balsamic vinegar
Salt and black pepper, to taste
Chopped basil, for garnish
8 ounces (227 g) pasta of choice, cooked

Directions:
Place a large stockpot over medium heat and add the olive oil. Once the oil is hot, add the onion and mushrooms. Cover and cook until both are soft, about 5 minutes. Add the tomato paste, garlic, and oregano and cook 2 minutes, stirring constantly.
Stir in the water and lentils. Bring to a boil, then reduce the heat to medium-low and cook covered for 5 minutes.
Add the tomatoes (and juice if using diced) and vinegar. Reduce the heat to low and cook until the lentils are tender, about 30 minutes. Remove from the heat and season with salt and pepper to taste. Garnish with the basil and serve over the cooked pasta.

Per Serving:
calories: 463 | fat: 15.9g | protein: 12.5g | carbs: 70.8g | fiber: 16.9g | sodium: 155mg

Asparagus and Broccoli Primavera Farfalle

Prep time: 15 minutes | Cook time: 12 minutes | Serves 4

Ingredients:
bunch asparagus, trimmed, cut into 1-inch pieces
cups broccoli florets
tablespoons olive oil
3 teaspoons salt
10 ounces (283 g) egg noodles
3 garlic cloves, minced
2½ cups vegetable stock
½ cup heavy cream
1 cup small tomatoes, halved
¼ cup chopped basil
½ cup grated Parmesan cheese

Directions:
Pour 2 cups of water, add the noodles, 2 tablespoons of olive oil, garlic and salt. Place a trivet over the water. Combine asparagus, broccoli, remaining olive oil and salt in a bowl. Place the vegetables on the trivet. Seal the lid and cook on Steam for 12 minutes on High. Do a quick release. Remove the vegetables to a plate. Stir the heavy cream and tomatoes in the pasta. Press Sauté and simmer the cream until desired consistency. Gently mix in the asparagus and broccoli. Garnish with basil and Parmesan, to serve.

Per Serving:
calories: 544 | fat: 23.8g | protein: 18.5g | carbs: 66.1g | fiber: 6.0g | sodium: 2354mg

Super Cheesy Tagliatelle

Prep time: 10 minutes | Cook time: 20 minutes | Serves 6

Ingredients:
¼ cup goat cheese, chevre
¼ cup grated Pecorino cheese
½ cup grated Parmesan
cup heavy cream
½ cup grated Gouda
tablespoons olive oil
1 tablespoon Italian Seasoning mix
1 cup vegetable broth
1 pound (454 g) tagliatelle

Directions:
In a bowl, mix goat cheese, pecorino, Parmesan, and heavy cream. Stir in Italian seasoning. Transfer to your instant pot. Stir in the broth and olive oil.

Seal the lid and cook on High Pressure for 4 minutes. Do a quick release. Meanwhile, drop the tagliatelle in boiling water and cook for 6 minutes.

Remove the instant pot's lid and stir in the tagliatelle. Top with grated gouda and let simmer for about 10 minutes on Sauté mode.

Per Serving:
calories: 511 | fat: 22.0g | protein: 14.5g | carbs: 65.7g | fiber: 9.0g | sodium: 548mg

Chickpea Curry

Prep time: 10 minutes | Cook time: 24 minutes | Serves 4

Ingredients:
½ cup raw chickpeas
1½ tablespoons cooking oil
½ cup chopped onions
1 bay leaf
½ tablespoon grated garlic
¼ tablespoon grated ginger
¾ cup water
1 cup fresh tomato purée
½ green chili, finely chopped
¼ teaspoon turmeric
½ teaspoon coriander powder
1 teaspoon chili powder
1 cup chopped baby spinach
Salt, to taste
Boiled white rice, for serving

Directions:
Add the oil and onions to the Instant Pot. Sauté for 5 minutes.
Stir in ginger, garlic paste, green chili and bay leaf. Cook for 1 minute, then add all the spices. Add the chickpeas, tomato purée and the water to the pot. Cover and secure the lid. Turn its pressure release handle to the sealing position. Cook on the Manual function with High Pressure for 15 minutes. After the beep, do a Natural release for 20 minutes.
Stir in spinach and cook for 3 minutes on the Sauté setting.
Serve hot with boiled white rice.

Per Serving:
calories: 176 | fat: 6.8g | protein: 6.7g | carbs: 24.1g | fiber: 5.1g | sodium: 185mg

Red Bean Curry

Prep time: 10 minutes | Cook time: 24 minutes | Serves 4

Ingredients:

½ cup raw red beans
1½ tablespoons cooking oil
½ cup chopped onions
1 bay leaf
½ tablespoon grated garlic
¼ tablespoon grated ginger
¾ cup water
1 cup fresh tomato purée
½ green chili, finely chopped
¼ teaspoon turmeric
½ teaspoon coriander powder
1 teaspoon chili powder
1 cup chopped baby spinach
Salt, to taste
Boiled white rice or quinoa, for serve

Directions:

Add the oil and onions to the Instant Pot. Sauté for 5 minutes.
Stir in ginger, garlic paste, green chili and bay leaf. Cook for 1 minute, then add all the spices. Add the red beans, tomato purée and water to the pot. Cover and secure the lid. Turn its pressure release handle to the sealing position. Cook on the Manual function with High Pressure for 15 minutes. After the beep, do a Natural release for 20 minutes. Stir in spinach and cook for 3 minutes on the Sauté setting.
Serve hot with boiled white rice or quinoa.

Per Serving:

calories: 159 | fat: 5.6g | protein: 6.8g | carbs: 22.5g | fiber: 5.5g |
sodium: 182mg

Shrimp and Asparagus Risotto

Prep time: 15 minutes | Cook time: 58 minutes | Serves 4

Ingredients:
1 tablespoon olive oil
1 pound (454 g) asparagus, trimmed and roughly chopped
1 cup spinach, chopped
1½ cups mushrooms, chopped
1 cup rice, rinsed and drained
1¼ cups chicken broth
¾ cup milk
1 tablespoon coconut oil
16 shrimp, cleaned and deveined
Salt and ground black pepper, to taste
¾ cup Parmesan cheese, shredded

Directions:
Warm the oil on Sauté. Add spinach, mushrooms and asparagus and Sauté for 10 minutes until cooked through. Press Cancel. Add rice, milk and chicken broth to the pot as you stir.
Seal the lid, press Multigrain and cook for 40 minutes on High Pressure. Do a quick release, open the lid and put the rice on a serving plate.
Take back the empty pot to the pressure cooker, add coconut oil and press Sauté. Add shrimp and cook each side for 4 minutes until cooked through and turns pink. Set shrimp over rice, add pepper and salt for seasoning. Serve topped with shredded Parmesan cheese.

Per Serving: calories: 385 | fat: 14.3g | protein: 16.5g | carbs: 48.4g | fiber: 4.1g | sodium: 771mg

Pancetta with Garbanzo Beans

Prep time: 10 minutes | Cook time: 38 minutes | Serves 6

Ingredients:

3 strips pancetta
1 onion, diced
15 ounces (425 g) canned garbanzo beans
2 cups water
cup apple cider
garlic cloves, minced
½ cup ketchup
¼ cup sugar
1 teaspoon ground mustard powder
1 teaspoon salt
1 teaspoon black pepper
Fresh parsley, for garnish

Directions:

Cook pancetta for 5 minutes, until crispy, on Sauté mode. Add onion and garlic, and cook for 3 minutes until soft. Mix in garbanzo beans, ketchup, sugar, salt, apple cider, mustard powder, water, and pepper. Seal the lid, press Bean/Chili and cook on High Pressure for 30 minutes. Release pressure naturally for 10 minutes. Serve in bowls garnished with parsley.

Per Serving:

calories: 163 | fat: 5.7g | protein: 5.4g | carbs: 22.1g | fiber: 3.7g | sodium: 705mg

Rigatoni and Zucchini Minestrone

Prep time: 20 minutes | Cook time: 7 minutes | Serves 4

Ingredients:
3 tablespoons olive oil
1 onion, diced
1 celery stalk, diced
1 large carrot, peeled and diced
14 ounces (397 g) canned chopped tomatoes
4 ounces (113 g) rigatoni
3 cups water
1 cup chopped zucchini 1 bay leaf
1 teaspoon mixed herbs
¼ teaspoon cayenne pepper
½ teaspoon salt
¼ cup shredded Pecorino Romano cheese
1 garlic clove, minced
⅓ cup olive oil based pesto

Directions:
Heat oil on Sauté and cook onion, celery, garlic, and carrot for 3 minutes, stirring occasionally until the vegetables are softened. Stir in rigatoni, tomatoes, water, zucchini, bay leaf, herbs, cayenne, and salt. Seal the lid and cook on High for 4 minutes. Do a natural pressure release for 5 minutes. Adjust the taste of the soup with salt and black pepper, and remove the bay leaf.
Ladle the soup into serving bowls and drizzle the pesto over. Serve with the garlic toasts.

Per Serving:
calories: 278 | fat: 23.4g | protein: 6.7g | carbs: 12.2g | fiber: 3.5g | sodium: 793mg

Vegetable Mains

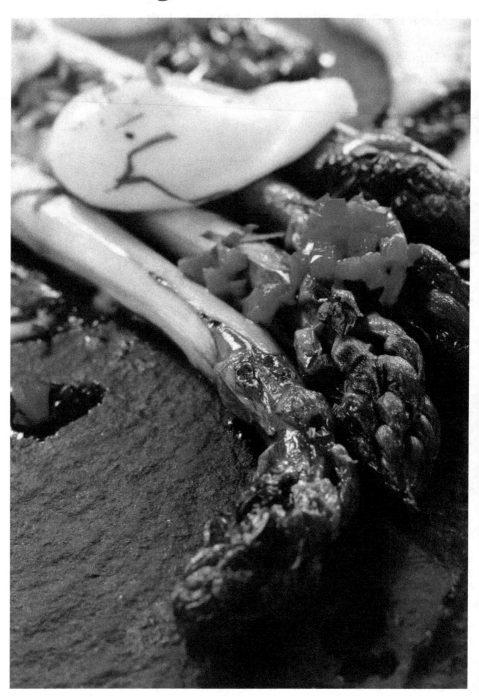

Zoodles with Walnut Pesto

Prep time: 10 minutes | Cook time: 10 minutes | Serves 4

Ingredients:
4 medium zucchini, spiralized
¼ cup extra-virgin olive oil, divided
teaspoon minced garlic, divided
½ teaspoon crushed red pepper
¼ teaspoon freshly ground black pepper, divided
¼ teaspoon kosher salt, divided
tablespoons grated Parmesan cheese, divided
1 cup packed fresh basil leaves
¾ cup walnut pieces, divided

Directions:

In a large bowl, stir together the zoodles, 1 tablespoon of the olive oil, ½ teaspoon of the minced garlic, red pepper, ⅛ teaspoon of the black pepper and ⅛ teaspoon of the salt. Set aside.

Heat ½ tablespoon of the oil in a large skillet over medium-high heat. Add half of the zoodles to the skillet and cook for 5 minutes, stirring constantly. Transfer the cooked zoodles into a bowl. Repeat with another ½ tablespoon of the oil and the remaining zoodles. When done, add the cooked zoodles to the bowl.

Make the pesto: In a food processor, combine the remaining ½ teaspoon of the minced garlic, ⅛ teaspoon of the black pepper and ⅛ teaspoon of the salt, 1 tablespoon of the Parmesan, basil leaves and ¼ cup of the walnuts. Pulse until smooth and then slowly drizzle the remaining 2 tablespoons of the oil into the pesto. Pulse again until well combined.

Add the pesto to the zoodles along with the remaining 1 tablespoon of the Parmesan and the remaining ½ cup of the walnuts. Toss to coat well.

Serve immediately.

Per Serving:

calories: 166 | fat: 16.0g | protein: 4.0g | carbs: 3.0g | fiber: 2.0g | sodium: 307mg

Cheesy Sweet Potato Burgers

Prep time: 10 minutes | Cook time: 19 to 20 minutes | Serves 4

Ingredients:
large sweet potato (about 8 ounces / 227 g)
tablespoons extra-virgin olive oil, divided
1 cup chopped onion
1 large egg
1 garlic clove
1 cup old-fashioned rolled oats
1 tablespoon dried oregano
1 tablespoon balsamic vinegar
¼ teaspoon kosher salt
½ cup crumbled Gorgonzola cheese

Directions:
Using a fork, pierce the sweet potato all over and microwave on high for 4 to 5 minutes, until softened in the center. Cool slightly before slicing in half. Meanwhile, in a large skillet over medium-high heat, heat 1 tablespoon of the olive oil. Add the onion and sauté for 5 minutes. Spoon the sweet potato flesh out of the skin and put the flesh in a food processor. Add the cooked onion, egg, garlic, oats, oregano, vinegar and salt. Pulse until smooth. Add the cheese and pulse four times to barely combine. Form the mixture into four burgers. Place the burgers on a plate, and press to flatten each to about ¾-inch thick. Wipe out the skillet with a paper towel. Heat the remaining 1 tablespoon of the oil over medium-high heat for about 2 minutes. Add the burgers to the hot oil, then reduce the heat to medium. Cook the burgers for 5 minutes per side.
Transfer the burgers to a plate and serve.

Per Serving:
calories: 290 | fat: 12.0g | protein: 12.0g | carbs: 43.0g | fiber: 8.0g | sodium: 566mg

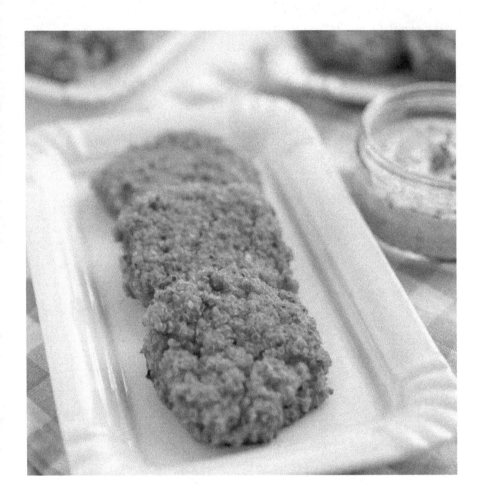

Eggplant and Zucchini Gratin

Prep time: 10 minutes | Cook time: 19 minutes | Serves 6

Ingredients:
2 large zucchini, finely chopped
1 large eggplant, finely chopped
¼ teaspoon kosher salt
¼ teaspoon freshly ground black pepper
3 tablespoons extra-virgin olive oil, divided
¾ cup unsweetened almond milk
1 tablespoon all-purpose flour
⅓ cup plus 2 tablespoons grated Parmesan cheese, divided
1 cup chopped tomato
1 cup diced fresh Mozzarella
¼ cup fresh basil leaves

Directions:

Preheat the oven to 425°F (220°C).

In a large bowl, toss together the zucchini, eggplant, salt and pepper.

In a large skillet over medium-high heat, heat 1 tablespoon of the oil. Add half of the veggie mixture to the skillet. Stir a few times, then cover and cook for about 4 minutes, stirring occasionally. Pour the cooked veggies into a baking dish. Place the skillet back on the heat, add 1 tablespoon of the oil and repeat with the remaining veggies. Add the veggies to the baking dish.

Meanwhile, heat the milk in the microwave for 1 minute. Set aside.

Place a medium saucepan over medium heat. Add the remaining 1 tablespoon of the oil and flour to the saucepan. Whisk together until well blended.

Slowly pour the warm milk into the saucepan, whisking the entire time. Continue to whisk frequently until the mixture thickens a bit. Add ⅓ cup

of the Parmesan cheese and whisk until melted. Pour the cheese sauce over the vegetables in the baking dish and mix well.

Fold in the tomatoes and Mozzarella cheese. Roast in the oven for 10 minutes, or until the gratin is almost set and not runny.

Top with the fresh basil leaves and the remaining 2 tablespoons of the Parmesan cheese before serving.

Per Serving:

calories: 122 | fat: 5.0g | protein: 10.0g | carbs: 11.0g | fiber: 4.0g | sodium: 364mg

Veggie-Stuffed Portabello Mushrooms

Prep time: 5 minutes | Cook time: 24 to 25 minutes | Serves 6

Ingredients:
3 tablespoons extra-virgin olive oil, divided
cup diced onion
garlic cloves, minced
1 large zucchini, diced
3 cups chopped mushrooms
1 cup chopped tomato
1 teaspoon dried oregano
¼ teaspoon kosher salt
¼ teaspoon crushed red pepper
6 large portabello mushrooms, stems and gills removed
Cooking spray
4 ounces (113 g) fresh Mozzarella cheese, shredded

Directions:

In a large skillet over medium heat, heat 2 tablespoons of the oil. Add the onion and sauté for 4 minutes. Stir in the garlic and sauté for 1 minute.

Stir in the zucchini, mushrooms, tomato, oregano, salt and red pepper. Cook for 10 minutes, stirring constantly. Remove from the heat.

Meanwhile, heat a grill pan over medium-high heat.

Brush the remaining 1 tablespoon of the oil over the portabello mushroom caps. Place the mushrooms, bottom-side down, on the grill pan. Cover with a sheet of aluminum foil sprayed with nonstick cooking spray. Cook for 5 minutes.

Flip the mushroom caps over, and spoon about ½ cup of the cooked vegetable mixture into each cap. Top each with about 2½ tablespoons of the Mozzarella.

Cover and grill for 4 to 5 minutes, or until the cheese is melted.

Using a spatula, transfer the portabello mushrooms to a plate. Let cool for about 5 minutes before serving.

Per Serving:

calories: 111 | fat: 4.0g | protein: 11.0g | carbs: 11.0g | fiber: 4.0g | sodium: 314mg

Fried Eggplant Rolls

Prep time: 20 minutes | Cook time: 10 minutes | Serves 4 to 6

Ingredients:
2 large eggplants, trimmed and cut lengthwise into ¼-inch-thick slices
1 teaspoon salt
1 cup ricotta cheese
4 ounces (113 g) goat cheese, shredded
¼ cup finely chopped fresh basil
½ teaspoon freshly ground black pepper
Olive oil spray

Directions:
Add the eggplant slices to a colander and season with salt. Set aside for 15 to 20 minutes.

Mix together the ricotta and goat cheese, basil, and black pepper in a large bowl and stir to combine. Set aside.

Dry the eggplant slices with paper towels and lightly mist them with olive oil spray.

Heat a large skillet over medium heat and lightly spray it with olive oil spray.

Arrange the eggplant slices in the skillet and fry each side for 3 minutes until golden brown.

Remove from the heat to a paper towel-lined plate and rest for 5 minutes.

Make the eggplant rolls: Lay the eggplant slices on a flat work surface and top each slice with a tablespoon of the prepared cheese mixture. Roll them up and serve immediately.

Per Serving:
calories: 254 | fat: 14.9g | protein: 15.3g | carbs: 18.6g | fiber: 7.1g | sodium: 745mg

Stir-Fry Baby Bok Choy

Prep time: 12 minutes | Cook time: 10 to 13 minutes | Serves 6

Ingredients:

2 tablespoons coconut oil

1 large onion, finely diced 2 teaspoons ground cumin

1-inch piece fresh ginger, grated

1 teaspoon ground turmeric

½ teaspoon salt

12 baby bok choy heads, ends trimmed and sliced lengthwise

Water, as needed

3 cups cooked brown rice

Directions:

Heat the coconut oil in a large pan over medium heat.

Saut é the onion for 5 minutes, stirring occasionally, or until the onion is translucent.

Fold in the cumin, ginger, turmeric, and salt and stir to coat well.

Add the bok choy and cook for 5 to 8 minutes, stirring occasionally, or until the bok choy is tender but crisp. You can add 1 tablespoon of water at a time, if the skillet gets dry until you finish sautéing.

Transfer the bok choy to a plate and serve over the cooked brown rice.

Per Serving:

calories: 443 | fat: 8.8g | protein: 30.3g | carbs: 75.7g | fiber: 19.0g | sodium: 1289mg

Brussels Sprouts Linguine

Prep time: 5 minutes | Cook time: 25 minutes | Serves 4

Ingredients:

8 ounces (227 g) whole-wheat linguine
⅓ cup plus 2 tablespoons extra-virgin olive oil, divided
medium sweet onion, diced
to 3 garlic cloves, smashed
8 ounces (227 g) Brussels sprouts, chopped
½ cup chicken stock
⅓ cup dry white wine
½ cup shredded Parmesan cheese
1 lemon, quartered

Directions:

Bring a large pot of water to a boil and cook the pasta for about 5 minutes, or until al dente. Drain the pasta and reserve 1 cup of the pasta water. Mix the cooked pasta with 2 tablespoons of the olive oil. Set aside. In a large skillet, heat the remaining ⅓ cup of the olive oil over medium heat. Add the onion to the skillet and sauté for about 4 minutes, or until tender. Add the smashed garlic cloves and sauté for 1 minute, or until fragrant. Stir in the Brussels sprouts and cook covered for 10 minutes. Pour in the chicken stock to prevent burning. Once the Brussels sprouts have wilted and are fork-tender, add white wine and cook for about 5 minutes, or until reduced. Add the pasta to the skillet and add the pasta water as needed. Top with the Parmesan cheese and squeeze the lemon over the dish right before eating.

Per Serving:

calories: 502 | fat: 31.0g | protein: 15.0g | carbs: 50.0g | fiber: 9.0g | sodium: 2

Roasted Cauliflower and Carrots

Prep time: 10 minutes | Cook time: 30 minutes | Serves 2

Ingredients:
4 cups cauliflower florets (about ½ small head)
2 medium carrots, peeled, halved, and then sliced into quarters lengthwise
2 tablespoons olive oil, divided
½ teaspoon salt, divided
½ teaspoon garlic powder, divided
2 teaspoons za'atar spice mix, divided
1 (15-ounce / 425-g) can chickpeas, drained, rinsed, and patted dry
¾ cup plain Greek yogurt
1 teaspoon harissa spice paste, plus additional as needed

Directions:
Preheat the oven to 400°F (205°C). Line a sheet pan with foil or parchment paper. Put the cauliflower and carrots in a large bowl. Drizzle with 1 tablespoon of olive oil and sprinkle with ¼ teaspoon of salt, ¼ teaspoon of garlic powder, and 1 teaspoon of za'atar. Toss to combine well. Spread the vegetables onto one half of the prepared sheet pan in a single layer. Put the chickpeas in the same bowl and season with the remaining 1 tablespoon of olive oil, ¼ teaspoon of salt, ¼ teaspoon of garlic powder, and the remaining 1 teaspoon of za'atar. Toss to combine well. Spread the chickpeas onto the other half of the sheet pan. Roast in the preheated oven for 30 minutes, or until the vegetables are crisp-tender. Flip the vegetables halfway through and give the chickpeas a stir so they cook evenly. Meanwhile, whisk the yogurt and harissa together in a small bowl. Taste and add additional harissa as needed.
Serve the vegetables and chickpeas with the yogurt mixture on the side.

Per Serving: calories: 468 | fat: 23.0g | protein: 18.1g | carbs: 54.1g | fiber: 13.8g | sodium: 631mg

Zucchini Crisp

Prep time: 10 minutes | Cook time: 20 minutes | Serves 2

Ingredients:
4 zucchini, sliced into ½-inch rounds
½ cup unsweetened almond milk
1 teaspoon fresh lemon juice
1 teaspoon arrowroot powder
½ teaspoon salt, divided
½ cup whole wheat bread crumbs
¼ cup nutritional yeast
¼ cup hemp seeds
½ teaspoon garlic powder
¼ teaspoon crushed red pepper
¼ teaspoon black pepper

Directions:
Preheat the oven to 375°F (190°C). Line two baking sheets with parchment paper and set aside.
Put the zucchini in a medium bowl with the almond milk, lemon juice, arrowroot powder, and ¼ teaspoon of salt. Stir to mix well.
In a large bowl with a lid, thoroughly combine the bread crumbs, nutritional yeast, hemp seeds, garlic powder, crushed red pepper and black pepper. Add the zucchini in batches and shake until the slices are evenly coated.
Arrange the zucchini on the prepared baking sheets in a single layer. Bake in the preheated oven for about 20 minutes, or until the zucchini slices are golden brown.
Season with the remaining ¼ teaspoon of salt before serving.

Per Serving:
calories: 255 | fat: 11.3g | protein: 8.6g | carbs: 31.9g | fiber: 3.8g | sodium: 826mg

Creamy Sweet Potatoes and Collards

Prep time: 20 minutes | Cook time: 35 minutes | Serves 2

Ingredients:

1 tablespoon avocado oil
3 garlic cloves, chopped
1 yellow onion, diced
½ teaspoon crushed red pepper flakes
large sweet potato, peeled and diced
bunches collard greens (about 2 pounds/907 g), stemmed, leaves choppedinto 1-inch squares
1 (14.5-ounce / 411-g) can diced tomatoes with juice
1 (15-ounce / 425-g) can red kidney beans or chickpeas, drained and rinsed
1½ cups water
½ cup unsweetened coconut milk
Salt and black pepper, to taste

Directions:

In a large, deep skillet over medium heat, melt the avocado oil.
Add the garlic, onion, and red pepper flakes and cook for 3 minutes.
Stir in the sweet potato and collards.
Add the tomatoes with their juice, beans, water, and coconut milk and mix well. Bring the mixture just to a boil.
Reduce the heat to medium-low, cover, and simmer for about 30 minutes, or until softened.
Season to taste with salt and pepper and serve.

Per Serving:

calories: 445 | fat: 9.6g | protein: 18.1g | carbs: 73.1g | fiber: 22.1g | sodium: 703mg

Paprika Cauliflower Steaks with Walnut Sauce

Prep time: 5 minutes | Cook time: 30 minutes | Serves 2

Ingredients:
Walnut Sauce:
½ cup raw walnut halves
2 tablespoons virgin olive oil, divided
1 clove garlic, chopped
small yellow onion, chopped
½ cup unsweetened almond milk
tablespoons fresh lemon juice
Salt and pepper, to taste Paprika Cauliflower:
1 medium head cauliflower
1 teaspoon sweet paprika
1 teaspoon minced fresh thyme leaves (about 2 sprigs)

Directions:

Preheat the oven to 350°F (180°C).

Make the walnut sauce: Toast the walnuts in a large, ovenproof skillet over medium heat until fragrant and slightly darkened, about 5 minutes. Transfer the walnuts to a blender.

Heat 1 tablespoon of olive oil in the skillet. Add the garlic and onion and sauté for about 2 minutes, or until slightly softened. Transfer the garlic and onion into the blender, along with the almond milk, lemon juice, salt, and pepper. Blend the ingredients until smooth and creamy. Keep the sauce warm while you prepare the cauliflower.

Make the paprika cauliflower: Cut two 1-inch-thick "steaks" from the center of the cauliflower. Lightly moisten the steaks with water and season both sides with paprika, thyme, salt, and pepper.

Heat the remaining 1 tablespoon of olive oil in the skillet over mediumhigh heat. Add the cauliflower steaks and sear for about 3 minutes until evenly browned. Flip the cauliflower steaks and transfer the skillet to the oven.

Roast in the preheated oven for about 20 minutes until crisp-tender. Serve the cauliflower steaks warm with the walnut sauce on the side.

Per Serving:

calories: 367 | fat: 27.9g | protein: 7.0g | carbs: 22.7g | fiber: 5.8g | sodium: 173mg 46mg

Cabbage Stuffed Acorn Squash

Prep time: 15 minutes | Cook time: 23 minutes | Serves 4

Ingredients:
½ tablespoon olive oil
2 medium Acorn squashes
¼ small yellow onion, chopped
1 jalapeño pepper, chopped
½ cup green onions, chopped
½ cup carrots, chopped
¼ cup cabbage, chopped
garlic clove, minced
½ (6-ounce / 170-g) can sugar-free tomato sauce
½ tablespoon chili powder
½ tablespoon ground cumin
Salt and freshly ground black pepper to taste
cups water
¼ cup Cheddar cheese, shredded

Directions:
Pour the water into the instant pot and place the trivet inside.
Slice the squash into 2 halves and remove the seeds.
Place over the trivet, skin side down, and sprinkle some salt and pepper over it. Secure the lid and cook on Manual for 15 minutes at High Pressure. Release the pressure naturally and remove the lid. Empty the pot into a bowl. Now add the oil, onion, and garlic in the instant pot and Sauté for 5 minutes. Stir in the remaining vegetables and stir-fry for 3 minutes. Add the remaining ingredients and secure the lid.
Cook on Manual function for 2 minutes at High Pressure.
After the beep, natural release the pressure and remove the lid.
Stuff the squashes with the prepared mixture and serve warm.

Per Serving: calories: 163 | fat: 5.1g | protein: 4.8g | carbs: 28.4g | fiber: 4.9g | sodium: 146mg

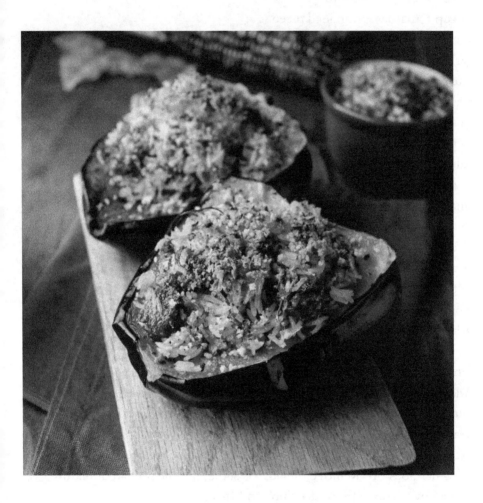

Black Bean and Corn Tortilla Bowls

Prep time: 10 minutes | Cook time: 8 minutes | Serves 4

Ingredients:
1½ cups vegetable broth
½ cup tomatoes, undrained diced
small onion, diced
garlic cloves, finely minced
1 teaspoon chili powder
teaspoon cumin
½ teaspoon paprika
½ teaspoon ground coriander
Salt and pepper to taste
½ cup carrots, diced
small potatoes, cubed
½ cup bell pepper, chopped
½ can black beans, drained and rinsed
cup frozen corn kernels
½ tablespoon lime juice
tablespoons cilantro for topping, chopped
Whole-wheat tortilla chips

Directions:
Add the oil and all the vegetables into the instant pot and Sauté for 3 minutes. Add all the spices, corn, lime juice, and broth, along with the beans, to the pot. Seal the lid and cook on Manual setting at High Pressure for 5 minutes. Once done, natural release the pressure when the timer goes off. Remove the lid. To serve, put the prepared mixture into a bowl. Top with tortilla chips and fresh cilantro.
Serve.

Per Serving: calories: 183 | fat: 0.9g | protein: 7.1g | carbs: 39.8g | fiber: 8.3g | sodium: 387mg

Cauliflower and Broccoli Bowls

Prep time: 5 minutes | Cook time: 7 minutes | Serves 3

Ingredients:
½ medium onion, diced
2 teaspoons olive oil
garlic clove, minced
½ cup tomato paste
½ pound (227 g) frozen cauliflower
½ pound (227 g) broccoli florets
½ cup vegetable broth
½ teaspoon paprika
¼ teaspoon dried thyme
pinches sea salt

Directions:
Add the oil, onion and garlic into the instant pot and Sauté for 2 minutes.
Add the broth, tomato paste, cauliflower, broccoli, and all the spices, to the pot.
Secure the lid. Cook on the Manual setting at with pressure for 5 minutes.
After the beep, Quick release the pressure and remove the lid.
Stir well and serve hot.

Per Serving:
calories: 109 | fat: 3.8g | protein: 6.1g | carbs: 16.7g | fiber: 6.1g | sodium: 265mg

Italian Zucchini Pomodoro

Prep time: 10 minutes | Cook time: 12 minutes | Serves 4

Ingredients:
1 tablespoon avocado oil
1 large onion, peeled and diced
3 cloves garlic, minced
1 (28-ounce / 794-g) can diced tomatoes, including juice
½ cup water
1 tablespoon Italian seasoning
teaspoon sea salt
½ teaspoon ground black pepper
medium zucchini, spiraled

Directions:
Press Sauté button on the Instant Pot. Heat avocado oil. Add onions and stir-fry for 3 to 5 minutes until translucent. Add garlic and cook for an additional minute. Add tomatoes, water, Italian seasoning, salt, and pepper. Add zucchini and toss to combine. Lock lid.
Press the Manual button and adjust time to 1 minute. When timer beeps, let pressure release naturally for 5 minutes. Quick release any additional pressure until float valve drops and then unlock lid. Transfer zucchini to four bowls. Press Sauté button, press Adjust button to change the temperature to Less, and simmer sauce in the Instant Pot unlidded for 5 minutes. Ladle over zucchini and serve immediately.

Per Serving:
calories: 92 | fat: 4.1g | protein: 2.5g | carbs: 13.1g | fiber: 5.1g | sodium: 980mg

Potato Curry

Prep time: 10 minutes | Cook time: 30 minutes | Serves 2

Ingredients:
2 large potatoes, peeled and diced
1 small onion, peeled and diced
8 ounces (227 g) fresh tomatoes
1 tablespoon olive oil
cup water
tablespoons garlic cloves, grated
½ tablespoon rosemary
½ tablespoon cayenne pepper
1½ tablespoons thyme
Salt and pepper, to taste

Directions:
Pour a cup of water into the instant pot and place the steamer trivet inside.
Place the potatoes and half the garlic over the trivet and sprinkle some salt and pepper on top.
Secure the lid and cook on Steam function for 20 minutes.
After the beep, natural release the pressure and remove the lid.
Put the potatoes to one side and empty the pot.
Add the remaining ingredients to the cooker and Sauté for 10 minutes.
Use an immerse blender to purée the cooked mixture.
Stir in the steamed potatoes and serve hot.

Per Serving:
calories: 398 | fat: 7.6g | protein: 9.6g | carbs: 76.2g | fiber: 10.9g | sodium: 111mg

Mushroom Swoodles

Prep time: 5 minutes | Cook time: 3 minutes | Serves 4

Ingredients:

2 tablespoons coconut aminos

tablespoon white vinegar

teaspoons olive oil

1 teaspoon sesame oil

1 tablespoon honey

¼ teaspoon red pepper flakes

3 cloves garlic, minced

1 large sweet potato, peeled and spiraled

1 pound (454 g) shiitake mushrooms, sliced

1 cup vegetable broth

¼ cup chopped fresh parsley

Directions:

In a large bowl, whisk together coconut aminos, vinegar, olive oil, sesame oil, honey, red pepper flakes, and garlic.

Toss sweet potato and shiitake mushrooms in sauce. Refrigerate covered for 30 minutes.

Pour vegetable broth into Instant Pot. Add trivet. Lower steamer basket onto trivet and add the sweet potato mixture to the basket. Lock lid.

Press the Manual button and adjust time to 3 minutes. When timer beeps, let pressure release naturally for 5 minutes. Quick release any additional pressure until float valve drops and then unlock lid.

Remove basket from the Instant Pot and distribute sweet potatoes and mushrooms evenly among four bowls; pour liquid from the Instant Pot over bowls and garnish with chopped parsley.

Per Serving:

calories: 127 | fat: 4.0g | protein: 4.2g | carbs: 20.9g | fiber: 4.1g | sodium: 671mg

Stuffed Portobello Mushroom with Tomatoes

Prep time: 10 minutes | Cook time: 15 minutes | Serves 4

Ingredients:
4 large portobello mushroom caps
tablespoons extra-virgin olive oil
Salt and freshly ground black pepper, to taste
sun-dried tomatoes
1 cup shredded mozzarella cheese, divided
½ to ¾ cup low-sodium tomato sauce

Directions:
Preheat the broiler to High.
Arrange the mushroom caps on a baking sheet and drizzle with olive oil. Sprinkle with salt and pepper.
Broil for 1o minutes, flipping the mushroom caps halfway through, until browned on the top.
Remove from the broil. Spoon 1 tomato, 2 tablespoons of cheese, and 2 to 3 tablespoons of sauce onto each mushroom cap.
Return the mushroom caps to the broiler and continue broiling for 2 to 3 minutes.
Cool for 5 minutes before serving.

Per Serving:
calories: 217 | fat: 15.8g | protein: 11.2g | carbs: 11.7g | fiber: 2.0g | sodium: 243mg

Vegetable and Tofu Scramble

Prep time: 5 minutes | Cook time: 10 minutes | Serves 2

Ingredients:
2 tablespoons extra-virgin olive oil
½ red onion, finely chopped
1 cup chopped kale
8 ounces (227 g) mushrooms, sliced
8 ounces (227 g) tofu, cut into pieces
2 garlic cloves, minced
Pinch red pepper flakes
½ teaspoon sea salt
⅛ teaspoon freshly ground black pepper

Directions:
Heat the olive oil in a medium nonstick skillet over medium-high heat until shimmering.
Add the onion, kale, and mushrooms to the skillet and cook for about 5 minutes, stirring occasionally, or until the vegetables start to brown.
Add the tofu and stir-fry for 3 to 4 minutes until softened.
Stir in the garlic, red pepper flakes, salt, and black pepper and cook for 30 seconds.
Let the mixture cool for 5 minutes before serving.

Per Serving:
calories: 233 | fat: 15.9g | protein: 13.4g | carbs: 11.9g | fiber: 2.0g | sodium: 672mg

Zoodles

Prep time: 10 minutes | Cook time: 5 minutes | Serves 2

Ingredients:
2 tablespoons avocado oil
2 medium zucchini, spiralized
¼ teaspoon salt
Freshly ground black pepper, to taste

Directions:
Heat the avocado oil in a large skillet over medium heat until it shimmers.
Add the zucchini noodles, salt, and black pepper to the skillet and toss to coat. Cook for 1 to 2 minutes, stirring constantly, until tender.
Serve warm.

Per Serving:
calories: 128 | fat: 14.0g | protein: 0.3g | carbs: 0.3g | fiber: 0.1g | sodium: 291mg

Lentil and Tomato Collard Wraps

Prep time: 15 minutes | Cook time: 0 minutes | Serves 4

Ingredients:
2 cups cooked lentils
5 Roma tomatoes, diced
½ cup crumbled feta cheese
10 large fresh basil leaves, thinly sliced
¼ cup extra-virgin olive oil
tablespoon balsamic vinegar
garlic cloves, minced
½ teaspoon raw honey
½ teaspoon salt
¼ teaspoon freshly ground black pepper
4 large collard leaves, stems removed

Directions:
Combine the lentils, tomatoes, cheese, basil leaves, olive oil, vinegar, garlic, honey, salt, and black pepper in a large bowl and stir until well blended.
Lay the collard leaves on a flat work surface. Spoon the equal-sized amounts of the lentil mixture onto the edges of the leaves. Roll them up and slice in half to serve.

Per Serving:
calories: 318 | fat: 17.6g | protein: 13.2g | carbs: 27.5g | fiber: 9.9g | sodium: 475mg

Radish and Cabbage Congee

Prep time: 5 minutes | Cook time: 20 minutes | Serves 3

Ingredients:
1 cup carrots, diced
½ cup radish, diced
6 cups vegetable broth
Salt, to taste
1½ cups short grain rice, rinsed
1 tablespoon grated fresh ginger
4 cups cabbage, shredded
Green onions for garnishing, chopped

Directions:
Add all the ingredients, except the cabbage and green onions, into the instant pot.
Select the Porridge function and cook on the default time and settings.
After the beep, Quick release the pressure and remove the lid
Stir in the shredded cabbage and cover with the lid.
Serve after 10 minutes with chopped green onions on top.

Per Serving:
calories: 438 | fat: 0.8g | protein: 8.7g | carbs: 98.4g | fiber: 6.7g | sodium: 1218mg

Potato and Broccoli Medley

Prep time: 10 minutes | Cook time: 20 minutes | Serves 3

Ingredients:
1 tablespoon olive oil
½ white onion, diced
1½ cloves garlic, finely chopped
1 pound (454 g) potatoes, cut into chunks
1 pound (454 g) broccoli florets, diced
1 pound (454 g) baby carrots, cut in half
¼ cup vegetable broth
½ teaspoon Italian seasoning
½ teaspoon Spike original seasoning
Fresh parsley for garnishing

Directions:
Put the oil and onion into the instant pot and Sauté for 5 minutes.
Stir in the carrots, and garlic and stir-fry for 5 minutes.
Add the remaining ingredients and secure the lid.
Cook on the Manual function for 10 minutes at High Pressure.
After the beep, Quick release the pressure and remove the lid.
Stir gently and garnish with fresh parsley , then serve.

Per Serving:
calories: 256 | fat: 5.6g | protein: 9.1g | carbs: 46.1g | fiber: 12.2g | sodium: 274mg

Mushroom and Potato Oat Burgers

Prep time: 20 minutes | Cook time: 21 minutes | Serves 5

Ingredients:
½ cup minced onion
1 teaspoon grated fresh ginger
½ cup minced mushrooms
½ cup red lentils, rinsed
¾ sweet potato, peeled and diced
cup vegetable stock
tablespoons hemp seeds
2 tablespoons chopped parsley
2 tablespoons chopped cilantro
1 tablespoon curry powder 1 cup quick oats
Brown rice flour, optional
5 tomato slices
Lettuce leaves
5 whole-wheat buns

Directions:
Add the oil, ginger, mushrooms and onion into the instant pot and Sauté for 5 minutes. Stir in the lentils, stock, and the sweet potatoes. Secure the lid and cook on the Manual function for 6 minutes at High Pressure. After the beep, natural release the pressure and remove the lid. Meanwhile, heat the oven to 375°F (190°C) and line a baking tray with parchment paper. Mash the prepared lentil mixture with a potato masher. Add the oats and the remaining spices. Put in some brown rice flour if the mixture is not thick enough. Wet your hands and prepare 5 patties, using the mixture, and place them on the baking tray. Bake the patties for 10 minutes in the preheated oven. Slice the buns in half and stack each with a tomato slice, a vegetable patty and lettuce leaves. Serve and enjoy.

Per Serving: calories: 266 | fat: 5.3g | protein: 14.5g | carbs: 48.7g | fiber: 9.6g | sodium: 276mg

Potato, Corn, and Spinach Medley

Prep time: 10 minutes | Cook time: 10 minutes | Serves 6

Ingredients:
1 tablespoon olive oil
3 scallions, chopped
½ cup onion, chopped
2 large white potatoes, peeled and diced
1 tablespoon ginger, grated
3 cups frozen corn kernels
1 cup vegetable stock
tablespoon fish sauce
tablespoons light soy sauce
2 large cloves garlic, diced
⅓ teaspoon white pepper
1 teaspoon salt
3-4 handfuls baby spinach leaves
Juice of ½ lemon

Directions:
Put the oil, ginger, garlic and onions in the instant pot and Sauté for 5 minutes.
Add all the remaining ingredients except the spinach leaves and lime juice
Secure the lid and cook on the Manual setting for 5 minutes at High Pressure.
After the beep, Quick release the pressure and remove the lid.
Add the spinach and cook for 3 minutes on Sauté
Drizzle the lime juice over the dish and serve hot.

Per Serving:
calories: 217 | fat: 3.4g | protein: 6.5g | carbs: 44.5g | fiber: 6.3g | sodium: 892mg

Braised Cauliflower with White Wine

Prep time: 10 minutes | Cook time: 12 to 16 minutes | Serves 4 to 6

Ingredients:
3 tablespoons plus 1 teaspoon extra-virgin olive oil, divided
3 garlic cloves, minced
⅛ teaspoon red pepper flakes
head cauliflower (2 pounds / 907 g), cored and cut into 1½-inch florets
¼ teaspoon salt, plus more for seasoning
Black pepper, to taste
⅓ cup vegetable broth
⅓ cup dry white wine
tablespoons minced fresh parsley

Directions:
Combine 1 teaspoon of the oil, garlic and pepper flakes in small bowl. Heat the remaining 3 tablespoons of the oil in a skillet over medium-high heat until shimmering. Add the cauliflower and ¼ teaspoon of the salt and cook for 7 to 9 minutes, stirring occasionally, or until florets are golden brown.
Push the cauliflower to sides of the skillet. Add the garlic mixture to the center of the skillet. Cook for about 30 seconds, or until fragrant. Stir the garlic mixture into the cauliflower.
Pour in the broth and wine and bring to simmer. Reduce the heat to medium-low. Cover and cook for 4 to 6 minutes, or until the cauliflower is crisp-tender. Off heat, stir in the parsley and season with salt and pepper.
Serve immediately.

Per Serving:
calories: 143 | fat: 11.7g | protein: 3.1g | carbs: 8.7g | fiber: 3.1g | sodium: 263mg

Cauliflower Steaks with Arugula

Prep time: 5 minutes | Cook time: 20 minutes | Serves 4

Ingredients:
Cauliflower:
1 head cauliflower
Cooking spray
½ teaspoon garlic powder
4 cups arugula Dressing:
1½ tablespoons extra-virgin olive oil
1½ tablespoons honey mustard
1 teaspoon freshly squeezed lemon juice

Directions:
Preheat the oven to 425°F (220°C).
Remove the leaves from the cauliflower head, and cut it in half
lengthwise. Cut 1½-inch-thick steaks from each half.
Spritz both sides of each steak with cooking spray and season both
sides with the garlic powder.
Place the cauliflower steaks on a baking sheet, cover with foil, and roast
in the oven for 10 minutes.
Remove the baking sheet from the oven and gently pull back the foil to
avoid the steam. Flip the steaks, then roast uncovered for 10 minutes
more.
Meanwhile, make the dressing: Whisk together the olive oil, honey
mustard and lemon juice in a small bowl.
When the cauliflower steaks are done, divide into four equal portions.
Top each portion with one-quarter of the arugula and dressing.
Serve immediately.

Per Serving:
calories: 115 | fat: 6.0g | protein: 5.0g | carbs: 14.0g | fiber: 4.0g |
sodium: 97mg

Mushrooms Ragu with Cheesy Polenta
Prep time: 20 minutes | Cook time: 30 minutes | Serves 2

Ingredients:
½ ounce (14 g) dried porcini mushrooms

pound (454 g) baby bella (cremini) mushrooms, quartered

tablespoons olive oil

1 garlic clove, minced

1 large shallot, minced

tablespoon flour

teaspoons tomato paste

½ cup red wine

cup mushroom stock (or reserved liquid from soaking the porcinimushrooms, if using) 1 fresh rosemary sprig

½ teaspoon dried thyme

1½ cups water

½ teaspoon salt, plus more as needed

⅓ cup instant polenta

tablespoons grated Parmesan cheese

Directions:

Soak the dried porcini mushrooms in 1 cup of hot water for about 15 minutes to soften them. When ready, scoop them out of the water, reserving the soaking liquid. Mince the porcini mushrooms.

Heat the olive oil in a large sauté pan over medium-high heat. Add the mushrooms, garlic, and shallot and sauté for 10 minutes, or until the vegetables are beginning to caramelize.

Stir in the flour and tomato paste and cook for an additional 30 seconds. Add the red wine, mushroom stock, rosemary, and thyme. Bring the mixture to a boil, stirring constantly, or until it has thickened. Reduce the heat and allow to simmer for 10 minutes.

Meanwhile, bring the water to a boil in a saucepan and sprinkle with the salt.

Add the instant polenta and stir quickly while it thickens. Scatter with the grated Parmesan cheese. Taste and season with more salt as needed. Serve warm.

Per Serving:

calories: 450 | fat: 16.0g | protein: 14.1g | carbs: 57.8g | fiber: 5.0g | sodium: 165mg

Veggie Rice Bowls with Pesto Sauce

Prep time: 15 minutes | Cook time: 1 minute | Serves 2

Ingredients:
2 cups water
cup arborio rice, rinsed
Salt and ground black pepper, to taste
eggs
1 cup broccoli florets
½ pound (227 g) Brussels sprouts
1 carrot, peeled and chopped
1 small beet, peeled and cubed
¼ cup pesto sauce
Lemon wedges, for serving

Directions:
Combine the water, rice, salt, and pepper in the Instant Pot. Insert a trivet over rice and place a steamer basket on top. Add the eggs, broccoli, Brussels sprouts, carrots, beet cubes, salt, and pepper to the steamer basket.
Lock the lid. Select the Manual mode and set the cooking time for 1 minute at High Pressure.
When the timer beeps, perform a natural pressure release for 10 minutes, then release any remaining pressure. Carefully open the lid. Remove the steamer basket and trivet from the pot and transfer the eggs to a bowl of ice water. Peel and halve the eggs. Use a fork to fluff the rice.
Divide the rice, broccoli, Brussels sprouts, carrot, beet cubes, and eggs into two bowls. Top with a dollop of pesto sauce and serve with the lemon wedges.

Per Serving:
calories: 590 | fat: 34.1g | protein: 21.9g | carbs: 50.0g | fiber: 19.6g | sodium: 670m

Roasted Vegetables

Prep time: 20 minutes | Cook time: 35 minutes | Serves 2

Ingredients:
6 teaspoons extra-virgin olive oil, divided
12 to 15 Brussels sprouts, halved
medium sweet potato, peeled and cut into 2-inch cubes
cups fresh cauliflower florets
1 medium zucchini, cut into 1-inch rounds
1 red bell pepper, cut into 1-inch slices
Salt, to taste

Directions:
Preheat the oven to 425°F (220°C).
Add 2 teaspoons of olive oil, Brussels sprouts, sweet potato, and salt to a large bowl and toss until they are completely coated.
Transfer them to a large roasting pan and roast for 10 minutes, or until the Brussels sprouts are lightly browned.
Meantime, combine the cauliflower florets with 2 teaspoons of olive oil and salt in a separate bowl.
Remove from the oven. Add the cauliflower florets to the roasting pan and roast for 10 minutes more.
Meanwhile, toss the zucchini and bell pepper with the remaining olive oil in a medium bowl until well coated. Season with salt.
Remove the roasting pan from the oven and stir in the zucchini and bell pepper. Continue roasting for 15 minutes, or until the vegetables are forktender.
Divide the roasted vegetables between two plates and serve warm.

Per Serving:
calories: 333 | fat: 16.8g | protein: 12.2g | carbs: 37.6g | fiber: 11.0g | sodium: 329mg

Ratatouille

Prep time: 10 minutes | Cook time: 30 minutes | Serves 4

Ingredients:
4 tablespoons extra-virgin olive oil, divided
cup diced zucchini
cups diced eggplant
1 cup diced onion
1 cup chopped green bell pepper
1 (15-ounce / 425-g) can no-salt-added diced tomatoes
½ teaspoon garlic powder
1 teaspoon ground thyme
Salt and freshly ground black pepper, to taste

Directions:
Heat 2 tablespoons of olive oil in a large saucepan over medium heat until it shimmers.
Add the zucchini and eggplant and sauté for 10 minutes, stirring occasionally. If necessary, add the remaining olive oil.
Stir in the onion and bell pepper and sauté for 5 minutes until softened.
Add the diced tomatoes with their juice, garlic powder, and thyme and stir to combine. Continue cooking for 15 minutes until the vegetables are cooked through, stirring occasionally. Sprinkle with salt and black pepper.
Remove from the heat and serve on a plate.

Per Serving:
calories: 189 | fat: 13.7g | protein: 3.1g | carbs: 14.8g | fiber: 4.0g | sodium: 27mg

Zoodles with Beet Pesto

Prep time: 10 minutes | Cook time: 50 minutes | Serves 2

Ingredients:
1 medium red beet, peeled, chopped
½ cup walnut pieces
½ cup crumbled goat cheese
3 garlic cloves
2 tablespoons freshly squeezed lemon juice
2 tablespoons plus 2 teaspoons extra-virgin olive oil, divided
¼ teaspoon salt
4 small zucchini, spiralized

Directions:
Preheat the oven to 375°F (190°C).
Wrap the chopped beet in a piece of aluminum foil and seal well.
Roast in the preheated oven for 30 to 40 minutes until tender.
Meanwhile, heat a skillet over medium-high heat until hot. Add the walnuts and toast for 5 to 7 minutes, or until fragrant and lightly browned.
Remove the cooked beets from the oven and place in a food processor. Add the toasted walnuts, goat cheese, garlic, lemon juice, 2 tablespoons of olive oil, and salt. Pulse until smoothly blended. Set aside.
Heat the remaining 2 teaspoons of olive oil in a large skillet over medium heat. Add the zucchini and toss to coat in the oil. Cook for 2 to 3 minutes, stirring gently, or until the zucchini is softened.
Transfer the zucchini to a serving plate and toss with the beet pesto, then serve.

Per Serving:
calories: 423 | fat: 38.8g | protein: 8.0g | carbs: 17.1g | fiber: 6.0g | sodium: 338mg

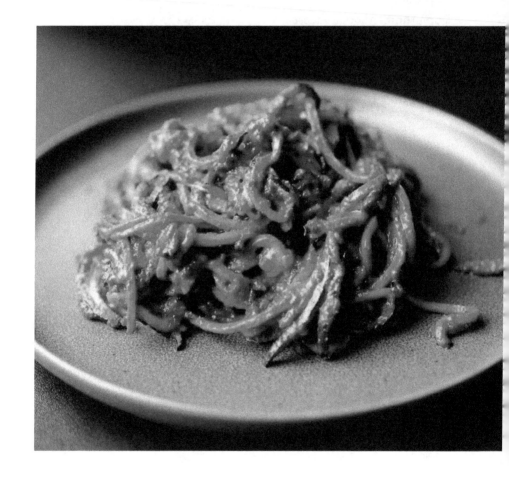

Sweet Potato Chickpea Buddha Bowl

Prep time: 10 minutes | Cook time: 10 to 15 minutes | Serves 2

Sauce:
tablespoon tahini
tablespoons plain Greek yogurt
2 tablespoons hemp seeds
1 garlic clove, minced
Pinch salt
Freshly ground black pepper, to taste
Bowl:
1 small sweet potato, peeled and finely diced
1 teaspoon extra-virgin olive oil
cup from 1 (15-ounce / 425-g) can low-sodium chickpeas, drained
andrinsed
cups baby kale

Directions:
Make the Sauce
Whisk together the tahini and yogurt in a small bowl.
Stir in the hemp seeds and minced garlic. Season with salt pepper. Add
2 to 3 tablespoons water to create a creamy yet pourable consistency
and set aside.
Make the Bowl
Preheat the oven to 425°F (220°C). Line a baking sheet with parchment
paper. Place the sweet potato on the prepared baking sheet and drizzle
with the olive oil. Toss well Roast in the preheated oven for 10 to 15
minutes, stirring once during cooking, or until fork-tender and
browned. In each of 2 bowls, place ½ cup of chickpeas, 1 cup of baby
kale, and half of the cooked sweet potato. Serve drizzled with half of
the prepared sauce.

Per Serving: calories: 323 | fat: 14.1g | protein: 17.0g | carbs: 36.0 g |
fiber: 7.9g | sodium: 304mg

Mushroom Tacos

Prep time: 10 minutes | Cook time: 13 minutes | Serves 3

Ingredients:
4 large guajillo chilies
2 teaspoons oil
2 bay leaves
2 large onions, sliced
2 garlic cloves
2 chipotle chillies in adobo sauce
2 teaspoons ground cumin
1 teaspoon dried oregano
1 teaspoon smoked hot paprika
½ teaspoon ground cinnamon,
Salt, to taste
¾ cup vegetable broth
1 teaspoon apple cider vinegar
3 teaspoons lime juice
¼ teaspoon sugar
8 ounces (227 g) mushrooms chopped
Whole-wheat tacos, for serving

Directions:
Put the oil, onion, garlic, salt and bay leaves into the instant pot and
Sauté for 5 minutes. Blend the half of this mixture, in a blender, with
all the spices and chillies. Add the mushrooms to the remaining onions
and Sauté for 3 minutes. Pour the blended mixture into the pot and
secure the lid. Cook on Manual function for 5 minutes at High
Pressure. Once done, Quick release the pressure and remove the lid.
Stir well and serve with tacos.

Per Serving:
calories: 138 | fat: 4.1g | protein: 5.7g | carbs: 23.8g | fiber: 4.8g |
sodium: 208mg

Lentils and Eggplant Curry

Prep time: 10 minutes | Cook time: 22 minutes | Serves 4

Ingredients:
¾ cup lentils, soaked and rinsed
1 teaspoon olive oil
½ onion, chopped
4 garlic cloves, chopped
1 teaspoon ginger, chopped
hot green chili, chopped
¼ teaspoon turmeric
½ teaspoon ground cumin
tomatoes, chopped
1 cup eggplant, chopped
cup sweet potatoes, cubed
¾ teaspoon salt
cups water
1 cup baby spinach leaves
Cayenne and lemon/lime to taste
Pepper flakes (garnish)

Directions:
Add the oil, garlic, ginger, chili and salt into the instant pot and Sauté for 3 minutes. Stir in the tomatoes and all the spices. Cook for 5 minutes. Add all the remaining ingredients, except the spinach leaves and garnish. Secure the lid and cook on Manual function for 12 minutes at High Pressure. After the beep, release the pressure naturally and remove the lid. Stir in the spinach leaves and let the pot simmer for 2 minutes on Sauté.
Garnish with the pepper flakes and serve warm.

Per Serving:
calories: 88 | fat: 1.5g | protein: 3.4g | carbs: 17.4g | fiber: 3.3g | sodium: 470mg

Cauliflower Hash with Carrots

Prep time: 10 minutes | Cook time: 10 minutes | Serves 4

Ingredients:
3 tablespoons extra-virgin olive oil
1 large onion, chopped
tablespoon minced garlic
cups diced carrots
4 cups cauliflower florets
½ teaspoon ground cumin
1 teaspoon salt

Directions:
In a large skillet, heat the olive oil over medium heat.
Add the onion and garlic and sauté for 1 minute. Stir in the carrots and stir-fry for 3 minutes.
Add the cauliflower florets, cumin, and salt and toss to combine.
Cover and cook for 3 minutes until lightly browned. Stir well and cook, uncovered, for 3 to 4 minutes, until softened.
Remove from the heat and serve warm.

Per Serving:
calories: 158 | fat: 10.8g | protein: 3.1g | carbs: 14.9g | fiber: 5.1g | sodium: 656mg

Garlicky Zucchini Cubes with Mint

Prep time: 5 minutes | Cook time: 10 minutes | Serves 4

Ingredients:
3 large green zucchini, cut into ½-inch cubes
3 tablespoons extra-virgin olive oil
1 large onion, chopped
3 cloves garlic, minced
1 teaspoon salt
1 teaspoon dried mint

Directions:
Heat the olive oil in a large skillet over medium heat.
Add the onion and garlic and saut é for 3 minutes, stirring constantly, or until softened.
Stir in the zucchini cubes and salt and cook for 5 minutes, or until the zucchini is browned and tender.
Add the mint to the skillet and toss to combine, then continue cooking for 2 minutes.
Serve warm.

Per Serving:
calories: 146 | fat: 10.6g | protein: 4.2g | carbs: 11.8g | fiber: 3.0g | sodium: 606mg

Stuffed Portobello Mushrooms with Spinach

Prep time: 5 minutes | Cook time: 20 minutes | Serves 4

Ingredients:
8 large portobello mushrooms, stems removed
3 teaspoons extra-virgin olive oil, divided
1 medium red bell pepper, diced
4 cups fresh spinach
¼ cup crumbled feta cheese

Directions:
Preheat the oven to 450°F (235°C).
Using a spoon to scoop out the gills of the mushrooms and discard them. Brush the mushrooms with 2 teaspoons of olive oil.
Arrange the mushrooms (cap-side down) on a baking sheet. Roast in the preheated oven for 20 minutes.
Meantime, in a medium skillet, heat the remaining olive oil over medium heat until it shimmers.
Add the bell pepper and spinach and saut é for 8 to 10 minutes, stirring occasionally, or until the spinach is wilted.
Remove the mushrooms from the oven to a paper towel-lined plate. Using a spoon to stuff each mushroom with the bell pepper and spinach mixture. Scatter the feta cheese all over.
Serve immediately.

Per Serving: (2 mushrooms)
calories: 115 | fat: 5.9g | protein: 7.2g | carbs: 11.5g | fiber: 4.0g | sodium: 125mg

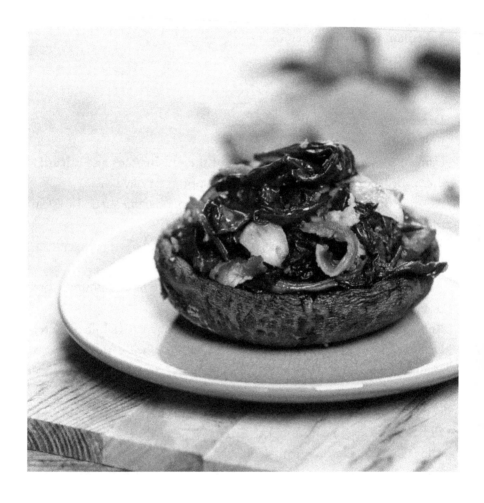

Chickpea Lettuce Wraps with Celery

Prep time: 10 minutes | Cook time: 0 minutes | Serves 4

Ingredients:
1 (15-ounce / 425-g) can low-sodium chickpeas, drained and rinsed
celery stalk, thinly sliced
tablespoons finely chopped red onion
tablespoons unsalted tahini
tablespoons honey mustard
1 tablespoon capers, undrained
12 butter lettuce leaves

Directions:
In a bowl, mash the chickpeas with a potato masher or the back of a
fork until mostly smooth.
Add the celery, red onion, tahini, honey mustard, and capers to the
bowl and stir until well incorporated.
For each serving, place three overlapping lettuce leaves on a plate and
top with ¼ of the mashed chickpea filling, then roll up. Repeat with the
remaining lettuce leaves and chickpea mixture.

Per Serving:
calories: 182 | fat: 7.1g | protein: 10.3g | carbs: 19.6g | fiber: 3.0g |
sodium: 171mg

Parmesan Stuffed Zucchini Boats

Prep time: 5 minutes | Cook time: 15 minutes | Serves 4

Ingredients:
1 cup canned low-sodium chickpeas, drained and rinsed
cup no-sugar-added spaghetti sauce
zucchinis
¼ cup shredded Parmesan cheese

Directions:
Preheat the oven to 425°F (220°C).
In a medium bowl, stir together the chickpeas and spaghetti sauce.
Cut the zucchini in half lengthwise and scrape a spoon gently down the length of each half to remove the seeds.
Fill each zucchini half with the chickpea sauce and top with one-quarter of the Parmesan cheese.
Place the zucchini halves on a baking sheet and roast in the oven for 15 minutes.
Transfer to a plate. Let rest for 5 minutes before serving.

Per Serving:
calories: 139 | fat: 4.0g | protein: 8.0g | carbs: 20.0g | fiber: 5.0g | sodium: 344mg

Baby Kale and Cabbage Salad

Prep time: 10 minutes | Cook time: 0 minutes | Serves 6

Ingredients:
2 bunches baby kale, thinly sliced
½ head green savoy cabbage, cored and thinly sliced
1 medium red bell pepper, thinly sliced
1 garlic clove, thinly sliced
1 cup toasted peanuts Dressing:
Juice of 1 lemon
¼ cup apple cider vinegar
1 teaspoon ground cumin
¼ teaspoon smoked paprika

Directions:
In a large mixing bowl, toss together the kale and cabbage.
Make the dressing: Whisk together the lemon juice, vinegar, cumin and paprika in a small bowl.
Pour the dressing over the greens and gently massage with your hands.
Add the pepper, garlic and peanuts to the mixing bowl. Toss to combine.
Serve immediately.

Per Serving:
calories: 199 | fat: 12.0g | protein: 10.0g | carbs: 17.0g | fiber: 5.0g | sodium: 46mg

Zucchini and Artichokes Bowl with Farro

Prep time: 15 minutes | Cook time: 10 minutes | Serves 4 to 6

Ingredients:

⅓ cup extra-virgin olive oil
⅓ cup chopped red onions
½ cup chopped red bell pepper
2 garlic cloves, minced
1 cup zucchini, cut into ½-inch-thick slices
½ cup coarsely chopped artichokes
½ cup canned chickpeas, drained and rinsed
3 cups cooked farro
Salt and freshly ground black pepper, to taste
½ cup crumbled feta cheese, for serving (optional)
¼ cup sliced olives, for serving (optional)
tablespoons fresh basil, chiffonade, for serving (optional)
tablespoons balsamic vinegar, for serving (optional)

Directions:

Heat the olive oil in a large skillet over medium heat until it shimmers.
Add the onions, bell pepper, and garlic and sauté for 5 minutes,
stirring occasionally, until softened.
Stir in the zucchini slices, artichokes, and chickpeas and sauté for
about 5 minutes until slightly tender.
Add the cooked farro and toss to combine until heated through.
Sprinkle the salt and pepper to season.
Divide the mixture into bowls. Top each bowl evenly with feta cheese,
olive slices, and basil and sprinkle with the balsamic vinegar, if desired.

Per Serving:

calories: 366 | fat: 19.9g | protein: 9.3g | carbs: 50.7g | fiber: 9.0g |
sodium: 86mg

Zucchini Fritters

Prep time: 15 minutes | Cook time: 5 minutes | Makes 14 fritters

Ingredients:
4 cups grated zucchini
Salt, to taste
2 large eggs, lightly beaten
⅓ cup sliced scallions (green and white parts)
⅔ all-purpose flour
⅛ teaspoon black pepper
2 tablespoons olive oil

Directions:
Put the grated zucchini in a colander and lightly season with salt. Set aside to rest for 10 minutes. Squeeze out as much liquid from the grated zucchini as possible.
Pour the grated zucchini into a bowl. Fold in the beaten eggs, scallions, flour, salt, and pepper and stir until everything is well combined.
Heat the olive oil in a large skillet over medium heat until hot.
Drop 3 tablespoons mounds of the zucchini mixture onto the hot skillet to make each fritter, pressing them lightly into rounds and spacing them about 2 inches apart.
Cook for 2 to 3 minutes. Flip the zucchini fritters and cook for 2 minutes more, or until they are golden brown and cooked through.
Remove from the heat to a plate lined with paper towels. Repeat with the remaining zucchini mixture.
Serve hot.

Per Serving: (2 fritters)
calories: 113 | fat: 6.1g | protein: 4.0g | carbs: 12.2g | fiber: 1.0g | sodium: 25mg

Creamy Cauliflower Chickpea Curry

Prep time: 5 minutes | Cook time: 15 minutes | Serves 4

Ingredients:

3 cups fresh or frozen cauliflower florets

2 cups unsweetened almond milk

1 (15-ounce / 425-g) can low-sodium chickpeas, drained and rinsed

1 (15-ounce / 425-g) can coconut milk

1 tablespoon curry powder

¼ teaspoon garlic powder

¼ teaspoon ground ginger

⅛ teaspoon onion powder

¼ teaspoon salt

Directions:

Add the cauliflower florets, almond milk, chickpeas, coconut milk, curry powder, garlic powder, ginger, and onion powder to a large stockpot and stir to combine.

Cover and cook over medium-high heat for 10 minutes, stirring occasionally.

Reduce the heat to low and continue cooking uncovered for 5 minutes, or until the cauliflower is tender.

Sprinkle with the salt and stir well. Serve warm.

Per Serving:

calories: 409 | fat: 29.6g | protein: 10.0g | carbs: 29.8g | fiber: 9.1g | sodium: 117mg

Cauliflower Rice Risotto with Mushrooms

Prep time: 5 minutes | Cook time: 10 minutes | Serves 4

Ingredients:
1 teaspoon extra-virgin olive oil
½ cup chopped portobello mushrooms
4 cups cauliflower rice
½ cup plain Greek yogurt
¼ cup low-sodium vegetable broth
1 cup shredded Parmesan cheese

Directions:
In a medium skillet, heat the olive oil over medium-low heat until shimmering.
Add the mushrooms and stir-fry for 3 minutes.
Stir in the cauliflower rice, yogurt, and vegetable broth. Cover and bring to a boil over high heat for 5 minutes, stirring occasionally.
Add the Parmesan cheese and stir to combine. Continue cooking for an additional 3 minutes until the cheese is melted.
Divide the mixture into four bowls and serve warm.

Per Serving:
calories: 167 | fat: 10.7g | protein: 12.1g | carbs: 8.1g | fiber: 3.0g | sodium: 326mg

Grilled Romaine Lettuce

Prep time: 5 minutes | Cook time: 3 to 5 minutes | Serves 4

Ingredients:
2 heads romaine lettuce, halved lengthwise
2 tablespoons extra-virgin olive oil Dressing:
½ cup unsweetened almond milk
1 tablespoon extra-virgin olive oil
¼ bunch fresh chives, thinly chopped
1 garlic clove, pressed
1 pinch red pepper flakes

Directions:
Heat a grill pan over medium heat.
Brush each lettuce half with the olive oil. Place the lettuce halves,
flatside down, on the grill. Grill for 3 to 5 minutes, or until the lettuce
slightly wilts and develops light grill marks.
Meanwhile, whisk together all the ingredients for the dressing in a small
bowl.
Drizzle 2 tablespoons of the dressing over each romaine half and serve.

Per Serving:
calories: 126 | fat: 11.0g | protein: 2.0g | carbs: 7.0g | fiber: 1.0g |
sodium: 41mg

Mini Crustless Spinach Quiches

Prep time: 10 minutes | Cook time: 20 minutes | Serves 6

Ingredients:
2 tablespoons extra-virgin olive oil
onion, finely chopped
cups baby spinach
2 garlic cloves, minced
8 large eggs, beaten
¼ cup unsweetened almond milk
½ teaspoon sea salt
¼ teaspoon freshly ground black pepper
1 cup shredded Swiss cheese
Cooking spray

Directions:
Preheat the oven to 375°F (190°C). Spritz a 6-cup muffin tin with
cooking spray. Set aside.
In a large skillet over medium-high heat, heat the olive oil until
shimmering. Add the onion and cook for about 4 minutes, or until
soft. Add the spinach and cook for about 1 minute, stirring constantly,
or until the spinach softens. Add the garlic and sauté for 30 seconds.
Remove from the heat and let cool.
In a medium bowl, whisk together the eggs, milk, salt and pepper.
Stir the cooled vegetables and the cheese into the egg mixture. Spoon
the mixture into the prepared muffin tins. Bake for about 15 minutes,
or until the eggs are set.
Let rest for 5 minutes before serving.

Per Serving:
calories: 218 | fat: 17.0g | protein: 14.0g | carbs: 4.0g | fiber: 1.0g |
sodium: 237mg

Roasted Veggies and Brown Rice Bowl

Prep time: 15 minutes | Cook time: 20 minutes | Serves 4

Ingredients:
2 cups cauliflower florets
2 cups broccoli florets
1 (15-ounce / 425-g) can chickpeas, drained and rinsed
cup carrot slices (about 1 inch thick)
to 3 tablespoons extra-virgin olive oil, divided
Salt and freshly ground black pepper, to taste
Nonstick cooking spray
2 cups cooked brown rice
to 3 tablespoons sesame seeds, for garnishDressing:
to 4 tablespoons tahini
2 tablespoons honey
1 lemon, juiced
1 garlic clove, minced
Salt and freshly ground black pepper, to taste

Directions:
Preheat the oven to 400°F (205°C). Spritz two baking sheets with
nonstick cooking spray. Spread the cauliflower and broccoli on the first
baking sheet and the second with the chickpeas and carrot slices.
Drizzle each sheet with half of the olive oil and sprinkle with salt and
pepper. Toss to coat well. Roast the chickpeas and carrot slices in the
preheated oven for 10 minutes, leaving the carrots tender but crisp, and
the cauliflower and broccoli for 20 minutes until fork-tender. Stir them
once halfway through the cooking time. Meanwhile, make the dressing:
Whisk together the tahini, honey, lemon juice, garlic, salt, and pepper in
a small bowl. Divide the cooked brown rice among four bowls. Top
each bowl evenly with roasted vegetables and dressing. Sprinkle the
sesame seeds on top for garnish before serving.
Per Serving: calories: 453 | fat: 17.8g | protein: 12.1g | carbs: 61.8g |
fiber: 11.2g | sodium: 60mg

Moroccan Tagine with Vegetables

Prep time: 20 minutes | Cook time: 40 minutes | Serves 2

Ingredients:
2 tablespoons olive oil
½ onion, diced
garlic clove, minced
cups cauliflower florets
1 medium carrot, cut into 1-inch pieces
1 cup diced eggplant
1 (28-ounce / 794-g) can whole tomatoes with their juices
(15-ounce / 425-g) can chickpeas, drained and rinsed
small red potatoes, cut into 1-inch pieces
1 cup water
1 teaspoon pure maple syrup
½ teaspoon cinnamon
½ teaspoon turmeric
1 teaspoon cumin
½ teaspoon salt
1 to 2 teaspoons harissa paste

Directions:
In a Dutch oven, heat the olive oil over medium-high heat. Saut é the onion for 5 minutes, stirring occasionally, or until the onion is translucent. Stir in the garlic, cauliflower florets, carrot, eggplant, tomatoes, and potatoes. Using a wooden spoon or spatula to break up the tomatoes into smaller pieces. Add the chickpeas, water, maple syrup, cinnamon, turmeric, cumin, and salt and stir to incorporate. Bring the mixture to a boil. Once it starts to boil, reduce the heat to medium-low. Stir in the harissa paste, cover, allow to simmer for about 40 minutes, or until the vegetables are softened. Taste and adjust seasoning as needed. Let the mixture cool for 5 minutes before serving.
Per Serving: calories: 293 | fat: 9.9g | protein: 11.2g | carbs: 45.5g | fiber: 12.1g | sodium: 337mg

Garlicky Broccoli Rabe

Prep time: 10 minutes | Cook time: 5 to 6 minutes | Serves 4

Ingredients:
14 ounces (397 g) broccoli rabe, trimmed and cut into 1-inch pieces
2 teaspoons salt, plus more for seasoning
Black pepper, to taste
tablespoons extra-virgin olive oil
garlic cloves, minced
¼ teaspoon red pepper flakes

Directions:
Bring 3 quarts water to a boil in a large saucepan. Add the broccoli rabe and 2 teaspoons of the salt to the boiling water and cook for 2 to 3 minutes, or until wilted and tender.
Drain the broccoli rabe. Transfer to ice water and let sit until chilled. Drain again and pat dry.
In a skillet over medium heat, heat the oil and add the garlic and red pepper flakes. Sauté for about 2 minutes, or until the garlic begins to sizzle.
Increase the heat to medium-high. Stir in the broccoli rabe and cook for about 1 minute, or until heated through, stirring constantly. Season with salt and pepper.
Serve immediately.

Per Serving:
calories: 87 | fat: 7.3g | protein: 3.4g | carbs: 4.0g | fiber: 2.9g | sodium: 1196mg

Sautéed Cabbage with Parsley

Prep time: 10 minutes | Cook time: 12 to 14 minutes | Serves 4 to 6

Ingredients:

small head green cabbage (about 1¼ pounds / 567 g), cored and sliced thin

tablespoons extra-virgin olive oil, divided

1 onion, halved and sliced thin

¾ teaspoon salt, divided

¼ teaspoon black pepper

¼ cup chopped fresh parsley 1½ teaspoons lemon juice

Directions:

Place the cabbage in a large bowl with cold water. Let sit for 3 minutes. Drain well.

Heat 1 tablespoon of the oil in a skillet over medium-high heat until shimmering. Add the onion and ¼ teaspoon of the salt and cook for 5 to 7 minutes, or until softened and lightly browned. Transfer to a bowl. Heat the remaining 1 tablespoon of the oil in now-empty skillet over medium-high heat until shimmering. Add the cabbage and sprinkle with the remaining ½ teaspoon of the salt and black pepper. Cover and cook for about 3 minutes, without stirring, or until cabbage is wilted and lightly browned on bottom.

Stir and continue to cook for about 4 minutes, uncovered, or until the cabbage is crisp-tender and lightly browned in places, stirring once halfway through cooking. Off heat, stir in the cooked onion, parsley and lemon juice.

Transfer to a plate and serve.

Per Serving:

calories: 117 | fat: 7.0g | protein: 2.7g | carbs: 13.4g | fiber: 5.1g | sodium: 472mg

Quick Steamed Broccoli

Prep time: 5 minutes | Cook time: 0 minutes | Serves 2

Ingredients:
¼ cup water
3 cups broccoli florets
Salt and ground black pepper, to taste

Directions:
Pour the water into the Instant Pot and insert a steamer basket. Place the broccoli florets in the basket.

Secure the lid. Select the Manual mode and set the cooking time for 0 minutes at High Pressure.

Once cooking is complete, do a quick pressure release. Carefully open the lid.

Transfer the broccoli florets to a bowl with cold water to keep bright green color.

Season the broccoli with salt and pepper to taste, then serve.

Per Serving:
calories: 16 | fat: 0.2g | protein: 1.9g | carbs: 1.7g | fiber: 1.6g | sodium: 292mg

Garlic-Butter Asparagus with Parmesan

Prep time: 5 minutes | Cook time: 8 minutes | Serves 2

Ingredients:
1 cup water
pound (454 g) asparagus, trimmed
cloves garlic, chopped
tablespoons almond butter
Salt and ground black pepper, to taste
3 tablespoons grated Parmesan cheese

Directions:
Pour the water into the Instant Pot and insert a trivet.
Put the asparagus on a tin foil add the butter and garlic. Season to taste with salt and pepper.
Fold over the foil and seal the asparagus inside so the foil doesn't come open. Arrange the asparagus on the trivet.
Secure the lid. Select the Manual mode and set the cooking time for 8 minutes at High Pressure.
Once cooking is complete, do a quick pressure release. Carefully open the lid.
Unwrap the foil packet and serve sprinkled with the Parmesan cheese.

Per Serving:
calories: 243 | fat: 15.7g | protein: 12.3g | carbs: 15.3g | fiber: 7.3g | sodium: 435mg

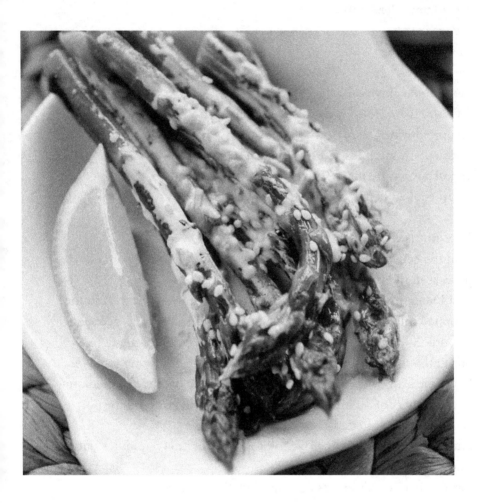

Vegan Lentil Bolognese

Prep time: 15 minutes | Cook time: 50 minutes | Serves 2

Ingredients:
1 medium celery stalk
1 large carrot
½ large onion
garlic clove
tablespoons olive oil
1 (28-ounce / 794-g) can crushed tomatoes
1 cup red wine
½ teaspoon salt, plus more as needed
½ teaspoon pure maple syrup
1 cup cooked lentils (prepared from ½ cup dry)

Directions:
Add the celery, carrot, onion, and garlic to a food processor and process until everything is finely chopped.

In a Dutch oven, heat the olive oil over medium-high heat. Add the chopped mixture and saut é for about 10 minutes, stirring occasionally, or until the vegetables are lightly browned.

Stir in the tomatoes, wine, salt, and maple syrup and bring to a boil. Once the sauce starts to boil, cover, and reduce the heat to medium-low. Simmer for 30 minutes, stirring occasionally, or until the vegetables are softened.

Stir in the cooked lentils and cook for an additional 5 minutes until warmed through.

Taste and add additional salt, if needed. Serve warm.

Per Serving:
calories: 367 | fat: 15.0g | protein: 13.7g | carbs: 44.5g | fiber: 17.6g | sodium: 1108mg

Grilled Vegetable Skewers

Prep time: 15 minutes | Cook time: 10 minutes | Serves 4

Ingredients:
4 medium red onions, peeled and sliced into 6 wedges
4 medium zucchini, cut into 1-inch-thick slices
2 beefsteak tomatoes, cut into quarters
4 red bell peppers, cut into 2-inch squares
2 orange bell peppers, cut into 2-inch squares
2 yellow bell peppers, cut into 2-inch squares 2 tablespoons plus 1 teaspoon olive oil, divided
Special Equipment:
4 wooden skewers, soaked in water for at least 30 minutes

Directions:
Preheat the grill to medium-high heat.
Skewer the vegetables by alternating between red onion, zucchini, tomatoes, and the different colored bell peppers. Brush them with 2 tablespoons of olive oil.
Oil the grill grates with 1 teaspoon of olive oil and grill the vegetable skewers for 5 minutes. Flip the skewers and grill for 5 minutes more, or until they are cooked to your liking.
Let the skewers cool for 5 minutes before serving.

Per Serving:
calories: 115 | fat: 3.0g | protein: 3.5g | carbs: 18.7g | fiber: 4.7g | sodium: 12mg

Butternut Noodles with Mushrooms

Prep time: 10 minutes | Cook time: 12 minutes | Serves 4

Ingredients:
¼ cup extra-virgin olive oil
1 pound (454 g) cremini mushrooms, sliced
½ red onion, finely chopped
1 teaspoon dried thyme
½ teaspoon sea salt
garlic cloves, minced
½ cup dry white wine
Pinch of red pepper flakes
cups butternut noodles
4 ounces (113 g) grated Parmesan cheese

Directions:
In a large skillet over medium-high heat, heat the olive oil until shimmering. Add the mushrooms, onion, thyme, and salt to the skillet. Cook for about 6 minutes, stirring occasionally, or until the mushrooms start to brown. Add the garlic and sauté for 30 seconds. Stir in the white wine and red pepper flakes.
Fold in the noodles. Cook for about 5 minutes, stirring occasionally, or until the noodles are tender.
Serve topped with the grated Parmesan.

Per Serving:
calories: 244 | fat: 14.0g | protein: 4.0g | carbs: 22.0g | fiber: 4.0g | sodium: 159mg

Potato Tortilla with Leeks and Mushrooms

Prep time: 30 minutes | Cook time: 50 minutes | Serves 2

Ingredients:
1 tablespoon olive oil
1 cup thinly sliced leeks
4 ounces (113 g) baby bella (cremini) mushrooms, stemmed and sliced
1 small potato, peeled and sliced ¼-inch thick
½ cup unsweetened almond milk
5 large eggs, beaten
1 teaspoon Dijon mustard
½ teaspoon salt
½ teaspoon dried thyme
Pinch freshly ground black pepper
3 ounces (85 g) Gruyère cheese, shredded

Directions:
Preheat the oven to 350°F (180°C).
In a large sauté pan over medium-high heat, heat the olive oil. Add the leeks, mushrooms, and potato and sauté for about 10 minutes, or until the potato starts to brown. Reduce the heat to medium-low, cover, and cook for an additional 10 minutes, or until the potato begins to soften. Add 1 to 2 tablespoons of water to prevent sticking to the bottom of the pan, if needed. Meanwhile, whisk together the milk, beaten eggs, mustard, salt, thyme, black pepper, and cheese in a medium bowl until combined. When the potatoes are fork-tender, turn off the heat. Transfer the cooked vegetables to an oiled nonstick ovenproof pan and arrange them in a nice layer along the bottom and slightly up the sides of the pan. Pour the milk mixture evenly over the vegetables.
Bake in the preheated oven for 25 to 30 minutes, or until the eggs are completely set and the top is golden and puffed. Remove from the oven and cool for 5 minutes before cutting and serving.
Per Serving: calories: 541 | fat: 33.1g | protein: 32.8g | carbs: 31.0g | fiber: 4.0g | sodium: 912mg

Ratatouille

Prep time: 10 minutes | Cook time: 6 minutes | Serves 4

Ingredients:
2 large zucchinis, sliced
2 medium eggplants, sliced
4 medium tomatoes, sliced
2 small red onions, sliced
4 cloves garlic, chopped
2 tablespoons thyme leaves
2 teaspoons sea salt
teaspoon black pepper
tablespoons balsamic vinegar
4 tablespoons olive oil
2 cups water

Directions:
Line a springform pan with foil and place the chopped garlic in the bottom.
Now arrange the vegetable slices, alternately, in circles.
Sprinkle the thyme, pepper and salt over the vegetables. Top with oil and vinegar.
Pour a cup of water into the instant pot and place the trivet inside.
Secure the lid and cook on Manual function for 6 minutes at High Pressure.
Release the pressure naturally and remove the lid.
Remove the vegetables along with the tin foil.
Serve on a platter and enjoy.

Per Serving:
calories: 240 | fat: 14.3g | protein: 4.7g | carbs: 27.5g | fiber: 10.8g | sodium: 1181mg

Mushroom and Potato Teriyaki

Prep time: 10 minutes | Cook time: 18 minutes | Serves 4

Ingredients:
¾ large yellow or white onion, chopped
1½ medium carrots, diced
1½ ribs celery, chopped
medium portabella mushroom, diced
¾ tablespoon garlic, chopped
cups water
pound (454 g) white potatoes, peeled and diced
¼ cup tomato paste
½ tablespoon sesame oil
teaspoons sesame seeds
½ tablespoon paprika
1 teaspoon fresh rosemary
¾ cups peas
¼ cup fresh parsley for garnishing, chopped

Directions:
Add the oil, sesame seeds, and all the vegetables in the instant pot and Sauté for 5 minutes.
Stir in the remaining ingredients and secure the lid.
Cook on Manual function for 13 minutes at High Pressure.
After the beep, natural release the pressure and remove the lid.
Garnish with fresh parsley and serve hot.

Per Serving:
calories: 160 | fat: 3.0g | protein: 4.7g | carbs: 30.6g | fiber: 5.5g | sodium: 52mg

Wilted Dandelion Greens with Sweet Onion

Prep time: 15 minutes | Cook time: 15 minutes | Serves 4

Ingredients:
tablespoon extra-virgin olive oil
garlic cloves, minced
Vidalia onion, thinly sliced
½ cup low-sodium vegetable broth
bunches dandelion greens, roughly chopped
Freshly ground black pepper, to taste

Directions:
Heat the olive oil in a large skillet over low heat.
Add the garlic and onion and cook for 2 to 3 minutes, stirring
occasionally, or until the onion is translucent.
Fold in the vegetable broth and dandelion greens and cook for 5 to 7
minutes until wilted, stirring frequently.
Sprinkle with the black pepper and serve on a plate while warm.

Per Serving:
calories: 81 | fat: 3.9g | protein: 3.2g | carbs: 10.8g | fiber: 4.0g |
sodium: 72mg

Celery and Mustard Greens

Prep time: 10 minutes | Cook time: 15 minutes | Serves 4

Ingredients:
½ cup low-sodium vegetable broth
celery stalk, roughly chopped
½ sweet onion, chopped
½ large red bell pepper, thinly sliced
garlic cloves, minced
1 bunch mustard greens, roughly chopped

Directions:
Pour the vegetable broth into a large cast iron pan and bring it to a simmer over medium heat.

Stir in the celery, onion, bell pepper, and garlic. Cook uncovered for about 3 to 5 minutes, or until the onion is softened.

Add the mustard greens to the pan and stir well. Cover, reduce the heat to low, and cook for an additional 10 minutes, or until the liquid is evaporated and the greens are wilted.

Remove from the heat and serve warm.

Per Serving: (1 cup)
calories: 39 | fat: 0g | protein: 3.1g | carbs: 6.8g | fiber: 3.0g | sodium: 120mg

Saut é ed Green Beans with Tomatoes

Prep time: 10 minutes | Cook time: 20 minutes | Serves 4

Ingredients:

¼ cup extra-virgin olive oil

1 large onion, chopped

4 cloves garlic, finely chopped

1 pound (454 g) green beans, fresh or frozen, cut into 2-inch pieces

1½ teaspoons salt, divided

1 (15-ounce / 425-g) can diced tomatoes

½ teaspoon freshly ground black pepper

Directions:

Heat the olive oil in a large skillet over medium heat.

Add the onion and garlic and saut é for 1 minute until fragrant.

Stir in the green beans and saut é for 3 minutes. Sprinkle with ½ teaspoon of salt.

Add the tomatoes, remaining salt, and pepper and stir to mix well.

Cook for an additional 12 minutes, stirring occasionally, or until the green beans are crisp and tender.

Remove from the heat and serve warm.

Per Serving:

calories: 219 | fat: 13.9g | protein: 4.0g | carbs: 17.7g | fiber: 6.2g | sodium: 843mg

Baked Tomatoes and Chickpeas

Prep time: 15 minutes | Cook time: 40 to 45 minutes | Serves 4

Ingredients:
1 tablespoon extra-virgin olive oil
½ medium onion, chopped
3 garlic cloves, chopped
¼ teaspoon ground cumin
2 teaspoons smoked paprika
2 (15-ounce / 425-g) cans chickpeas, drained and rinsed
4 cups halved cherry tomatoes
½ cup plain Greek yogurt, for serving
1 cup crumbled feta cheese, for serving

Directions:
Preheat the oven to 425°F (220°C).
Heat the olive oil in an ovenproof skillet over medium heat.
Add the onion and garlic and saut é for about 5 minutes, stirring occasionally, or until tender and fragrant.
Add the paprika and cumin and cook for 2 minutes. Stir in the chickpeas and tomatoes and allow to simmer for 5 to 10 minutes.
Transfer the skillet to the preheated oven and roast for 25 to 30 minutes, or until the mixture bubbles and thickens.
Remove from the oven and serve topped with yogurt and crumbled feta cheese.

Per Serving:
calories: 411 | fat: 14.9g | protein: 20.2g | carbs: 50.7g | fiber: 13.3g | sodium: 443mg

Stir-Fried Eggplant

Prep time: 25 minutes | Cook time: 15 minutes | Serves 2

Ingredients:

1 cup water, plus more as needed
½ cup chopped red onion
1 tablespoon finely chopped garlic
1 tablespoon dried Italian herb seasoning
1 teaspoon ground cumin
1 small eggplant (about 8 ounces / 227 g), peeled and cut into ½-inch cubes
medium carrot, sliced
cups green beans, cut into 1-inch pieces
2 ribs celery, sliced
cup corn kernels
tablespoons almond butter
2 medium tomatoes, chopped

Directions:

Heat 1 tablespoon of water in a large soup pot over medium-high heat until it sputters. Cook the onion for 2 minutes, adding a little more water as needed. Add the garlic, Italian seasoning, cumin, and eggplant and stir-fry for 2 to 3 minutes, adding a little more water as needed. Add the carrot, green beans, celery, corn kernels, and ½ cup of water and stir well. Reduce the heat to medium, cover, and cook for 8 to 10 minutes, stirring occasionally, or until the vegetables are tender. Meanwhile, in a bowl, stir together the almond butter and ½ cup of water. Remove the vegetables from the heat and stir in the almond butter mixture and chopped tomatoes. Cool for a few minutes before serving.

Per Serving:

calories: 176 | fat: 5.5g | protein: 5.8g | carbs: 25.4g | fiber: 8.6g | sodium: 198mg

---

Honey-Glazed Baby Carrots

Prep time: 5 minutes | Cook time: 6 minutes | Serves 2

Ingredients:

⅔ cup water

1½ pounds (680 g) baby carrots

4 tablespoons almond butter

½ cup honey

1 teaspoon dried thyme 1½ teaspoons dried dill

Salt, to taste

Directions:

Pour the water into the Instant Pot and add a steamer basket. Place the baby carrots in the basket.

Secure the lid. Select the Manual mode and set the cooking time for 4 minutes at High Pressure.

Once cooking is complete, do a quick pressure release. Carefully open the lid.

Transfer the carrots to a plate and set aside.

Pour the water out of the Instant Pot and dry it.

Press the Sauté button on the Instant Pot and heat the almond butter. Stir in the honey, thyme, and dill.

Return the carrots to the Instant Pot and stir until well coated. Sauté for another 1 minute.

Taste and season with salt as needed. Serve warm.

Per Serving:

calories: 575 | fat: 23.5g | protein: 2.8g | carbs: 90.6g | fiber: 10.3g | sodium: 547mg

Sweet Pepper Stew

Prep time: 20 minutes | Cook time: 50 minutes | Serves 2

Ingredients:
2 tablespoons olive oil
2 sweet peppers, diced (about 2 cups)
½ large onion, minced
1 garlic clove, minced
1 tablespoon gluten-free Worcestershire sauce
1 teaspoon oregano
1 cup low-sodium tomato juice
1 cup low-sodium vegetable stock
¼ cup brown rice
¼ cup brown lentils
Salt, to taste

Directions:
In a Dutch oven, heat the olive oil over medium-high heat.
Sauté the sweet peppers and onion for 10 minutes, stirring occasionally, or until the onion begins to turn golden and the peppers are wilted.
Stir in the garlic, Worcestershire sauce, and oregano and cook for 30 seconds more. Add the tomato juice, vegetable stock, rice, and lentils to the Dutch oven and stir to mix well.
Bring the mixture to a boil and then reduce the heat to medium-low. Let it simmer covered for about 45 minutes, or until the rice is cooked through and the lentils are tender.
Sprinkle with salt and serve warm.

Per Serving:
calories: 378 | fat: 15.6g | protein: 11.4g | carbs: 52.8g | fiber: 7.0g | sodium: 391mg

Vegetable and Red Lentil Stew

Prep time: 10 minutes | Cook time: 35 minutes | Serves 6

Ingredients:
tablespoon extra-virgin olive oil
onions, peeled and finely diced
6½ cups water
2 zucchini, finely diced
4 celery stalks, finely diced
3 cups red lentils
1 teaspoon dried oregano
1 teaspoon salt, plus more as needed

Directions:
Heat the olive oil in a large pot over medium heat.
Add the onions and saut é for about 5 minutes, stirring constantly, or until the onions are softened.
Stir in the water, zucchini, celery, lentils, oregano, and salt and bring the mixture to a boil.
Reduce the heat to low and let simmer covered for 30 minutes, stirring occasionally, or until the lentils are tender.
Taste and adjust the seasoning as needed.

Per Serving:
calories: 387 | fat: 4.4g | protein: 24.0g | carbs: 63.7g | fiber: 11.7g | sodium: 418mg

Saut é ed Spinach and Leeks

Prep time: 5 minutes | Cook time: 8 minutes | Serves 2

Ingredients:
3 tablespoons olive oil
2 garlic cloves, crushed
2 leeks, chopped
2 red onions, chopped
9 ounces (255 g) fresh spinach
1 teaspoon kosher salt
½ cup crumbled goat cheese

Directions:
Coat the bottom of the Instant Pot with the olive oil.
Add the garlic, leek, and onions and stir-fry for about 5 minutes, on
Sauté mode.
Stir in the spinach. Sprinkle with the salt and sauté for an additional 3
minutes, stirring constantly.
Transfer to a plate and scatter with the goat cheese before serving.

Per Serving:
calories: 447 | fat: 31.2g | protein: 14.6g | carbs: 28.7g | fiber: 6.3g |
sodium: 937mg

Zucchini Patties

Prep time: 15 minutes | Cook time: 5 minutes | Serves 2

Ingredients:
2 medium zucchini, shredded
teaspoon salt, divided
eggs
2 tablespoons chickpea flour
1 tablespoon chopped fresh mint
scallion, chopped
tablespoons extra-virgin olive oil

Directions:
Put the shredded zucchini in a fine-mesh strainer and season with ½ teaspoon of salt. Set aside.
Beat together the eggs, chickpea flour, mint, scallion, and remaining ½ teaspoon of salt in a medium bowl.
Squeeze the zucchini to drain as much liquid as possible. Add the zucchini to the egg mixture and stir until well incorporated.
Heat the olive oil in a large skillet over medium-high heat.
Drop the zucchini mixture by spoonfuls into the skillet. Gently flatten the zucchini with the back of a spatula.
Cook for 2 to 3 minutes or until golden brown. Flip and cook for an additional 2 minutes.
Remove from the heat and serve on a plate.

Per Serving:
calories: 264 | fat: 20.0g | protein: 9.8g | carbs: 16.1g | fiber: 4.0g | sodium: 1780mg

Creamy Potato Curry

Prep time: 10 minutes | Cook time: 18 minutes | Serves 4

Ingredients:

¾ large yellow or white onion, chopped

1½ ribs celery, chopped

¼ cup carrots, diced

¼ cup green onions

½ cup coconut milk

¾ tablespoon garlic, chopped

1½ cups water

pound (454 g) white potatoes, peeled and diced

¼ cup heavy cream

¼ teaspoon thyme

¼ teaspoon rosemary

½ tablespoon black pepper

¾ cup peas

Salt, to taste

tablespoons fresh cilantro for garnishing, chopped

Directions:

Add the oil and all the vegetables in the instant pot and Sauté for 5 minutes.

Stir in the remaining ingredients and secure the lid.

Cook on Manual function for 13 minutes at High Pressure.

Once it beeps, natural release the pressure and remove the lid.

Garnish with fresh cilantro and serve hot.

Per Serving:

calories: 210 | fat: 10.1g | protein: 4.1g | carbs: 27.6g | fiber: 4.7g | sodium: 74mg

Mushroom and Spinach Stuffed Peppers

Prep time: 15 minutes | Cook time: 8 minutes | Serves 7

Ingredients:

7 mini sweet peppers
1 cup button mushrooms, minced
5 ounces (142 g) organic baby spinach
½ teaspoon fresh garlic
½ teaspoon coarse sea salt
¼ teaspoon cracked mixed pepper
2 tablespoons water
1 tablespoon olive oil
Organic Mozzarella cheese, diced

Directions:

Put the sweet peppers and water in the instant pot and Sauté for 2 minutes.

Remove the peppers and put the olive oil into the pot.

Stir in the mushrooms, garlic, spices and spinach.

Cook on Sauté until the mixture is dry.

Stuff each sweet pepper with the cheese and spinach mixture.

Bake the stuffed peppers in an oven for 6 minutes at 400°F (205°C).

Once done, serve hot.

Per Serving: calories: 81 | fat: 2.4g | protein: 4.1g | carbs: 13.2g | fiber: 2.4g | sodium: 217mg

Carrot and Turnip Purée

Prep time: 10 minutes | Cook time: 10 minutes | Serves 6

Ingredients:
tablespoons olive oil, divided
large turnips, peeled and quartered
large carrots, peeled and cut into 2-inch pieces
2 cups vegetable broth
teaspoon salt
½ teaspoon ground nutmeg
tablespoons sour cream

Directions:
Press the Sauté button on Instant Pot. Heat 1 tablespoon olive oil.
Toss turnips and carrots in oil for 1 minute. Add broth. Lock lid.
Press the Manual button and adjust time to 8 minutes. When timer
beeps, quick release pressure until float valve drops and then unlock
lid.
Drain vegetables and reserve liquid; set liquid aside. Add 2 tablespoons
of reserved liquid plus remaining ingredients to vegetables in the
Instant Pot. Use an immersion blender to blend until desired
smoothness. If too thick, add more liquid 1 tablespoon at a time. Serve
warm.

Per Serving:
calories: 95 | fat: 5.2g | protein: 1.4g | carbs: 11.8g | fiber: 3.0g |
sodium: 669mg

Potato and Kale Bowls

Prep time: 10 minutes | Cook time: 10 minutes | Serves 4

Ingredients:

1 tablespoon olive oil
1 small onion, peeled and diced
stalk celery, diced
cloves garlic, minced
4 medium potatoes, peeled and diced
2 bunches kale, washed, deveined, and chopped
1½ cups vegetable broth
2 teaspoons salt
½ teaspoon ground black pepper ¼ teaspoon caraway seeds
1 tablespoon apple cider vinegar
4 tablespoons sour cream

Directions:

Press the Sauté button on Instant Pot. Heat oil. Add onion and celery and stir-fry for 3 to 5 minutes until onions are translucent. Add garlic and cook for an additional minute. Add potatoes in an even layer. Add chopped kale in an even layer. Add broth. Lock lid.
Press the Manual button and adjust time to 5 minutes. Let the pressure release naturally for 10 minutes. Quick release any additional pressure until float valve drops and then unlock lid; then drain broth.
Stir in salt, pepper, caraway seeds, and vinegar; slightly mash the potatoes in the Instant Pot. Garnish each serving with 1 tablespoon sour cream.

Per Serving:

calories: 259 | fat: 5.5g | protein: 7.9g | carbs: 47.6g | fiber: 7.6g | sodium: 1422mg

Eggplant and Millet Pilaf

Prep time: 5 minutes | Cook time: 17 minutes | Serves 4

Ingredients:
1 tablespoon olive oil
¼ cup peeled and diced onion
1 cup peeled and diced eggplant
1 small Roma tomato, seeded and diced
cup millet
cups vegetable broth
1 teaspoon sea salt
¼ teaspoon ground black pepper
⅛ teaspoon saffron
⅛ teaspoon cayenne pepper
1 tablespoon chopped fresh chives

Directions:
Press Sauté button on Instant Pot. Add the olive oil. Add onion and cook for 3 to 5 minutes until translucent. Toss in eggplant and stir-fry for 2 more minutes. Add diced tomato.
Add millet to Instant Pot in an even layer. Gently pour in broth. Lock lid.
Press the Rice button (the Instant Pot will determine the time, about 10 minutes pressurized cooking time). When timer beeps, let pressure release naturally for 5 minutes. Quick release any additional pressure until float valve drops and then unlock lid.
Transfer pot ingredients to a serving bowl. Season with salt, pepper, saffron, and cayenne pepper. Garnish with chives.

Per Serving:
calories: 238 | fat: 5.6g | protein: 6.0g | carbs: 40.8g | fiber: 5.3g | sodium: 861mg

Poultry and Meats

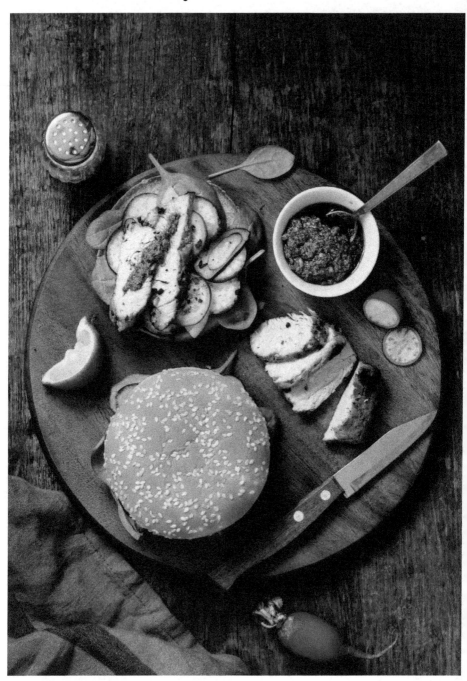

Ground Beef, Tomato, and Kidney Bean Chili

Prep time: 10 minutes | Cook time: 15 minutes | Serves 4

Ingredients:
1 tablespoon extra-virgin olive oil
1 pound (454 g) extra-lean ground beef
onion, chopped
(14-ounce / 397-g) cans kidney beans
2 (28-ounce / 794-g) cans chopped tomatoes, juice reserved Chili

Spice:
1 teaspoon garlic powder
1 tablespoon chili powder
½ teaspoon sea salt

Directions:
Heat the olive oil in a pot over medium-high heat until shimmering.
Add the beef and onion to the pot and sauté for 5 minutes or until the
beef is lightly browned and the onion is translucent.
Add the remaining ingredients. Bring to a boil. Reduce the heat to
medium and cook for 10 more minutes. Keep stirring during the
cooking.
Pour them in a large serving bowl and serve immediately.

Per Serving:
calories: 891 | fat: 20.1g | protein: 116.3g | carbs: 62.9g | fiber: 17.0g
| sodium: 561mg

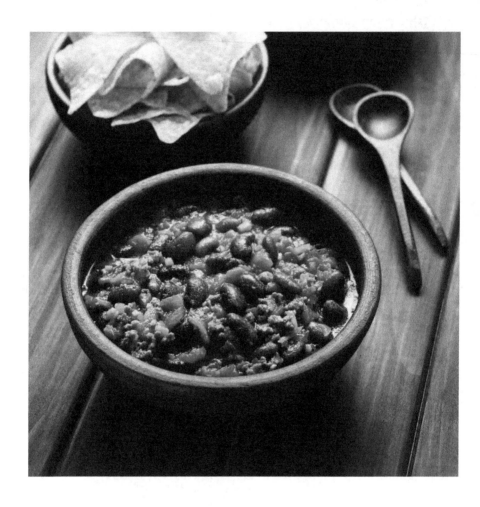

Lamb Tagine with Couscous and Almonds

Prep time: 15 minutes | Cook time: 7 hours 7 minutes | Serves 6

Ingredients:
2 tablespoons almond flour
Juice and zest of 1 navel orange
2 tablespoons extra-virgin olive oil
2 pounds (907 g) boneless lamb leg, fat trimmed and cut into 1½-inch cubes
½ cup low-sodium chicken stock
2 large white onions, chopped
1 teaspoon pumpkin pie spice
¼ teaspoon crushed saffron threads
teaspoon ground cumin
¼ teaspoon ground red pepper flakes
½ teaspoon sea salt
tablespoons raw honey
1 cup pitted dates
3 cups cooked couscous, for serving
2 tablespoons toasted slivered almonds, for serving

Directions:

Combine the almond flour with orange juice in a large bowl. Stir until smooth, then mix in the orange zest. Set aside.

Heat the olive oil in a nonstick skillet over medium-high heat until shimmering. Add the lamb cubes and sauté for 7 minutes or until lightly browned.

Pour in the flour mixture and chicken stock, then add the onions, pumpkin pie spice, saffron, cumin, ground red pepper flakes, and salt. Stir to mix well.

Pour them in the slow cooker.

Cover and cook on low for 6 hours or until the internal temperature of the lamb reaches at least 145°F (63°C).

When the cooking is complete, mix in the honey and dates, then cook for another an hour.

Put the couscous in a tagine bowl or a large bowl, then top with lamb mixture. Scatter with slivered almonds and serve immediately.

Per Serving:

calories: 447 | fat: 10.2g | protein: 36.3g | carbs: 53.5g | fiber: 4.9g | sodium: 329mg

Beef Kebabs with Onion and Pepper

Prep time: 15 minutes | Cook time: 10 minutes | Serves 6

Ingredients:
2 pounds (907 g) beef fillet
1½ teaspoons salt
1 teaspoon freshly ground black pepper
½ teaspoon ground nutmeg
½ teaspoon ground allspice
⅓ cup extra-virgin olive oil
1 large onion, cut into 8 quarters
1 large red bell pepper, cut into 1-inch cubes

Directions:
Preheat the grill to high heat.
Cut the beef into 1-inch cubes and put them in a large bowl.
In a small bowl, mix together the salt, black pepper, allspice, and nutmeg.
Pour the olive oil over the beef and toss to coat. Evenly sprinkle the seasoning over the beef and toss to coat all pieces.
Skewer the beef, alternating every 1 or 2 pieces with a piece of onion or bell pepper.
To cook, place the skewers on the preheated grill, and flip every 2 to 3 minutes until all sides have cooked to desired doneness, 6 minutes for medium-rare, 8 minutes for well done. Serve hot.

Per Serving:
calories: 485 | fat: 36.0g | protein: 35.0g | carbs: 4.0g | fiber: 1.0g | sodium: 1453mg

Grilled Pork Chops

Prep time: 20 minutes | Cook time: 10 minutes | Serves 4

Ingredients:
¼ cup extra-virgin olive oil
2 tablespoons fresh thyme leaves
1 teaspoon smoked paprika
1 teaspoon salt
4 pork loin chops, ½-inch-thick

Directions:
In a small bowl, mix together the olive oil, thyme, paprika, and salt.
Put the pork chops in a plastic zip-top bag or a bowl and coat them with the spice mix. Let them marinate for 15 minutes.
Preheat the grill to high heat. Cook the pork chops for 4 minutes on each side until cooked through.
Serve warm.

Per Serving:
calories: 282 | fat: 23.0g | protein: 21.0g | carbs: 1.0g | fiber: 0g | sodium: 832mg

Baked Teriyaki Turkey Meatballs

Prep time: 20 minutes | Cook time: 20 minutes | Serves 6

Ingredients:
1 pound (454 g) lean ground turkey
egg, whisked
¼ cup finely chopped scallions, both white and green parts
garlic cloves, minced
2 tablespoons reduced-sodium tamari or gluten-free soy sauce
1 teaspoon grated fresh ginger
tablespoon honey
teaspoons mirin
1 teaspoon olive oil

Directions:
Preheat the oven to 400°F (205°C). Line a baking sheet with parchment paper and set aside.

Mix together the ground turkey, whisked egg, scallions, garlic, tamari, ginger, honey, mirin, and olive oil in a large bowl, and stir until well blended.

Using a tablespoon to scoop out rounded heaps of the turkey mixture, and then roll them into balls with your hands. Transfer the balls to the prepared baking sheet.

Bake in the preheated oven for 20 minutes, flipping the balls with a spatula halfway through, or until the meatballs are browned and cooked through.

Serve warm.

Per Serving:
calories: 158 | fat: 8.6g | protein: 16.2g | carbs: 4.0g | fiber: 0.2g | sodium: 269mg

Beef, Tomato, and Lentils Stew

Prep time: 10 minutes | Cook time: 10 minutes | Serves 4

Ingredients:
1 tablespoon extra-virgin olive oil
1 pound (454 g) extra-lean ground beef
1 onion, chopped
1 (14-ounce / 397-g) can chopped tomatoes with garlic and basil, drained
1 (14-ounce / 397-g) can lentils, drained ½ teaspoon sea salt
⅛ teaspoon freshly ground black pepper

Directions:
Heat the olive oil in a pot over medium-high heat until shimmering.
Add the beef and onion to the pot and sauté for 5 minutes or until the beef is lightly browned.
Add the remaining ingredients. Bring to a boil. Reduce the heat to medium and cook for 4 more minutes or until the lentils are tender. Keep stirring during the cooking.
Pour them in a large serving bowl and serve immediately.

Per Serving:
calories: 460 | fat: 14.8g | protein: 44.2g | carbs: 36.9g | fiber: 17.0g | sodium: 320mg

Spiced Roast Chicken

Prep time: 10 minutes | Cook time: 35 minutes | Serves 6

Ingredients:
1 teaspoon garlic powder
1 teaspoon ground paprika
½ teaspoon ground cumin
½ teaspoon ground coriander
½ teaspoon salt
¼ teaspoon ground cayenne pepper
6 chicken legs
1 teaspoon extra-virgin olive oil

Directions:
Preheat the oven to 400°F (205°C).
Combine the garlic powder, paprika, cumin, coriander, salt, and cayenne pepper in a small bowl.
On a clean work surface, rub the spices all over the chicken legs until completely coated.
Heat the olive oil in an ovenproof skillet over medium heat.
Add the chicken thighs and sear each side for 8 to 10 minutes, or until the skin is crispy and browned.
Transfer the skillet to the preheated oven and continue cooking for 10 to 15 minutes, or until the juices run clear and it registers an internal temperature of 165°F (74°C).
Remove from the heat and serve on plates.

Per Serving:
calories: 275 | fat: 15.6g | protein: 30.3g | carbs: 0.9g | fiber: 0g | sodium: 255mg

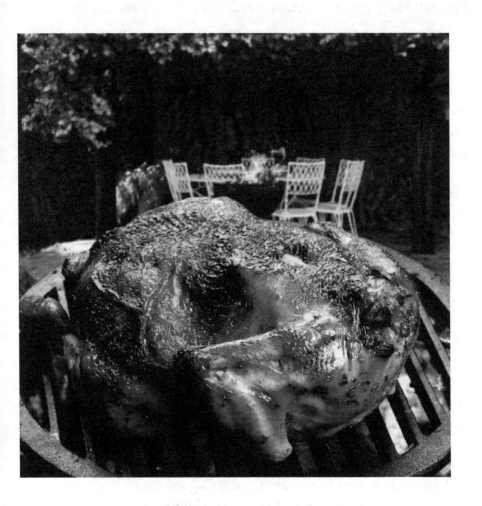

Yogurt Chicken Breasts

Prep time: 10 minutes | Cook time: 10 minutes | Serves 4

Ingredients:
1 pound (454 g) boneless, skinless chicken breasts, cut into 2-inch strips
tablespoon extra-virgin olive oil
Yogurt Sauce:
½ cup plain Greek yogurt
tablespoons water
Pinch saffron (3 or 4 threads)
garlic cloves, minced
½ onion, chopped
2 tablespoons chopped fresh cilantro
Juice of ½ lemon
½ teaspoon salt

Directions:
Make the yogurt sauce: Place the yogurt, water, saffron, garlic, onion, cilantro, lemon juice, and salt in a blender, and pulse until completely mixed.
Transfer the yogurt sauce to a large bowl, along with the chicken strips. Toss to coat well.
Cover with plastic wrap and marinate in the refrigerator for at least 1 hour, or up to overnight.
When ready to cook, heat the olive oil in a large skillet over medium heat.
Add the chicken strips to the skillet, discarding any excess marinade.
Cook each side for 5 minutes, or until cooked through.
Let the chicken cool for 5 minutes before serving.

Per Serving:
calories: 154 | fat: 4.8g | protein: 26.3g | carbs: 2.9g | fiber: 0g | sodium: 500mg

Greek-Style Lamb Burgers

Prep time: 10 minutes | Cook time: 10 minutes | Serves 4

Ingredients:
1 pound (454 g) ground lamb
½ teaspoon salt
½ teaspoon freshly ground black pepper
4 tablespoons crumbled feta cheese
Buns, toppings, and tzatziki, for serving (optional)

Directions:
Preheat the grill to high heat.
In a large bowl, using your hands, combine the lamb with the salt and pepper.
Divide the meat into 4 portions. Divide each portion in half to make a top and a bottom. Flatten each half into a 3-inch circle. Make a dent in the center of one of the halves and place 1 tablespoon of the feta cheese in the center. Place the second half of the patty on top of the feta cheese and press down to close the 2 halves together, making it resemble a round burger.
Grill each side for 3 minutes, for medium-well. Serve on a bun with your favorite toppings and tzatziki sauce, if desired.

Per Serving:
calories: 345 | fat: 29.0g | protein: 20.0g | carbs: 1.0g | fiber: 0g | sodium: 462mg

Chicken Bruschetta Burgers

Prep time: 10 minutes | Cook time: 16 minutes | Serves 2

Ingredients:
tablespoon olive oil
garlic cloves, minced
tablespoons finely minced onion
1 teaspoon dried basil
3 tablespoons minced sun-dried tomatoes packed in olive oil
8 ounces (227 g) ground chicken breast
¼ teaspoon salt
3 pieces small Mozzarella balls, minced

Directions:
Heat the olive oil in a nonstick skillet over medium-high heat. Add the garlic and onion and sauté for 5 minutes until tender. Stir in the basil. Remove from the skillet to a medium bowl.
Add the tomatoes, ground chicken, and salt and stir until incorporated. Mix in the Mozzarella balls.
Divide the chicken mixture in half and form into two burgers, each about ¾-inch thick.
Heat the same skillet over medium-high heat and add the burgers. Cook each side for 5 to 6 minutes, or until they reach an internal temperature of 165°F (74°C).
Serve warm.

Per Serving:
calories: 300 | fat: 17.0g | protein: 32.2g | carbs: 6.0g | fiber: 1.1g | sodium: 724mg

Herbed-Mustard-Coated Pork Tenderloin

Prep time: 10 minutes | Cook time: 15 minutes | Serves 4

Ingredients:
3 tablespoons fresh rosemary leaves
¼ cup Dijon mustard
½ cup fresh parsley leaves
6 garlic cloves
½ teaspoon sea salt
¼ teaspoon freshly ground black pepper
1 tablespoon extra-virgin olive oil
1 (1½-pound / 680-g) pork tenderloin

Directions:
Preheat the oven to 400°F (205°C).
Put all the ingredients, except for the pork tenderloin, in a food processor. Pulse until it has a thick consistency.
Put the pork tenderloin on a baking sheet, then rub with the mixture to coat well.
Put the sheet in the preheated oven and bake for 15 minutes or until the internal temperature of the pork reaches at least 165°F (74°C). Flip the tenderloin halfway through the cooking time.
Transfer the cooked pork tenderloin to a large plate and allow to cool for 5 minutes before serving.

Per Serving:
calories: 363 | fat: 18.1g | protein: 2.2g | carbs: 4.9g | fiber: 2.0g | sodium: 514mg

Grilled Lemon Chicken

Prep time: 10 minutes | Cook time: 12 to 14 minutes | Serves 2

Ingredients:

2 (4-ounce / 113-g) boneless, skinless chicken breasts Marinade:
4 tablespoons freshly squeezed lemon juice
2 tablespoons olive oil, plus more for greasing the grill grates
1 teaspoon dried basil
1 teaspoon paprika
½ teaspoon dried thyme
¼ teaspoon salt
¼ teaspoon garlic powder

Directions:

Make the marinade: Whisk together the lemon juice, olive oil, basil, paprika, thyme, salt, and garlic powder in a large bowl until well combined.
Add the chicken breasts to the bowl and let marinate for at least 30 minutes.
When ready to cook, preheat the grill to medium-high heat. Lightly grease the grill grates with the olive oil.
Discard the marinade and arrange the chicken breasts on the grill grates.
Grill for 12 to 14 minutes, flipping the chicken halfway through, or until a meat thermometer inserted in the center of the chicken reaches 165°F (74°C).
Let the chicken cool for 5 minutes and serve warm.

Per Serving:

calories: 251 | fat: 15.5g | protein: 27.3g | carbs: 1.9g | fiber: 1.0g | sodium: 371mg

Quick Chicken Salad Wraps

Prep time: 15 minutes | Cook time: 0 minutes | Serves 2

Ingredients:
Tzatziki Sauce:
½ cup plain Greek yogurt
1 tablespoon freshly squeezed lemon juice
Pinch garlic powder
teaspoon dried dill
Salt and freshly ground black pepper, to taste Salad Wraps:
(8-inch) whole-grain pita bread
cup shredded chicken meat
cups mixed greens
2 roasted red bell peppers, thinly sliced
½ English cucumber, peeled if desired and thinly sliced
¼ cup pitted black olives
1 scallion, chopped

Directions:
Make the tzatziki sauce: In a bowl, whisk together the yogurt, lemon juice, garlic powder, dill, salt, and pepper until creamy and smooth.
Make the salad wraps: Place the pita bread on a clean work surface and spoon ¼ cup of the tzatziki sauce onto each piece of pita bread, spreading it all over. Top with the shredded chicken, mixed greens, red pepper slices, cucumber slices, black olives, finished by chopped scallion.
Roll the salad wraps and enjoy.

Per Serving:
calories: 428 | fat: 10.6g | protein: 31.1g | carbs: 50.9g | fiber: 6.0g | sodium: 675mg

Potato Lamb and Olive Stew

**Prep time: 20 minutes | Cook time: 3 hours 42 minutes |
Serves 10**

Ingredients:
4 tablespoons almond flour
¾ cup low-sodium chicken stock
1¼ pounds (567 g) small potatoes, halved
cloves garlic, minced
large shallots, cut into ½-inch wedges
3 sprigs fresh rosemary
tablespoon lemon zest
Coarse sea salt and black pepper, to taste
3½ pounds (1.6 kg) lamb shanks, fat trimmed and cut crosswise into
1½inch pieces
tablespoons extra-virgin olive oil
½ cup dry white wine
cup pitted green olives, halved
tablespoons lemon juice

Directions:

Combine 1 tablespoon of almond flour with chicken stock in a bowl. Stir to mix well.

Put the flour mixture, potatoes, garlic, shallots, rosemary, and lemon zest in the slow cooker. Sprinkle with salt and black pepper. Stir to mix well. Set aside.

Combine the remaining almond flour with salt and black pepper in a large bowl, then dunk the lamb shanks in the flour and toss to coat.

Heat the olive oil in a nonstick skillet over medium-high heat until shimmering.

Add the well-coated lamb and cook for 10 minutes or until golden brown.

Flip the lamb pieces halfway through the cooking time. Transfer the cooked lamb to the slow cooker.

Pour the wine in the same skillet, then cook for 2 minutes or until it reduces in half. Pour the wine in the slow cooker.

Put the slow cooker lid on and cook on high for 3 hours and 30 minutes or until the lamb is very tender.

In the last 20 minutes of the cooking, open the lid and fold in the olive halves to cook.

Pour the stew on a large plate, let them sit for 5 minutes, then skim any fat remains over the face of the liquid.

Drizzle with lemon juice and sprinkle with salt and pepper. Serve warm.

Per Serving:

calories: 309 | fat: 10.3g | protein: 36.9g | carbs: 16.1g | fiber: 2.2g | sodium: 239mg

Grilled Chicken and Zucchini Kebabs

Prep time: 10 minutes | Cook time: 20 minutes | Serves 4

Ingredients:
¼ cup extra-virgin olive oil
2 tablespoons balsamic vinegar
1 teaspoon dried oregano, crushed between your fingers
pound (454 g) boneless, skinless chicken breasts, cut into 1½-inch pieces
medium zucchini, cut into 1-inch pieces
½ cup Kalamata olives, pitted and halved
2 tablespoons olive brine
¼ cup torn fresh basil leaves
Nonstick cooking spray Special Equipment:
14 to 15 (12-inch) wooden skewers, soaked for at least 30 minutes

Directions:
Spray the grill grates with nonstick cooking spray. Preheat the grill to medium-high heat.
In a small bowl, whisk together the olive oil, vinegar, and oregano. Divide the marinade between two large plastic zip-top bags.
Add the chicken to one bag and the zucchini to another. Seal and massage the marinade into both the chicken and zucchini.
Thread the chicken onto 6 wooden skewers. Thread the zucchini onto 8 or 9 wooden skewers.
Cook the kebabs in batches on the grill for 5 minutes, flip, and grill for 5 minutes more, or until any chicken juices run clear.
Remove the chicken and zucchini from the skewers to a large serving bowl. Toss with the olives, olive brine, and basil and serve.

Per Serving:
calories: 283 | fat: 15.0g | protein: 11.0g | carbs: 26.0g | fiber: 3.0g | sodium: 575mg

Almond-Crusted Chicken Tenders with Honey

Prep time: 10 minutes | Cook time: 20 minutes | Serves 4

Ingredients:
1 tablespoon honey
1 tablespoon whole-grain or Dijon mustard
¼ teaspoon freshly ground black pepper
¼ teaspoon kosher or sea salt
1 pound (454 g) boneless, skinless chicken breast tenders or tenderloins
1 cup almonds, roughly chopped
Nonstick cooking spray

Directions:
Preheat the oven to 425°F (220°C). Line a large, rimmed baking sheet with parchment paper. Place a wire cooling rack on the parchment-lined baking sheet, and spray the rack well with nonstick cooking spray. In a large bowl, combine the honey, mustard, pepper, and salt. Add the chicken and toss gently to coat. Set aside.

Dump the almonds onto a large sheet of parchment paper and spread them out. Press the coated chicken tenders into the nuts until evenly coated on all sides. Place the chicken on the prepared wire rack.

Bake in the preheated oven for 15 to 20 minutes, or until the internal temperature of the chicken measures 165°F (74°C) on a meat thermometer and any juices run clear.

Cool for 5 minutes before serving.

Per Serving:
calories: 222 | fat: 7.0g | protein: 11.0g | carbs: 29.0g | fiber: 2.0g | sodium: 448mg

Roasted Chicken Thighs With Basmati Rice

Prep time: 15 minutes | Cook time: 50 to 55 minutes | Serves 2

Chicken:

½ teaspoon cumin

½ teaspoon cinnamon

½ teaspoon paprika

¼ teaspoon ginger powder

¼ teaspoon garlic powder

¼ teaspoon coriander

¼ teaspoon salt

⅛ teaspoon cayenne pepper

10 ounces (284 g) boneless, skinless chicken thighs (about 4 pieces)

Rice:

tablespoon olive oil

½ small onion, minced

½ cup basmati rice

pinches saffron

1 cup low-sodium chicken stock

¼ teaspoon salt

Directions:

Preheat the oven to 350°F (180°C).

Combine the cumin, cinnamon, paprika, ginger powder, garlic powder, coriander, salt, and cayenne pepper in a small bowl.

Using your hands to rub the spice mixture all over the chicken thighs.

Transfer the chicken thighs to a baking dish. Roast in the preheated oven for 35 to 40 minutes, or until the internal temperature reaches 165°F (74°C) on a meat thermometer.

Make the Rice

Meanwhile, heat the olive oil in a skillet over medium-high heat.

Sauté the onion for 5 minutes until fragrant, stirring occasionally.

Stir in the basmati rice, saffron, chicken stock, and salt. Reduce the heat to low, cover, and bring to a simmer for 15 minutes, until light and fluffy.

Remove the chicken from the oven to a plate and serve with the rice.

Per Serving:

calories: 400 | fat: 9.6g | protein: 37.2g | carbs: 40.7g | fiber: 2.1g | sodium: 714mg

Macadamia Pork

Prep time: 10 minutes | Cook time: 10 minutes | Serves 4

Ingredients:
1 (1-pound / 454-g) pork tenderloin, cut into ½-inch slices and pounded thin
1 teaspoon sea salt, divided
¼ teaspoon freshly ground black pepper, divided
½ cup macadamia nuts
1 cup unsweetened coconut milk
1 tablespoon extra-virgin olive oil

Directions:
Preheat the oven to 400°F (205°C).
On a clean work surface, rub the pork with ½ teaspoon of the salt and ⅛ teaspoon of the ground black pepper. Set aside.
Ground the macadamia nuts in a food processor, then combine with remaining salt and black pepper in a bowl. Stir to mix well and set aside.
Combine the coconut milk and olive oil in a separate bowl. Stir to mix well.
Dredge the pork chops into the bowl of coconut milk mixture, then dunk into the bowl of macadamia nut mixture to coat well. Shake the excess off.
Put the well-coated pork chops on a baking sheet, then bake for 10 minutes or until the internal temperature of the pork reaches at least 165°F (74°C).
Transfer the pork chops to a serving plate and serve immediately.

Per Serving:
calories: 436 | fat: 32.8g | protein: 33.1g | carbs: 5.9g | fiber: 3.0g | sodium: 310mg

Panko Grilled Chicken Patties

Prep time: 10 minutes | Cook time: 8 to 10 minutes | Serves 4

Ingredients:
1 pound (454 g) ground chicken
3 tablespoons crumbled feta cheese
3 tablespoons finely chopped red pepper
¼ cup finely chopped red onion
3 tablespoons panko bread crumbs
1 garlic clove, minced
1 teaspoon chopped fresh oregano
¼ teaspoon salt
⅛ teaspoon freshly ground black pepper
Cooking spray

Directions:
Mix together the ground chicken, feta cheese, red pepper, red onion, bread crumbs, garlic, oregano, salt, and black pepper in a large bowl, and stir to incorporate.

Divide the chicken mixture into 8 equal portions and form each portion into a patty with your hands.

Preheat a grill to medium-high heat and oil the grill grates with cooking spray.

Arrange the patties on the grill grates and grill each side for 4 to 5 minutes, or until the patties are cooked through.

Rest for 5 minutes before serving.

Per Serving:
calories: 241 | fat: 13.5g | protein: 23.2g | carbs:6.7g | fiber: 1.1g | sodium: 321mg

Chicken Gyros with Tzatziki Sauce

Prep time: 15 minutes | Cook time: 10 minutes | Serves 2

Ingredients:

2 tablespoons freshly squeezed lemon juice

2 tablespoons olive oil, divided, plus more for oiling the grill

1 teaspoon minced fresh oregano

½ teaspoon garlic powder

Salt, to taste

8 ounces (227 g) chicken tenders

1 small eggplant, cut into 1-inch strips lengthwise

1 small zucchini, cut into ½-inch strips lengthwise

½ red pepper, seeded and cut in half lengthwise

½ English cucumber, peeled and minced

¾ cup plain Greek yogurt

tablespoon minced fresh dill

(8-inch) pita breads

Directions:

Combine the lemon juice, 1 tablespoon of olive oil, oregano, garlic powder, and salt in a medium bowl. Add the chicken and let marinate for 30 minutes.

Place the eggplant, zucchini, and red pepper in a large mixing bowl and sprinkle with salt and the remaining 1 tablespoon of olive oil. Toss well to coat. Let the vegetables rest while the chicken is marinating.

Make the tzatziki sauce: Combine the cucumber, yogurt, salt, and dill in a medium bowl. Stir well to incorporate and set aside in the refrigerator.

When ready, preheat the grill to medium-high heat and oil the grill grates.

Drain any liquid from the vegetables and put them on the grill.

Remove the chicken tenders from the marinade and put them on the grill.

Grill the chicken and vegetables for 3 minutes per side, or until the chicken is no longer pink inside.

Remove the chicken and vegetables from the grill and set aside. On the grill, heat the pitas for about 30 seconds, flipping them frequently. Divide the chicken tenders and vegetables between the pitas and top each with ¼ cup of the prepared sauce. Roll the pitas up like a cone and serve.

Per Serving:

calories: 586 | fat: 21.9g | protein: 39.0g | carbs: 62.0g | fiber: 11.8g | sodium: 955mg

Crispy Pesto Chicken

Prep time: 15 minutes | Cook time: 50 minutes | Serves 2

Ingredients:

12 ounces (340 g) small red potatoes (3 or 4 potatoes), scrubbed and diced into 1-inch pieces 1 tablespoon olive oil

½ teaspoon garlic powder

¼ teaspoon salt

1 (8-ounce / 227-g) boneless, skinless chicken breast

3 tablespoons prepared pesto

Directions:

Preheat the oven to 425°F (220°C). Line a baking sheet with parchment paper.

Combine the potatoes, olive oil, garlic powder, and salt in a medium bowl. Toss well to coat.

Arrange the potatoes on the parchment paper and roast for 10 minutes. Flip the potatoes and roast for an additional 10 minutes.

Meanwhile, put the chicken in the same bowl and toss with the pesto, coating the chicken evenly.

Check the potatoes to make sure they are golden brown on the top and bottom. Toss them again and add the chicken breast to the pan.

Turn the heat down to 350°F (180°C) and roast the chicken and potatoes for 30 minutes. Check to make sure the chicken reaches an internal temperature of 165°F (74°C) and the potatoes are fork-tender. Let cool for 5 minutes before serving.

Per Serving:

calories: 378 | fat: 16.0g | protein: 29.8g | carbs: 30.1g | fiber: 4.0g | sodium: 425mg

Gyro Burgers with Tahini Sauce

Prep time: 15 minutes | Cook time: 10 minutes | Serves 4

Ingredients:
2 tablespoons extra-virgin olive oil
1 tablespoon dried oregano
1¼ teaspoons garlic powder, divided
1 teaspoon ground cumin
½ teaspoon freshly ground black pepper
¼ teaspoon kosher or sea salt
1 pound (454 g) beef flank steak, top round steak, or lamb leg steak, center cut, about 1 inch thick
medium green bell pepper, halved and seeded
tablespoons tahini or peanut butter
1 tablespoon hot water (optional)
½ cup plain Greek yogurt
1 tablespoon freshly squeezed lemon juice
1 cup thinly sliced red onion
4 (6-inch) whole-wheat pita breads, warmed
Nonstick cooking spray

Directions:

Set an oven rack about 4 inches below the broiler element. Preheat the oven broiler to high. Line a large, rimmed baking sheet with aluminum foil. Place a wire cooling rack on the foil, and spray the rack with nonstick cooking spray. Set aside.

In a small bowl, whisk together the olive oil, oregano, 1 teaspoon of garlic powder, cumin, pepper, and salt. Rub the oil mixture on all sides of the steak, reserving 1 teaspoon of the mixture. Place the steak on the prepared rack. Rub the remaining oil mixture on the bell pepper, and place on the rack, cut-side down. Press the pepper with the heel of your
hand to flatten.

Broil for 5 minutes. Flip the steak and the pepper pieces, and broil for 2 to 5 minutes more, until the pepper is charred and the internal temperature of the meat measures 145°F (63°C) on a meat thermometer. Put the pepper and steak on a cutting board to rest for 5 minutes.

Meanwhile, in a small bowl, whisk the tahini until smooth (adding 1 tablespoon of hot water if your tahini is sticky). Add the remaining ¼ teaspoon of garlic powder and the yogurt and lemon juice, and whisk thoroughly.

Slice the steak crosswise into ¼-inch-thick strips. Slice the bell pepper into strips. Divide the steak, bell pepper, and onion among the warm pita breads. Drizzle with tahini sauce and serve.

Per Serving:

calories: 348 | fat: 15.0g | protein: 33.0g | carbs: 20.0g | fiber: 3.0g | sodium: 530mg

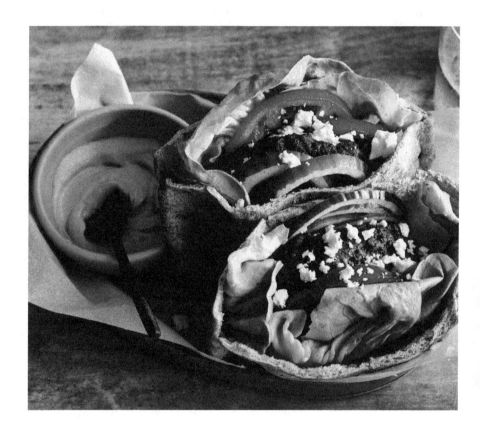

Coconut Chicken Tenders

Prep time: 10 minutes | Cook time: 15 to 20 minutes | Serves 6

Ingredients:
4 chicken breasts, each cut lengthwise into 3 strips
½ teaspoon salt
¼ teaspoon freshly ground black pepper
½ cup coconut flour
2 eggs
2 tablespoons unsweetened plain almond milk
1 cup unsweetened coconut flakes

Directions:
Preheat the oven to 400°F (205°C). Line a baking sheet with parchment paper.
On a clean work surface, season the chicken with salt and pepper.
In a small bowl, add the coconut flour. In a separate bowl, whisk the eggs with almond milk until smooth. Place the coconut flakes on a plate.
One at a time, roll the chicken strips in the coconut flour, then dredge them in the egg mixture, shaking off any excess, and finally in the coconut flakes to coat.
Arrange the coated chicken pieces on the baking skeet. Bake in the preheated oven for 15 to 20 minutes, flipping the chicken halfway through, or until the chicken is golden brown and cooked through. Remove from the oven and serve on plates.

Per Serving:
calories: 215 | fat: 12.6g | protein: 20.2g | carbs: 8.9g | fiber: 6.1g | sodium: 345mg

Sautéed Ground Turkey with Brown Rice

Prep time: 20 minutes | Cook time: 45 minutes | Serves 2

Ingredients:
tablespoon olive oil
½ medium onion, minced
garlic cloves, minced
8 ounces (227 g) ground turkey breast
½ cup chopped roasted red peppers, (about 2 jarred peppers)
¼ cup sun-dried tomatoes, minced
1¼ cups low-sodium chicken stock
½ cup brown rice
teaspoon dried oregano
Salt, to taste
cups lightly packed baby spinach

Directions:
In a skillet, heat the olive oil over medium heat. Sauté the onion for 5 minutes, stirring occasionally.
Stir in the garlic and sauté for 30 seconds more until fragrant.
Add the turkey breast and cook for about 7 minutes, breaking apart with a wooden spoon, until the turkey is no longer pink.
Stir in the roasted red peppers, tomatoes, chicken stock, brown rice, and oregano and bring to a boil.
When the mixture starts to boil, cover, and reduce the heat to mediumlow. Bring to a simmer until the rice is tender, stirring occasionally, about 30 minutes. Sprinkle with the salt.
Add the baby spinach and keep stirring until wilted.
Remove from the heat and serve warm.

Per Serving:
calories: 445 | fat: 16.8g | protein: 30.2g | carbs: 48.9g | fiber: 5.1g | sodium: 662

Chermoula Roasted Pork Tenderloin

Prep time: 15 minutes | Cook time: 20 minutes | Serves 2

Ingredients:
½ cup fresh cilantro
½ cup fresh parsley
6 small garlic cloves
3 tablespoons olive oil, divided
3 tablespoons freshly squeezed lemon juice
2 teaspoons cumin
1 teaspoon smoked paprika
½ teaspoon salt, divided
Pinch freshly ground black pepper
1 (8-ounce / 227-g) pork tenderloin

Directions:
Preheat the oven to 425°F (220°C).
In a food processor, combine the cilantro, parsley, garlic, 2 tablespoons of olive oil, lemon juice, cumin, paprika, and ¼ teaspoon of salt. Pulse 15 to 20 times, or until the mixture is fairly smooth. Scrape the sides down as needed to incorporate all the ingredients. Transfer the sauce to a small bowl and set aside.
Season the pork tenderloin on all sides with the remaining ¼ teaspoon of salt and a generous pinch of black pepper.
Heat the remaining 1 tablespoon of olive oil in a sauté pan.
Sear the pork for 3 minutes, turning often, until golden brown on all sides.
Transfer the pork to a baking dish and roast in the preheated oven for 15 minutes, or until the internal temperature registers 145°F (63°C).
Cool for 5 minutes before serving.

Per Serving:
calories: 169 | fat: 13.1g | protein: 11.0g | carbs: 2.9g | fiber: 1.0g | sodium: 332mg

Lamb Kofta (Spiced Meatballs)

Prep time: 15 minutes | Cook time: 30 minutes | Serves 2

Ingredients:
¼ cup walnuts
1 garlic clove
½ small onion
roasted piquillo pepper
tablespoons fresh mint
2 tablespoons fresh parsley
¼ teaspoon cumin
¼ teaspoon allspice
¼ teaspoon salt
Pinch cayenne pepper
8 ounces (227 g) lean ground lamb

Directions:
Preheat the oven to 350°F (180°C). Line a baking sheet with aluminum foil.

In a food processor, combine the walnuts, garlic, onion, roasted pepper, mint, parsley, cumin, allspice, salt, and cayenne pepper. Pulse about 10 times to combine everything.

Transfer the spice mixture to a large bowl and add the ground lamb. With your hands or a spatula, mix the spices into the lamb.

Roll the lamb into 1½-inch balls (about the size of golf balls).

Arrange the meatballs on the prepared baking sheet and bake for 30 minutes, or until cooked to an internal temperature of 165°F (74°C). Serve warm.

Per Serving:
calories: 409 | fat: 22.9g | protein: 22.0g | carbs: 7.1g | fiber: 3.0g | sodium: 428mg

Chicken Cacciatore

Prep time: 15 minutes | Cook time: 1 hour and 30 minutes | Serves 2

Ingredients:
1½ pounds (680 g) bone-in chicken thighs, skin removed and patted dry
Salt, to taste
2 tablespoons olive oil
½ large onion, thinly sliced
4 ounces (113 g) baby bella mushrooms, sliced
1 red sweet pepper, cut into 1-inch pieces
1 (15-ounce / 425-g) can crushed fire-roasted tomatoes
1 fresh rosemary sprig
½ cup dry red wine
1 teaspoon Italian herb seasoning
½ teaspoon garlic powder
3 tablespoons flour

Directions:

Season the chicken thighs with a generous pinch of salt.

Heat the olive oil in a Dutch oven over medium-high heat. Add the chicken and brown for 5 minutes per side.

Add the onion, mushrooms, and sweet pepper to the Dutch oven and sauté for another 5 minutes.

Add the tomatoes, rosemary, wine, Italian seasoning, garlic powder, and salt, stirring well.

Bring the mixture to a boil, then reduce the heat to low. Allow to simmer slowly for at least 1 hour, stirring occasionally, or until the chicken is tender and easily pulls away from the bone.

Measure out 1 cup of the sauce from the pot and put it into a bowl. Add the flour and whisk well to make a slurry.

Increase the heat to medium-high and slowly whisk the slurry into the pot. Stir until it comes to a boil and cook until the sauce is thickened.

Remove the chicken from the bones and shred it, and add it back to the sauce before serving, if desired.

Per Serving:

calories: 520 | fat: 23.1g | protein: 31.8g | carbs: 37.0g | fiber: 6.0g | sodium: 484mg

Slow Cook Lamb Shanks with Cannellini Beans Stew

Prep time: 20 minutes | Cook time: 10 hours 15 minutes | Serves 12

Ingredients:

1 (19-ounce / 539-g) can cannellini beans, rinsed and drained

large yellow onion, chopped

medium-sized carrots, diced

large stalk celery, chopped

cloves garlic, thinly sliced

4 (1½-pound / 680-g) lamb shanks, fat trimmed

2 teaspoons tarragon

½ teaspoon sea salt

¼ teaspoon ground black pepper

1 (28-ounce / 794-g) can diced tomatoes, with the juice

Directions:

Combine the beans, onion, carrots, celery, and garlic in the slow cooker. Stir to mix well. Add the lamb shanks and sprinkle with tarragon, salt, and ground black pepper. Pour in the tomatoes with juice, then cover the lid and cook on high for an hour. Reduce the heat to low and cook for 9 hours or until the lamb is super tender. Transfer the lamb on a plate, then pour the bean mixture in a colander over a separate bowl to reserve the liquid. Let the liquid sit for 5 minutes until set, then skim the fat from the surface of the liquid. Pour the bean mixture back to the liquid. Remove the bones from the lamb heat and discard the bones. Put the lamb meat and bean mixture back to the slow cooker. Cover and cook to reheat for 15 minutes or until heated through. Pour them on a large serving plate and serve immediately.

Per Serving: calories: 317 | fat: 9.7g | protein: 52.1g | carbs: 7.0g | fiber: 2.1g | sodium: 375m

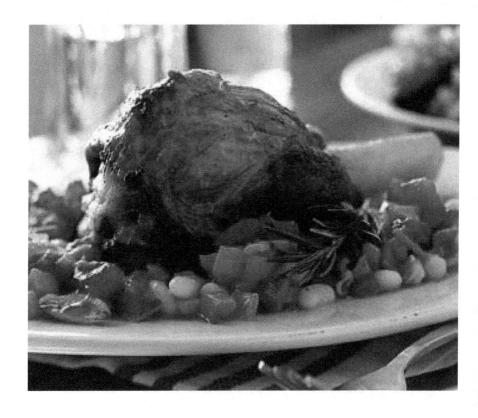

Parsley-Dijon Chicken and Potatoes

Prep time: 5 minutes | Cook time: 22 minutes | Serves 6

Ingredients:

tablespoon extra-virgin olive oil

1½ pounds (680 g) boneless, skinless chicken thighs, cut into 1-inch cubes, patted dry

1½ pounds (680 g) Yukon Gold potatoes, unpeeled, cut into ½-inch cubes

garlic cloves, minced

¼ cup dry white wine

1 cup low-sodium or no-salt-added chicken broth

1 tablespoon Dijon mustard

¼ teaspoon freshly ground black pepper

¼ teaspoon kosher or sea salt

1 cup chopped fresh flat-leaf (Italian) parsley, including stems

1 tablespoon freshly squeezed lemon juice

Directions:

In a large skillet over medium-high heat, heat the oil. Add the chicken and cook for 5 minutes, stirring only after the chicken has browned on one side. Remove the chicken and reserve on a plate.

Add the potatoes to the skillet and cook for 5 minutes, stirring only after the potatoes have become golden and crispy on one side. Push the potatoes to the side of the skillet, add the garlic, and cook, stirring constantly, for 1 minute. Add the wine and cook for 1 minute, until nearly evaporated. Add the chicken broth, mustard, salt, pepper, and reserved chicken. Turn the heat to high and bring to a boil.

Once boiling, cover, reduce the heat to medium-low, and cook for 10 to 12 minutes, until the potatoes are tender and the internal temperature of the chicken measures 165°F (74°C) on a meat thermometer and any juices run clear.

During the last minute of cooking, stir in the parsley. Remove from the heat, stir in the lemon juice, and serve.

Per Serving:

calories: 324 | fat: 9.0g | protein: 16.0g | carbs: 45.0g | fiber: 5.0g | sodium: 560mg

Beef Stew with Beans and Zucchini

Prep time: 20 minutes | Cook time: 6 to 8 hours | Serves 2

Ingredients:
1 (15-ounce / 425-g) can diced or crushed tomatoes with basil
teaspoon beef base
tablespoons olive oil, divided
8 ounces (227 g) baby bella (cremini) mushrooms, quartered
2 garlic cloves, minced
½ large onion, diced
1 pound (454 g) cubed beef stew meat
3 tablespoons flour
¼ teaspoon salt
Pinch freshly ground black pepper
¾ cup dry red wine
¼ cup minced brined olives
1 fresh rosemary sprig
1 (15-ounce / 425-g) can white cannellini beans, drained and rinsed
1 medium zucchini, cut in half lengthwise and then cut into 1-inch
pieces.

Directions:

Place the tomatoes into a slow cooker and set it to low heat. Add the beef base and stir to incorporate.

Heat 1 tablespoon of olive oil in a large sauté pan over medium heat. Add the mushrooms and onion and sauté for 10 minutes, stirring occasionally, or until they're golden.

Add the garlic and cook for 30 seconds more. Transfer the vegetables to the slow cooker.

In a plastic food storage bag, combine the stew meat with the flour, salt, and pepper. Seal the bag and shake well to combine.

Heat the remaining 1 tablespoon of olive oil in the sauté pan over high heat.

Add the floured meat and sear to get a crust on the outside edges. Deglaze the pan by adding about half of the red wine and scraping up any browned bits on the bottom. Stir so the wine thickens a bit and transfer to the slow cooker along with any remaining wine.

Stir the stew to incorporate the ingredients. Stir in the olives and rosemary, cover, and cook for 6 to 8 hours on Low.

About 30 minutes before the stew is finished, add the beans and zucchini to let them warm through. Serve warm.

Per Serving:

calories: 389 | fat: 15.1g | protein: 30.8g | carbs: 25.0g | fiber: 8.0g | sodium: 582mg

Greek Beef Kebabs

Prep time: 15 minutes | Cook time: 20 minutes | Serves 2

Ingredients:
6 ounces (170 g) beef sirloin tip, trimmed of fat and cut into 2-inch pieces
3 cups of any mixture of vegetables: mushrooms, summer squash, zucchini, onions, red peppers, cherry tomatoes
½ cup olive oil
¼ cup freshly squeezed lemon juice
2 tablespoons balsamic vinegar
2 teaspoons dried oregano
1 teaspoon garlic powder
1 teaspoon salt
1 teaspoon minced fresh rosemary
Cooking spray

Directions:
Put the beef in a plastic freezer bag.
Slice the vegetables into similar-size pieces and put them in a second freezer bag. Make the marinade: Mix the olive oil, lemon juice, balsamic vinegar, oregano, garlic powder, salt, and rosemary in a measuring cup. Whisk well to combine. Pour half of the marinade over the beef, and the other half over the vegetables. Put the beef and vegetables in the refrigerator to marinate for 4 hours. When ready, preheat the grill to medium-high heat and spray the grill grates with cooking spray. Thread the meat onto skewers and the vegetables onto separate skewers. Grill the meat for 3 minutes per side. They should only take 10 to 12 minutes to cook, depending on the thickness of the meat. Grill the vegetables for about 3 minutes per side, or until they have grill marks and are softened. Serve hot.

Per Serving: calories: 284 | fat: 18.2g | protein: 21.0g | carbs: 9.0g | fiber: 3.9g | sodium: 122mg

Fish and Seafood

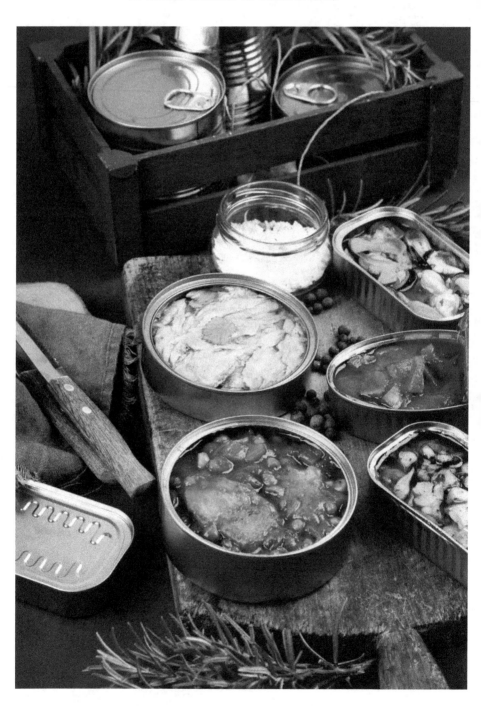

Glazed Broiled Salmon

Prep time: 5 minutes | Cook time: 5 to 10 minutes | Serves 4

Ingredients:
4 (4-ounce / 113-g) salmon fillets
3 tablespoons miso paste
2 tablespoons raw honey
1 teaspoon coconut aminos
1 teaspoon rice vinegar

Directions:
Preheat the broiler to High. Line a baking dish with aluminum foil and add the salmon fillets.
Whisk together the miso paste, honey, coconut aminos, and vinegar in a small bowl. Pour the glaze over the fillets and spread it evenly with a brush.
Broil for about 5 minutes, or until the salmon is browned on top and opaque. Brush any remaining glaze over the salmon and broil for an additional 5 minutes if needed. The cooking time depends on the thickness of the salmon.
Let the salmon cool for 5 minutes before serving.

Per Serving:
calories: 263 | fat: 8.9g | protein: 30.2g | carbs: 12.8g | fiber: 0.7g | sodium: 716mg

Baked Salmon with Basil and Tomato

Prep time: 10 minutes | Cook time: 20 minutes | Serves 2

Ingredients:
2 (6-ounce / 170-g) boneless salmon fillets
1 tablespoon dried basil
1 tomato, thinly sliced
tablespoon olive oil
tablespoons grated Parmesan cheese
Nonstick cooking spray

Directions:
Preheat the oven to 375°F (190°C). Line a baking sheet with a piece of aluminum foil and mist with nonstick cooking spray.
Arrange the salmon fillets onto the aluminum foil and scatter with basil. Place the tomato slices on top and drizzle with olive oil. Top with the grated Parmesan cheese.
Bake for about 20 minutes, or until the flesh is opaque and it flakes apart easily.
Remove from the oven and serve on a plate.

Per Serving:
calories: 403 | fat: 26.5g | protein: 36.3g | carbs: 3.8g | fiber: 0.1g | sodium: 179mg

Mediterranean Cod Stew

Prep time: 10 minutes | Cook time: 20 minutes | Serves 6

Ingredients:
2 tablespoons extra-virgin olive oil
2 cups chopped onion
2 garlic cloves, minced
¾ teaspoon smoked paprika
1 (14.5-ounce / 411-g) can diced tomatoes, undrained
1 (12-ounce / 340-g) jar roasted red peppers, drained and chopped
1 cup sliced olives, green or black
⅓ cup dry red wine
¼ teaspoon kosher or sea salt
¼ teaspoon freshly ground black pepper
1½ pounds (680 g) cod fillets, cut into 1-inch pieces
3 cups sliced mushrooms

Directions:
In a large stockpot over medium heat, heat the oil. Add the onion and cook for 4 minutes, stirring occasionally. Add the garlic and smoked paprika and cook for 1 minute, stirring often.
Mix in the tomatoes with their juices, roasted peppers, olives, wine, pepper, and salt, and turn the heat to medium-high. Bring the mixture to a boil. Add the cod fillets and mushrooms, and reduce the heat to medium.
Cover and cook for about 10 minutes, stirring a few times, until the cod is cooked through and flakes easily, and serve.

Per Serving:
calories: 167 | fat: 5.0g | protein: 19.0g | carbs: 11.0g | fiber: 5.0g | sodium: 846mg

Fennel Poached Cod with Tomatoes

Prep time: 10 minutes | Cook time: 20 minutes | Serves 4

Ingredients:
1 tablespoon olive oil
1 cup thinly sliced fennel
½ cup thinly sliced onion
1 tablespoon minced garlic
(15-ounce / 425-g) can diced tomatoes
cups chicken broth
½ cup white wine
Juice and zest of 1 orange
1 pinch red pepper flakes
1 bay leaf
1 pound (454 g) cod

Directions:
Heat the olive oil in a large skillet. Add the onion and fennel and cook
for 6 minutes, stirring occasionally, or until translucent. Add the garlic
and cook for 1 minute more.
Add the tomatoes, chicken broth, wine, orange juice and zest, red
pepper flakes, and bay leaf, and simmer for 5 minutes to meld the
flavors.
Carefully add the cod in a single layer, cover, and simmer for 6 to 7
minutes.
Transfer fish to a serving dish, ladle the remaining sauce over the fish,
and serve.

Per Serving:
calories: 336 | fat: 12.5g | protein: 45.1g | carbs:11.0g | fiber: 3.3g |
sodium: 982mg

Hazelnut Crusted Sea Bass

Prep time: 10 minutes | Cook time: 15 minutes | Serves 2

Ingredients:
2 tablespoons almond butter
2 sea bass fillets
⅓ cup roasted hazelnuts
A pinch of cayenne pepper

Directions:
Preheat the oven to 425°F (220°C). Line a baking dish with waxed paper.
Brush the almond butter over the fillets.
Pulse the hazelnuts and cayenne in a food processor. Coat the sea bass with the hazelnut mixture, then transfer to the baking dish.
Bake in the preheated oven for about 15 minutes. Cool for 5 minutes before serving.

Per Serving:
calories: 468 | fat: 30.8g | protein: 40.0g | carbs: 8.8g | fiber: 4.1g | sodium: 90mg

Mediterranean Braised Cod with Vegetables

Prep time: 10 minutes | Cook time: 18 minutes | Serves 2

Ingredients:
tablespoon olive oil
½ medium onion, minced
garlic cloves, minced
1 teaspoon oregano
1 (15-ounce / 425-g) can artichoke hearts in water, drained and halved
1 (15-ounce / 425-g) can diced tomatoes with basil
¼ cup pitted Greek olives, drained
10 ounces (284 g) wild cod
Salt and freshly ground black pepper, to taste

Directions:
In a skillet, heat the olive oil over medium-high heat.
Saut é the onion for about 5 minutes, stirring occasionally, or until tender.
Stir in the garlic and oregano and cook for 30 seconds more until fragrant.
Add the artichoke hearts, tomatoes, and olives and stir to combine. Top with the cod.
Cover and cook for 10 minutes, or until the fish flakes easily with a fork and juices run clean.
Sprinkle with the salt and pepper. Serve warm.

Per Serving:
calories: 332 | fat: 10.5g | protein: 29.2g | carbs: 30.7g | fiber: 8.0g | sodium: 1906mg

Lemon-Parsley Swordfish

Prep time: 10 minutes | Cook time: 17 to 20 minutes | Serves 4

Ingredients:
cup fresh Italian parsley
¼ cup lemon juice
¼ cup extra-virgin olive oil
¼ cup fresh thyme
cloves garlic
½ teaspoon salt
4 swordfish steaks
Olive oil spray

Directions:
Preheat the oven to 450°F (235°C). Grease a large baking dish generously with olive oil spray.
Place the parsley, lemon juice, olive oil, thyme, garlic, and salt in a food processor and pulse until smoothly blended.
Arrange the swordfish steaks in the greased baking dish and spoon the parsley mixture over the top.
Bake in the preheated oven for 17 to 20 minutes until flaky.
Divide the fish among four plates and serve hot.

Per Serving:
calories: 396 | fat: 21.7g | protein: 44.2g | carbs: 2.9g | fiber: 1.0g | sodium: 494mg

Spicy Grilled Shrimp with Lemon Wedges

Prep time: 15 minutes | Cook time: 6 minutes | Serves 6

Ingredients:
1 large clove garlic, crushed
1 teaspoon coarse salt
teaspoon paprika
½ teaspoon cayenne pepper
teaspoons lemon juice
2 tablespoons plus 1 teaspoon olive oil, divided
2 pounds (907 g) large shrimp, peeled and deveined
8 wedges lemon, for garnish

Directions:
Preheat the grill to medium heat.
Stir together the garlic, salt, paprika, cayenne pepper, lemon juice, and 2 tablespoons of olive oil in a small bowl until a paste forms. Add the shrimp and toss until well coated.
Grease the grill grates lightly with remaining 1 teaspoon of olive oil.
Grill the shrimp for 4 to 6 minutes, flipping the shrimp halfway through, or until the shrimp is totally pink and opaque.
Garnish the shrimp with lemon wedges and serve hot.

Per Serving:
calories: 163 | fat: 5.8g | protein: 25.2g | carbs: 2.8g | fiber: 0.4g | sodium: 585mg

Orange Flavored Scallops

Prep time: 10 minutes | Cook time: 10 minutes | Serves 4

Ingredients:
2 pounds (907 g) sea scallops, patted dry
Sea salt and freshly ground black pepper, to taste
2 tablespoons extra-virgin olive oil
1 tablespoon minced garlic
¼ cup freshly squeezed orange juice
teaspoon orange zest
teaspoons chopped fresh thyme, for garnish

Directions:
In a bowl, lightly season the scallops with salt and pepper. Set aside.
Heat the olive oil in a large skillet over medium-high heat until it shimmers.
Add the garlic and saut é for about 3 minutes, or until fragrant.
Stir in the seasoned scallops and sear each side for about 4 minutes, or until the scallops are browned.
Remove the scallops from the heat to a plate and set aside.
Add the orange juice and zest to the skillet, scraping up brown bits from bottom of skillet.
Drizzle the sauce over the scallops and garnish with the thyme before serving.

Per Serving:
calories: 266 | fat: 7.6g | protein: 38.1g | carbs: 7.9g | fiber: 0g | sodium: 360mg

Haddock with Cucumber Sauce

Prep time: 10 minutes | Cook time: 10 minutes | Serves 4

Ingredients:
¼ cup plain Greek yogurt
½ scallion, white and green parts, finely chopped
½ English cucumber, grated, liquid squeezed out
2 teaspoons chopped fresh mint
1 teaspoon honey
Sea salt and freshly ground black pepper, to taste
4 (5-ounce / 142-g) haddock fillets, patted dry
Nonstick cooking spray

Directions:
In a small bowl, stir together the yogurt, cucumber, scallion, mint, honey, and a pinch of salt. Set aside.
Season the fillets lightly with salt and pepper.
Place a large skillet over medium-high heat and spray lightly with cooking spray.
Cook the haddock, turning once, until it is just cooked through, about 5 minutes per side.
Remove the fish from the heat and transfer to plates.
Serve topped with the cucumber sauce.

Per Serving:
calories: 164 | fat: 2.0g | protein: 27.0g | carbs: 4.0g | fiber: 0g | sodium: 104mg

Cod with Parsley Pistou

Prep time: 15 minutes | Cook time: 10 minutes | Serves 4

Ingredients:
1 cup packed roughly chopped fresh flat-leaf Italian parsley
Zest and juice of 1 lemon
1 to 2 small garlic cloves, minced
1 teaspoon salt
½ teaspoon freshly ground black pepper
1 cup extra-virgin olive oil, divided
1 pound (454 g) cod fillets, cut into 4 equal-sized pieces

Directions:
Make the pistou: Place the parsley, lemon zest and juice, garlic, salt, and pepper in a food processor until finely chopped.
With the food processor running, slowly drizzle in ¾ cup of olive oil until a thick sauce forms. Set aside.
Heat the remaining ¼ cup of olive oil in a large skillet over medium-high heat.
Add the cod fillets, cover, and cook each side for 4 to 5 minutes, until browned and cooked through.
Remove the cod fillets from the heat to a plate and top each with generous spoonfuls of the prepared pistou. Serve immediately.

Per Serving:
calories: 580 | fat: 54.6g | protein: 21.1g | carbs: 2.8g | fiber: 1.0g | sodium: 651mg

Fried Cod Fillets

Prep time: 5 minutes | Cook time: 10 minutes | Serves 4

Ingredients:

½ cup all-purpose flour

1 teaspoon garlic powder

1 teaspoon salt

4 (4- to 5-ounce / 113- to 142-g) cod fillets

1 tablespoon extra-virgin olive oil

Directions:

Mix together the flour, garlic powder, and salt in a shallow dish.

Dredge each piece of fish in the seasoned flour until they are evenly coated.

Heat the olive oil in a medium skillet over medium-high heat.

Once hot, add the cod fillets and fry for 6 to 8 minutes, flipping the fish halfway through, or until the fish is opaque and flakes easily.

Remove from the heat and serve on plates.

Per Serving:

calories: 333 | fat: 18.8g | protein: 21.2g | carbs: 20.0g | fiber: 5.7g | sodium: 870mg

Canned Sardine Donburi (Rice Bowl)

Prep time: 10 minutes | Cook time: 40 to 50 minutes | Serves 4 to 6

Ingredients:
4 cups water
cups brown rice, rinsed well
½ teaspoon salt
(4-ounce / 113-g) cans sardines packed in water, drained
scallions, sliced thin
1-inch piece fresh ginger, grated
tablespoons sesame oil

Directions:
Place the water, brown rice, and salt to a large saucepan and stir to combine. Allow the mixture to boil over high heat.
Once boiling, reduce the heat to low, and cook covered for 45 to 50 minutes, or until the rice is tender.
Meanwhile, roughly mash the sardines with a fork in a medium bowl.
When the rice is done, stir in the mashed sardines, scallions, and ginger.
Divide the mixture into four bowls. Top each bowl with a drizzle of sesame oil. Serve warm.

Per Serving:
calories: 603 | fat: 23.6g | protein: 25.2g | carbs: 73.8g | fiber: 4.0g | sodium: 498mg

Baked Halibut Steaks with Vegetables

Prep time: 15 minutes | Cook time: 20 minutes | Serves 4

Ingredients:
2 teaspoon olive oil, divided
1 clove garlic, peeled and minced
½ cup minced onion
cup diced zucchini
cups diced fresh tomatoes
2 tablespoons chopped fresh basil
¼ teaspoon salt
¼ teaspoon ground black pepper
4 (6-ounce / 170-g) halibut steaks
⅓ cup crumbled feta cheese

Directions:
Preheat oven to 450°F (235°C). Coat a shallow baking dish lightly with 1 teaspoon of olive oil.

In a medium saucepan, heat the remaining 1 teaspoon of olive oil. Add the garlic, onion, and zucchini and mix well. Cook for 5 minutes, stirring occasionally, or until the zucchini is softened.

Remove the saucepan from the heat and stir in the tomatoes, basil, salt, and pepper.

Place the halibut steaks in the coated baking dish in a single layer. Spread the zucchini mixture evenly over the steaks. Scatter the top with feta cheese.

Bake in the preheated oven for about 15 minutes, or until the fish flakes when pressed lightly with a fork. Serve hot.

Per Serving:
calories: 258 | fat: 7.6g | protein: 38.6g | carbs: 6.5g | fiber: 1.2g | sodium: 384mg

Pesto Shrimp over Zoodles

Prep time: 15 minutes | Cook time: 10 minutes | Serves 4

Ingredients:
pound (454 g) fresh shrimp, peeled and deveined
Salt and freshly ground black pepper, to taste
tablespoons extra-virgin olive oil
½ small onion, slivered
8 ounces (227 g) store-bought jarred pesto
¾ cup crumbled goat or feta cheese, plus additional for serving
2 large zucchini, spiralized, for serving
¼ cup chopped flat-leaf Italian parsley, for garnish

Directions:
In a bowl, season the shrimp with salt and pepper. Set aside.
In a large skillet, heat the olive oil over medium-high heat. Sauté the onion until just golden, 5 to 6 minutes.
Reduce the heat to low and add the pesto and cheese, whisking to combine and melt the cheese. Bring to a low simmer and add the shrimp. Reduce the heat back to low and cover. Cook until the shrimp is cooked through and pink, about 3 to 4 minutes.
Serve the shrimp warm over zoodles, garnishing with chopped parsley and additional crumbled cheese.

Per Serving:
calories: 491 | fat: 35.0g | protein: 29.0g | carbs: 15.0g | fiber: 4.0g | sodium: 870mg

Salt and Pepper Calamari and Scallops

Prep time: 5 minutes | Cook time: 10 minutes | Serves 4

Ingredients:
8 ounces (227 g) calamari steaks, cut into ½-inch-thick rings
8 ounces (227 g) sea scallops
1½ teaspoons salt, divided
1 teaspoon garlic powder
teaspoon freshly ground black pepper
⅓ cup extra-virgin olive oil
tablespoons almond butter

Directions:
Place the calamari and scallops on several layers of paper towels and pat dry. Sprinkle with 1 teaspoon of salt and allow to sit for 15 minutes at room temperature. Pat dry with additional paper towels. Sprinkle with pepper and garlic powder.

In a deep medium skillet, heat the olive oil and butter over medium-high heat. When the oil is hot but not smoking, add the scallops and calamari in a single layer to the skillet and sprinkle with the remaining ½ teaspoon of salt. Cook for 2 to 4 minutes on each side, depending on the size of the scallops, until just golden but still slightly opaque in center.

Using a slotted spoon, remove from the skillet and transfer to a serving platter. Allow the cooking oil to cool slightly and drizzle over the seafood before serving.

Per Serving:
calories: 309 | fat: 25.0g | protein: 18.0g | carbs: 3.0g | fiber: 0g | sodium: 928mg

Baked Salmon with Tarragon Mustard Sauce

Prep time: 5 minutes | Cook time: 12 minutes | Serves 4

Ingredients:

1¼ pounds (567 g) salmon fillet (skin on or removed), cut into 4 equal pieces
¼ cup Dijon mustard
¼ cup avocado oil mayonnaise
Zest and juice of ½ lemon
2 tablespoons chopped fresh tarragon
½ teaspoon salt
¼ teaspoon freshly ground black pepper
4 tablespoons extra-virgin olive oil, for serving

Directions:

Preheat the oven to 425°F (220°C). Line a baking sheet with parchment paper.

Arrange the salmon pieces on the prepared baking sheet, skin-side down.

Stir together the mustard, avocado oil mayonnaise, lemon zest and juice, tarragon, salt, and pepper in a small bowl. Spoon the mustard mixture over the salmon.

Bake for 10 to 12 minutes, or until the top is golden and salmon is opaque in the center.

Divide the salmon among four plates and drizzle each top with 1 tablespoon of olive oil before serving.

Per Serving:

calories: 386 | fat: 27.7g | protein: 29.3g | carbs: 3.8g | fiber: 1.0g | sodium: 632mg

Baked Lemon Salmon

Prep time: 5 minutes | Cook time: 20 minutes | Serves 4

Ingredients:
¼ teaspoon dried thyme
Zest and juice of ½ lemon
¼ teaspoon salt
½ teaspoon freshly ground black pepper
1 pound (454 g) salmon fillet
Nonstick cooking spray

Directions:
Preheat the oven to 425°F (220°C). Coat a baking sheet with nonstick cooking spray.
Mix together the thyme, lemon zest and juice, salt, and pepper in a small bowl and stir to incorporate.
Arrange the salmon, skin-side down, on the coated baking sheet.
Spoon the thyme mixture over the salmon and spread it all over.
Bake in the preheated oven for about 15 to 20 minutes, or until the fish flakes apart easily. Serve warm.

Per Serving:
calories: 162 | fat: 7.0g | protein: 23.1g | carbs: 1.0g | fiber: 0g | sodium: 166mg

Lemon Grilled Shrimp

Prep time: 20 minutes | Cook time: 4 to 6 minutes | Serves 4

Ingredients:
tablespoons garlic, minced
tablespoons fresh Italian parsley, finely chopped
¼ cup extra-virgin olive oil
½ cup lemon juice
teaspoon salt
pounds (907 g) jumbo shrimp (21 to 25), peeled and deveinedSpecial
Equipment:
4 wooden skewers, soaked in water for at least 30 minutes

Directions:
Whisk together the garlic, parsley, olive oil, lemon juice, and salt in a
large bowl.
Add the shrimp to the bowl and toss well, making sure the shrimp are
coated in the marinade. Set aside to sit for 15 minutes.
When ready, skewer the shrimps by piercing through the center. You
can place about 5 to 6 shrimps on each skewer.
Preheat the grill to high heat.
Grill the shrimp for 4 to 6 minutes, flipping the shrimp halfway
through, or until the shrimp are pink on the outside and opaque in the
center.
Serve hot.

Per Serving:
calories: 401 | fat: 17.8g | protein: 56.9g | carbs: 3.9g | fiber: 0g |
sodium: 1223mg

Garlic Shrimp with Mushrooms

Prep time: 10 minutes | Cook time: 15 minutes | Serves 4

Ingredients:
1 pound (454 g) fresh shrimp, peeled, deveined, and patted dry
1 teaspoon salt
1 cup extra-virgin olive oil
8 large garlic cloves, thinly sliced
4 ounces (113 g) sliced mushrooms (shiitake, baby bella, or button)
½ teaspoon red pepper flakes
¼ cup chopped fresh flat-leaf Italian parsley

Directions:
In a bowl, season the shrimp with salt. Set aside.
Heat the olive oil in a large skillet over medium-low heat.
Add the garlic and cook for 3 to 4 minutes until fragrant, stirring occasionally.
Saut é the mushrooms for 5 minutes, or until they start to exude their juices.
Stir in the shrimp and sprinkle with red pepper flakes and saut é for 3 to 4 minutes more, or until the shrimp start to turn pink.
Remove the skillet from the heat and add the parsley. Stir to combine and serve warm.

Per Serving:
calories: 619 | fat: 55.5g | protein: 24.1g | carbs: 3.7g | fiber: 0g | sodium: 735mg

Steamed Bass

Prep time: 10 minutes | Cook time: 8 minutes | Serves 4

Ingredients:
1½ cups water
1 lemon, sliced
4 sea bass fillets
4 sprigs thyme
white onion, cut into thin rings
turnips, chopped
2 pinches salt
pinch ground black pepper
teaspoons olive oil

Directions:
Add water and set a rack into the pot.
Line a parchment paper to the bottom of the steamer basket. Place lemon slices in a single layer on the rack.
Arrange fillets on the top of the lemons, cover with onion and thyme sprigs. Top with turnip slices.
Drizzle pepper, salt, and olive oil over the mixture. Put steamer basket onto the rack.
Seal lid and cook on Low pressure for 8 minutes. Release the pressure quickly.
Serve over the delicate onion rings and thinly turnips.

Per Serving: calories: 177 | fat: 4.9g | protein: 24.7g | carbs: 7.8g | fiber: 2.0g | sodium: 209mg

Honey-Mustard Roasted Salmon

Prep time: 5 minutes | Cook time: 15 to 20 minutes | Serves 4

Ingredients:
2 tablespoons whole-grain mustard
2 garlic cloves, minced
1 tablespoon honey
¼ teaspoon salt
¼ teaspoon freshly ground black pepper
1 pound (454 g) salmon fillet
Nonstick cooking spray

Directions:
Preheat the oven to 425°F (220°C). Coat a baking sheet with nonstick cooking spray.
Stir together the mustard, garlic, honey, salt, and pepper in a small bowl.
Arrange the salmon fillet, skin-side down, on the coated baking sheet. Spread the mustard mixture evenly over the salmon fillet.
Roast in the preheated oven for 15 to 20 minutes, or until it flakes apart easily and reaches an internal temperature of 145°F (63°C). Serve hot.

Per Serving:
calories: 185 | fat: 7.0g | protein: 23.2g | carbs: 5.8g | fiber: 0g | sodium: 311mg

Salmon and Mushroom Hash with Pesto

Prep time: 15 minutes | Cook time: 20 minutes | Serves 6

Pesto:
¼ cup extra-virgin olive oil
bunch fresh basil
Juice and zest of 1 lemon
⅓ cup water
¼ teaspoon salt, plus additional as needed Hash:
tablespoons extra-virgin olive oil
6 cups mixed mushrooms (brown, white, shiitake, cremini, portobello, etc.), sliced
1 pound (454 g) wild salmon, cubed

Make the pesto:
Pulse the olive oil, basil, juice and zest, water, and salt in a blender or food processor until smoothly blended. Set aside.
Heat the olive oil in a large skillet over medium heat.
Stir-fry the mushrooms for 6 to 8 minutes, or until they begin to exude their juices.
Add the salmon and cook each side for 5 to 6 minutes until cooked through.
Fold in the prepared pesto and stir well. Taste and add additional salt as needed. Serve warm.

Per Serving:
calories: 264 | fat: 14.7g | protein: 7.0g | carbs: 30.9g | fiber: 4.0g | sodium: 480mg

Sole Piccata with Capers

Prep time: 10 minutes | Cook time: 17 minutes | Serves 4

Ingredients:
1 teaspoon extra-virgin olive oil
4 (5-ounce / 142-g) sole fillets, patted dry
3 tablespoons almond butter
2 teaspoons minced garlic
2 tablespoons all-purpose flour
2 cups low-sodium chicken broth
Juice and zest of ½ lemon
2 tablespoons capers

Directions:
Place a large skillet over medium-high heat and add the olive oil.
Sear the sole fillets until the fish flakes easily when tested with a fork, about 4 minutes on each side. Transfer the fish to a plate and set aside.
Return the skillet to the stove and add the butter.
Sauté the garlic until translucent, about 3 minutes.
Whisk in the flour to make a thick paste and cook, stirring constantly, until the mixture is golden brown, about 2 minutes.
Whisk in the chicken broth, lemon juice and zest.
Cook for about 4 minutes until the sauce is thickened.
Stir in the capers and serve the sauce over the fish.

Per Serving:
calories: 271 | fat:13.0g | protein: 30.0g | carbs: 7.0g | fiber: 0g | sodium: 413mg

Breaded Shrimp

Prep time: 10 minutes | Cook time: 4 to 6 minutes | Serves 4

Ingredients:
2 large eggs

tablespoon water

cups seasoned Italian bread crumbs

1 teaspoon salt

1 cup flour

1 pound (454 g) large shrimp (21 to 25), peeled and deveined

Extra-virgin olive oil, as needed

Directions:
In a small bowl, beat the eggs with the water, then transfer to a shallow dish.

Add the bread crumbs and salt to a separate shallow dish, then mix well.

Place the flour into a third shallow dish.

Coat the shrimp in the flour, then the beaten egg, and finally the bread crumbs. Place on a plate and repeat with all of the shrimp.

Heat a skillet over high heat. Pour in enough olive oil to coat the bottom of the skillet. Cook the shrimp in the hot skillet for 2 to 3 minutes on each side. Remove and drain on a paper towel. Serve warm.

Per Serving:
calories: 714 | fat: 34.0g | protein: 37.0g | carbs: 63.0g | fiber: 3.0g | sodium: 1727mg

Slow Cooker Salmon in Foil

Prep time: 5 minutes | Cook time: 2 hours | Serves 2

Ingredients:
2 (6-ounce / 170-g) salmon fillets
tablespoon olive oil
cloves garlic, minced
½ tablespoon lime juice
1 teaspoon finely chopped fresh parsley
¼ teaspoon black pepper

Directions:
Spread a length of foil onto a work surface and place the salmon fillets in the middle.
Mix together the olive oil, garlic, lime juice, parsley, and black pepper in a small bowl. Brush the mixture over the fillets. Fold the foil over and crimp the sides to make a packet.
Place the packet into the slow cooker, cover, and cook on High for 2 hours, or until the fish flakes easily with a fork.
Serve hot.

Per Serving:
calories: 446 | fat: 20.7g | protein: 65.4g | carbs: 1.5g | fiber: 0.2g | sodium: 240mg

Crispy Herb Crusted Halibut

Prep time: 10 minutes | Cook time: 20 minutes | Serves 4

Ingredients:
4 (5-ounce / 142-g) halibut fillets, patted dry
Extra-virgin olive oil, for brushing
½ cup coarsely ground unsalted pistachios
1 tablespoon chopped fresh parsley
1 teaspoon chopped fresh basil
1 teaspoon chopped fresh thyme
Pinch sea salt
Pinch freshly ground black pepper

Directions:
Preheat the oven to 350°F (180°C). Line a baking sheet with parchment paper.
Place the fillets on the baking sheet and brush them generously with olive oil.
In a small bowl, stir together the pistachios, parsley, basil, thyme, salt, and pepper.
Spoon the nut mixture evenly on the fish, spreading it out so the tops of the fillets are covered.
Bake in the preheated oven until it flakes when pressed with a fork, about 20 minutes.
Serve immediately.

Per Serving:
calories: 262 | fat: 11.0g | protein: 32.0g | carbs: 4.0g | fiber: 2.0g | sodium: 77mg

Asian-Inspired Tuna Lettuce Wraps

Prep time: 10 minutes | Cook time: 0 minutes | Serves 2

Ingredients:

⅓ cup almond butter

1 tablespoon freshly squeezed lemon juice

1 teaspoon low-sodium soy sauce

teaspoon curry powder

½ teaspoon sriracha, or to taste

½ cup canned water chestnuts, drained and chopped

(2.6-ounce / 74-g) package tuna packed in water, drained

2 large butter lettuce leaves

Directions:

Stir together the almond butter, lemon juice, soy sauce, curry powder, sriracha in a medium bowl until well mixed. Add the water chestnuts and tuna and stir until well incorporated.

Place 2 butter lettuce leaves on a flat work surface, spoon half of the tuna mixture onto each leaf and roll up into a wrap. Serve immediately.

Per Serving:

calories: 270 | fat: 13.9g | protein: 19.1g | carbs: 18.5g | fiber: 3.0g | sodium: 626mg

Braised Branzino with Wine Sauce

Prep time: 15 minutes | Cook time: 15 minutes | Serves 2 to 3

Ingredients:

¾ cup dry white wine

2 tablespoons white wine vinegar

2 tablespoons cornstarch

1 tablespoon honey Fish:

large branzino, butterflied and patted dry

tablespoons onion powder

2 tablespoons paprika

½ tablespoon salt

6 tablespoons extra-virgin olive oil, divided

4 garlic cloves, thinly sliced

4 scallions, both green and white parts, thinly sliced

1 large tomato, cut into ¼-inch cubes

4 kalamata olives, pitted and chopped

Directions:

Make the sauce: Mix together the white wine, vinegar, cornstarch, and honey in a bowl and keep stirring until the honey has dissolved. Set aside.

Make the fish: Place the fish on a clean work surface, skin-side down. Sprinkle the onion powder, paprika, and salt to season. Drizzle 2 tablespoons of olive oil all over the fish.

Heat 2 tablespoons of olive oil in a large skillet over high heat until it shimmers.

Add the fish, skin-side up, to the skillet and brown for about 2 minutes. Carefully flip the fish and cook for another 3 minutes. Remove from the heat to a plate and set aside.

Add the remaining 2 tablespoons olive oil to the skillet and swirl to coat. Stir in the garlic cloves, scallions, tomato, and kalamata olives and saut é for 5 minutes. Pour in the prepared sauce and stir to combine. Return the fish (skin-side down) to the skillet, flipping to coat in the sauce. Reduce the heat to medium-low, and cook for an additional 5 minutes until cooked through.

Using a slotted spoon, transfer the fish to a plate and serve warm.

Per Serving:

calories: 1059 | fat: 71.9g | protein: 46.2g | carbs: 55.8g | fiber: 5.1g | sodium: 2807mg

Peppercorn-Seared Tuna Steaks

Prep time: 5 minutes | Cook time: 10 minutes | Serves 2

Ingredients:
2 (5-ounce / 142-g) ahi tuna steaks
teaspoon kosher salt
¼ teaspoon cayenne pepper
tablespoons olive oil
1 teaspoon whole peppercorns

Directions:
On a plate, Season the tuna steaks on both sides with salt and cayenne
pepper.
In a skillet, heat the olive oil over medium-high heat until it shimmers.
Add the peppercorns and cook for about 5 minutes, or until they
soften and pop.
Carefully put the tuna steaks in the skillet and sear for 1 to 2 minutes
per side, depending on the thickness of the tuna steaks, or until the fish
is cooked to the desired level of doneness.
Cool for 5 minutes before serving.

Per Serving:
calories: 260 | fat: 14.3g | protein: 33.4g | carbs: 0.2g | fiber: 0.1g |
sodium: 1033mg

Grilled Lemon Pesto Salmon

Prep time: 5 minutes | Cook time: 6 to 10 minutes | Serves 2

Ingredients:
10 ounces (283 g) salmon fillet (1 large piece or 2 smaller ones)
Salt and freshly ground black pepper, to taste
2 tablespoons prepared pesto sauce
1 large fresh lemon, sliced
Cooking spray

Directions:
Preheat the grill to medium-high heat. Spray the grill grates with cooking spray.
Season the salmon with salt and black pepper. Spread the pesto sauce on top.
Make a bed of fresh lemon slices about the same size as the salmon fillet on the hot grill, and place the salmon on top of the lemon slices. Put any additional lemon slices on top of the salmon.
Grill the salmon for 6 to 10 minutes, or until the fish is opaque and flakes apart easily.
Serve hot.

Per Serving:
calories: 316 | fat: 21.1g | protein: 29.0g | carbs: 1.0g | fiber: 0g | sodium: 175mg

Steamed Trout with Lemon Herb Crust

Prep time: 10 minutes | Cook time: 15 minutes | Serves 2

Ingredients:
3 tablespoons olive oil
3 garlic cloves, chopped
2 tablespoons fresh lemon juice
1 tablespoon chopped fresh mint
1 tablespoon chopped fresh parsley
¼ teaspoon dried ground thyme
1 teaspoon sea salt
pound (454 g) fresh trout (2 pieces)
cups fish stock

Directions:
Stir together the olive oil, garlic, lemon juice, mint, parsley, thyme, and salt in a small bowl. Brush the marinade onto the fish.
Insert a trivet in the Instant Pot. Pour in the fish stock and place the fish on the trivet.
Secure the lid. Select the Steam mode and set the cooking time for 15 minutes at High Pressure.
Once cooking is complete, do a quick pressure release. Carefully open the lid. Serve warm.

Per Serving:
calories: 477 | fat: 29.6g | protein: 51.7g | carbs: 3.6g | fiber: 0.2g | sodium: 2011mg

Spicy Cumin Salmon

Prep time: 10 minutes | Cook time: 2 minutes | Serves 8

Ingredients:
2 cups water

2 garlic cloves, minced

2 teaspoons powdered stevia

8 lemon slices

2 tablespoons red chili powder

2 teaspoons ground cumin

Salt and freshly grated black pepper, to taste

2 pounds (907 g) salmon fillet, cut into 8 pieces

Directions:
Pour two cups of water in the insert of the Instant Pot. Set the trivet in it.

In a separate bowl, add all the ingredients except the lemon slices and mix them well.

Pour this mixture over the salmon fillets and rub it all over it.

Place the salmon slices over the trivet in a single layer.

Top each fillet with a lemon slice.

Secure the lid and select Steam function for 2 minutes.

After the beep, do a Quick release and then remove the lid.

Serve immediately.

Per Serving:
calories: 151 | fat: 4.7g | protein: 23.3g | carbs: 3.1g | fiber: 1.0g | sodium: 117mg

Mediterranean Grilled Sea Bass

Prep time: 20 minutes | Cook time: 20 minutes | Serves 6

Ingredients:
¼ teaspoon onion powder ¼ teaspoon garlic powder
¼ teaspoon paprika
Lemon pepper and sea salt to taste
pounds (907 g) sea bass
tablespoons extra-virgin olive oil, divided
2 large cloves garlic, chopped
1 tablespoon chopped Italian flat leaf parsley

Directions:
Preheat the grill to high heat.
Place the onion powder, garlic powder, paprika, lemon pepper, and sea salt in a large bowl and stir to combine.
Dredge the fish in the spice mixture, turning until well coated.
Heat 2 tablespoon of olive oil in a small skillet. Add the garlic and parsley and cook for 1 to 2 minutes, stirring occasionally. Remove the skillet from the heat and set aside.
Brush the grill grates lightly with remaining 1 tablespoon olive oil. Grill the fish for about 7 minutes. Flip the fish and drizzle with the garlic mixture and cook for an additional 7 minutes, or until the fish flakes when pressed lightly with a fork.
Serve hot.

Per Serving:
calories: 200 | fat: 10.3g | protein: 26.9g | carbs: 0.6g | fiber: 0.1g | sodium: 105mg

Spicy Haddock Stew

Prep time: 15 minutes | Cook time: 35 minutes | Serves 6

Ingredients:

¼ cup coconut oil
1 tablespoon minced garlic
onion, chopped
celery stalks, chopped
½ fennel bulb, thinly sliced
1 carrot, diced
1 sweet potato, diced
1 (15-ounce / 425-g) can low-sodium diced tomatoes
1 cup coconut milk
1 cup low-sodium chicken broth
¼ teaspoon red pepper flakes
12 ounces (340 g) haddock, cut into 1-inch chunks
2 tablespoons chopped fresh cilantro, for garnish

Directions:

In a large saucepan, heat the coconut oil over medium-high heat.
Add the garlic, onion, and celery and saut é for about 4 minutes,
stirring occasionally, or until they are tender. Stir in the fennel bulb,
carrot, and sweet potato and saut é for 4 minutes more. Add the diced
tomatoes, coconut milk, chicken broth, and red pepper flakes and stir
to incorporate, then bring the mixture to a boil. Once it starts to boil,
reduce the heat to low, and bring to a simmer for about 15 minutes, or
until the vegetables are fork-tender. Add the haddock chunks and
continue simmering for about 10 minutes, or until the fish is cooked
through. Sprinkle the cilantro on top for garnish before serving.

Per Serving:

calories: 276 | fat: 20.9g | protein: 14.2g | carbs: 6.8g | fiber: 3.0g |
sodium: 226mg

Roasted Trout Stuffed with Veggies

Prep time: 10 minutes | Cook time: 25 minutes | Serves 2

Ingredients:
2 (8-ounce / 227-g) whole trout fillets, dressed (cleaned but with bones and skin intact)
1 tablespoon extra-virgin olive oil
¼ teaspoon salt
⅛ teaspoon freshly ground black pepper
1 small onion, thinly sliced
½ red bell pepper, seeded and thinly sliced
poblano pepper, seeded and thinly sliced
or 3 shiitake mushrooms, sliced
1 lemon, sliced
Nonstick cooking spray

Directions:
Preheat the oven to 425°F (220°C). Spray a baking sheet with nonstick cooking spray.
Rub both trout fillets, inside and out, with the olive oil. Season with salt and pepper.
Mix together the onion, bell pepper, poblano pepper, and mushrooms in a large bowl. Stuff half of this mixture into the cavity of each fillet. Top the mixture with 2 or 3 lemon slices inside each fillet.
Place the fish on the prepared baking sheet side by side. Roast in the preheated oven for 25 minutes, or until the fish is cooked through and the vegetables are tender.
Remove from the oven and serve on a plate.

Per Serving:
calories: 453 | fat: 22.1g | protein: 49.0g | carbs: 13.8g | fiber: 3.0g | sodium: 356mg

Lemony Trout with Caramelized Shallots

Prep time: 10 minutes | Cook time: 20 minutes | Serves 2

Shallots:
teaspoon almond butter
shallots, thinly sliced
Dash salt
Trout:
tablespoon plus 1 teaspoon almond butter, divided
(4-ounce / 113-g) trout fillets
tablespoons capers
¼ cup freshly squeezed lemon juice
¼ teaspoon salt
Dash freshly ground black pepper
1 lemon, thinly sliced

Make the Shallots:
In a large skillet over medium heat, cook the butter, shallots, and salt
for 20 minutes, stirring every 5 minutes, or until the shallots are wilted
and caramelized.
Make the Trout
Meanwhile, in another large skillet over medium heat, heat 1 teaspoon
of almond butter.
Add the trout fillets and cook each side for 3 minutes, or until flaky.
Transfer to a plate and set aside.
In the skillet used for the trout, stir in the capers, lemon juice, salt, and
pepper, then bring to a simmer. Whisk in the remaining 1 tablespoon
of almond butter. Spoon the sauce over the fish.
Garnish the fish with the lemon slices and caramelized shallots before
serving.

Per Serving:
calories: 344 | fat: 18.4g | protein: 21.1g | carbs: 14.7g | fiber: 5.0g |
sodium: 1090mg

Rosemary Cod with Cherry Tomato

Prep time: 20 minutes | Cook time: 5 minutes | Serves 6

Ingredients:
1½ pounds (680 g) cherry tomatoes, halved
2½ tablespoons fresh rosemary, chopped
6 (4-ounce / 113-g) cod fillets
3 garlic cloves, minced
2 tablespoons olive oil
Salt and freshly ground black pepper, to taste

Directions:
Add the olive oil, half of the tomatoes and rosemary to the insert of the Instant Pot.
Place the cod fillets over these tomatoes. Then add more tomatoes to the pot.
Add the garlic to the pot. Then secure the lid.
Select the Manual function with High Pressure for 5 minutes.
After the beep, use the quick release to discharge all the steam.
Serve cod fillets with tomatoes and sprinkle a pinch of salt and pepper on top.

Per Serving:
calories: 143 | fat: 5.2g | protein: 18.8g | carbs: 5.0g | fiber: 1.5g | sodium: 358mg

Mussels with Onions

Prep time: 10 minutes | Cook time: 7 minutes | Serves 8

Ingredients:
2 tablespoons olive oil
2 medium yellow onions, chopped
teaspoon dried rosemary, crushed
garlic cloves, minced
2 cups chicken broth
4 pounds (1.8 kg) mussels, cleaned and debearded
¼ cup fresh lemon juice
Salt and ground black pepper as needed

Directions:
Put the oil to the Instant Pot and select the Sauté function for cooking.
Add the onions and cook for 5 minutes with occasional stirring.
Add the rosemary and garlic to the pot. Stir and cook for 1 minute.
Pour the chicken broth and lemon juice into the cooker, sprinkle some
salt and black pepper over it.
Place the trivet inside the cooker and arrange the mussels over it.
Select the Manual function at Low Pressure for 1 minute.
Secure the lid and let the mussels cook.
After the beep, do a Quick release then remove the lid.
Serve the mussels with its steaming hot soup in a bowl.

Per Serving:
calories: 249 | fat: 8.8g | protein: 28.5g | carbs: 11.9g | fiber: 0.5g |
sodium: 844mg

Cod Curry

Prep time: 5 minutes | Cook time: 12 minutes | Serves 8

Ingredients:
3 pounds (1.4 kg) cod fillets, cut into bite-sized pieces
2 tablespoons olive oil
4 curry leaves
4 medium onions, chopped
2 tablespoons fresh ginger, grated finely
4 garlic cloves, minced
4 tablespoons curry powder
4 teaspoons ground cumin
4 teaspoons ground coriander
2 teaspoons red chili powder
1 teaspoon ground turmeric
4 cups unsweetened coconut milk
2½ cups tomatoes, chopped
2 Serrano peppers, seeded and chopped
2 tablespoons fresh lemon juice

Directions:
Add the oil to the Instant Pot and select Sauté function for cooking.
Add the curry leaves and cook for 30 seconds. Stir the onion, garlic,
and ginger into the pot and cook 5 minutes. Add all the spices to the
mixture and cook for another 1½ minutes. Hit Cancel then add the
coconut milk, Serrano pepper, tomatoes, and fish to the pot.
Secure the lid and select the Manual settings with Low Pressure and 5
minutes cooking time. After the beep, do a Quick release and remove
the lid. Drizzle lemon juice over the curry then stir. Serve immediately.

Per Serving:
calories: 424 | fat: 29.1g | protein: 30.2g | carbs: 14.4g | fiber: 3.8g |
sodium: 559mg

Cioppino (Seafood Tomato Stew)

Prep time: 10 minutes | Cook time: 20 minutes | Serves 2

Ingredients:
2 tablespoons olive oil
½ small onion, diced
½ green pepper, diced
2 teaspoons dried basil
2 teaspoons dried oregano
½ cup dry white wine
1 (14.5-ounce / 411-g) can diced tomatoes with basil
1 (8-ounce / 227-g) can no-salt-added tomato sauce
1 (6.5-ounce / 184-g) can minced clams with their juice
8 ounces (227 g) peeled, deveined raw shrimp
4 ounces (113 g) any white fish (a thick piece works best)
3 tablespoons fresh parsley
Salt and freshly ground black pepper, to taste

Directions:
In a Dutch oven, heat the olive oil over medium heat.
Saut é the onion and green pepper for 5 minutes, or until tender.
Stir in the basil, oregano, wine, diced tomatoes, and tomato sauce and
bring to a boil.
Once boiling, reduce the heat to low and bring to a simmer for 5
minutes.
Add the clams, shrimp, and fish and cook for about 10 minutes, or
until the shrimp are pink and cooked through.
Scatter with the parsley and add the salt and black pepper to taste.
Remove from the heat and serve warm.

Per Serving:
calories: 221 | fat: 7.7g | protein: 23.1g | carbs: 10.9g | fiber: 4.2g |
sodium: 720mg

Lemony Shrimp with Orzo Salad

Prep time: 10 minutes | Cook time: 22 minutes | Serves 4

Ingredients:
1 cup orzo
hothouse cucumber, deseeded and chopped
½ cup finely diced red onion
tablespoons extra-virgin olive oil
pounds (907 g) shrimp, peeled and deveined
lemons, juiced
Salt and freshly ground black pepper, to taste
¾ cup crumbled feta cheese
2 tablespoons dried dill
1 cup chopped fresh flat-leaf parsley

Directions:
Bring a large pot of water to a boil. Add the orzo and cook covered for 15 to 18 minutes, or until the orzo is tender. Transfer to a colander to drain and set aside to cool.

Mix the cucumber and red onion in a bowl. Set aside.

Heat the olive oil in a medium skillet over medium heat until it shimmers.

Reduce the heat, add the shrimp, and cook each side for 2 minutes until cooked through.

Add the cooked shrimp to the bowl of cucumber and red onion. Mix in the cooked orzo and lemon juice and toss to combine. Sprinkle with salt and pepper. Scatter the top with the feta cheese and dill. Garnish with the parsley and serve immediately.

Per Serving:
calories: 565 | fat: 17.8g | protein: 63.3g | carbs: 43.9g | fiber: 4.1g | sodium: 2225mg

Avocado Shrimp Ceviche

Prep time: 15 minutes | Cook time: 0 minutes | Serves 4

Ingredients:
1 pound (454 g) fresh shrimp, peeled, deveined, and cut in half lengthwise
small red or yellow bell pepper, cut into ½-inch chunks
½ small red onion, cut into thin slivers
½ English cucumber, peeled and cut into ½-inch chunks
¼ cup chopped fresh cilantro
½ cup extra-virgin olive oil
⅓ cup freshly squeezed lime juice
tablespoons freshly squeezed clementine juice
2 tablespoons freshly squeezed lemon juice
teaspoon salt
½ teaspoon freshly ground black pepper
ripe avocados, peeled, pitted, and cut into ½-inch chunks

Directions:
Place the shrimp, bell pepper, red onion, cucumber, and cilantro in a large bowl and toss to combine.
In a separate bowl, stir together the olive oil, lime, clementine, and lemon juice, salt, and black pepper until smooth. Pour the mixture into the bowl of shrimp and vegetable mixture and toss until they are completely coated.
Cover the bowl with plastic wrap and transfer to the refrigerator to marinate for at least 2 hours, or up to 8 hours.
When ready, stir in the avocado chunks and toss to incorporate. Serve immediately.

Per Serving:
calories: 496 | fat: 39.5g | protein: 25.3g | carbs: 13.8g | fiber: 6.0g | sodium: 755mg

Garlic Skillet Salmon

Prep time: 5 minutes | Cook time: 14 to 16 minutes | Serves 4

Ingredients:
tablespoon extra-virgin olive oil
garlic cloves, minced
1 teaspoon smoked paprika
1½ cups grape or cherry tomatoes, quartered
1 (12-ounce / 340-g) jar roasted red peppers, drained and chopped
1 tablespoon water
¼ teaspoon freshly ground black pepper
¼ teaspoon kosher or sea salt
1 pound (454 g) salmon fillets, skin removed and cut into 8 pieces
1 tablespoon freshly squeezed lemon juice

Directions:
In a large skillet over medium heat, heat the oil. Add the garlic and smoked paprika and cook for 1 minute, stirring often. Add the tomatoes, roasted peppers, water, black pepper, and salt. Turn up the heat to medium-high, bring to a simmer, and cook for 3 minutes, stirring occasionally and smashing the tomatoes with a wooden spoon toward the end of the cooking time.
Add the salmon to the skillet, and spoon some of the sauce over the top. Cover and cook for 10 to 12 minutes, or until the salmon is cooked through and just starts to flake.
Remove the skillet from the heat, and drizzle lemon juice over the top of the fish. Stir the sauce, then break up the salmon into chunks with a fork. Serve hot.

Per Serving:
calories: 255 | fat: 11.7g | protein: 24.2g | carbs: 5.9g | fiber: 1.2g | sodium: 809mg

Baked Oysters with Vegetables

Prep time: 30 minutes | Cook time: 15 to 17 minutes | Serves 2

Ingredients:
2 cups coarse salt, for holding the oysters
1 dozen fresh oysters, scrubbed
1 tablespoon almond butter
¼ cup finely chopped scallions, both white and green parts
½ cup finely chopped artichoke hearts
¼ cup finely chopped red bell pepper
1 garlic clove, minced
1 tablespoon finely chopped fresh parsley
Zest and juice of ½ lemon
Pinch salt
Freshly ground black pepper, to taste

Directions:
Pour the salt into a baking dish and spread to evenly fill the bottom of the dish. Prepare a clean work surface to shuck the oysters. Using a shucking knife, insert the blade at the joint of the shell, where it hinges open and shut. Firmly apply pressure to pop the blade in, and work the knife around the shell to open. Discard the empty half of the shell. Using the knife, gently loosen the oyster, and remove any shell particles. Set the oysters in their shells on the salt, being careful not to spill the juices. Preheat the oven to 425°F (220°C). Heat the almond butter in a large skillet over medium heat. Add the scallions, artichoke hearts, and bell pepper, and cook for 5 to 7 minutes. Add the garlic and cook for 1 minute more. Remove from the heat and stir in the parsley, lemon zest and juice, and season to taste with salt and pepper. Divide the vegetable mixture evenly among the oysters. Bake in the preheated oven for 10 to 12 minutes, or until the vegetables are lightly browned. Serve warm.

Per Serving: calories: 135 | fat: 7.2g | protein: 6.0g | carbs: 10.7g | fiber: 2.0g | sodium: 280mg

Steamed Cod

Prep time: 15 minutes | Cook time: 7 minutes | Serves 4

Ingredients:
1 pound (454 g) cherry tomatoes, halved
1 bunch fresh thyme sprigs
4 fillets cod
1 teaspoon olive oil
1 clove garlic, pressed
3 pinches salt
2 cups water
1 cup white rice
cup Kalamata olives
tablespoons pickled capers1 tablespoon olive oil
1 pinch ground black pepper

Directions:
Line a parchment paper on the basket of your instant pot. Place about half the tomatoes in a single layer on the paper. Sprinkle with thyme, reserving some for garnish. Arrange cod fillets on top. Sprinkle with a little bit of olive oil. Spread the garlic, pepper, salt, and remaining tomatoes over the fish. In the pot, mix rice and water. Lay a trivet over the rice and water. Lower steamer basket onto the trivet. Seal the lid, and cook for 7 minutes on Low Pressure. Release the pressure quickly. Remove the steamer basket and trivet from the pot. Use a fork to fluff rice. Plate the fish fillets and apply a garnish of olives, reserved thyme, pepper, remaining olive oil, and capers. Serve with rice.

Per Serving:
calories: 352 | fat: 9.1g | protein: 22.2g | carbs: 44.7g | fiber: 3.9g | sodium: 827mg

Catfish and Shrimp Jambalaya

Prep time: 20 minutes | Cook time: 4 hours 45 minutes | Serves 3

Ingredients:

4 ounces (113 g) catfish (cut into 1-inch cubes)

4 ounces (113 g) shrimp (peeled and deveined)

tablespoon olive oil

bacon slices, chopped

1¼ cups vegetable broth

¾ cup sliced celery stalk

¼ teaspoon minced garlic

½ cup chopped onion

1 cup canned diced tomatoes

1 cup uncooked long-grain white rice

½ tablespoon Cajun seasoning

¼ teaspoon dried thyme

¼ teaspoon cayenne pepper

½ teaspoon dried oregano

Salt and freshly ground black pepper, to taste

Directions:

Select the Sauté function on your Instant Pot and add the oil into it. Put the onion, garlic, celery, and bacon to the pot and cook for 10 minutes. Add all the remaining ingredients to the pot except seafood. Stir well, then secure the cooker lid. Select the Slow Cook function on a medium mode. Keep the pressure release handle on venting position. Cook for 4 hours. Once done, remove the lid and add the seafood to the gravy. Secure the lid again, keep the pressure handle in the venting position. Cook for another 45 minutes then serve.

Per Serving:

calories: 437 | fat: 13.1g | protein: 21.3g | carbs: 56.7g | fiber: 2.6g | sodium: 502mg

Salmon and Potato Casserole

Prep time: 20 minutes | Cook time: 8 hours | Serves 4

Ingredients:

½ tablespoon olive oil

8 ounces (227 g) cream of mushroom soup

¼ cup water

3 medium potatoes (peeled and sliced)

3 tablespoons flour

1 (1-pound / 454-g) can salmon (drained and flaked)

½ cup chopped scallion

¼ teaspoon ground nutmeg

Salt and freshly ground black pepper, to taste

Directions:

Pour mushroom soup and water in a separate bowl and mix them well.

Add the olive oil to the Instant Pot and grease it lightly.

Place half of the potatoes in the pot and sprinkle salt, pepper, and half of the flour over it.

Now add a layer of half of the salmon over potatoes, then a layer of half of the scallions.

Repeat these layers and pour mushroom soup mix on top.

Top it with nutmeg evenly.

Secure the lid and set its pressure release handle to the venting position.

Select the Slow Cook function with Medium heat on your Instant Pot.

Let it cook for 8 hours then serve.

Per Serving:

calories: 388 | fat: 11.6g | protein: 34.6g | carbs: 37.2g | fiber: 4.4g | sodium: 842mg

Mahi-Mahi and Tomato Bowls

Prep time: 5 minutes | Cook time: 14 minutes | Serves 3

Ingredients:

3 (4-ounce / 113-g) mahi-mahi fillets

1½ tablespoons olive oil

½ yellow onion, sliced

½ teaspoon dried oregano

1 tablespoon fresh lemon juice

Salt and freshly ground black pepper, to taste

1 (14-ounce / 397-g) can sugar-free diced tomatoes

Directions:

Add the olive oil to the Instant Pot. Select the Sauté function on it.

Add all the ingredient to the pot except the fillets. Cook them for 10 minutes.

Press the Cancel key, then add the mahi-mahi fillets to the sauce.

Cover the fillets with sauce by using a spoon.

Secure the lid and set the Manual function at High Pressure for 4 minutes.

After the beep, do a Quick release then remove the lid.

Serve the fillets with their sauce, poured on top.

Per Serving:

calories: 265 | fat: 8.6g | protein: 39.1g | carbs: 7.0g | fiber: 3.1g | sodium: 393mg

Alfredo Tuscan Shrimp with Penne

Prep time: 5 minutes | Cook time: 5 minutes | Serves 3

Ingredients:
1 pound (454 g) shrimp
1 jar alfredo sauce
1½ cups fresh spinach
1 cup sun-dried tomatoes
1 box penne pasta
1½ teaspoons Tuscan seasoning
3 cups water

Directions:
Add the water and pasta to a pot over a medium heat, boil until it cooks completely. Then strain the pasta and keep it aside.
Select the Sauté function on your Instant Pot and add the tomatoes, shrimp, Tuscan seasoning, and alfredo sauce into it.
Stir and cook until shrimp turn pink in color.
Now add the spinach leaves to the pot and cook for 5 minutes.
Add the pasta to the pot and stir well.
Serve hot.

Per Serving:
calories: 1361 | fat: 70.1g | protein: 55.9g | carbs: 134.4g | fiber: 19.4g | sodium: 933mg

Tuna with Shirataki Noodles

Prep time: 5 minutes | Cook time: 4 minutes | Serves 2

Ingredients:
½ can tuna, drained
8 ounces (227 g) Shirataki noodles
½ cup frozen peas
(14-ounce / 397-g) can cream mushroom soup
ounces (57 g) shredded Cheddar cheese
1½ cups water

Directions:
Add the water with noodles to the base of your Instant Pot.
Place the tuna and peas over it. Then pour the mushroom soup on top.
Secure the lid and cook with the Manual function at High Pressure for
4 minutes.
After the beep, do a Quick release then remove the lid.
Stir in shredded cheese to the tuna mix.
Serve warm.

Per Serving:
calories: 362 | fat: 11.1g | protein: 19.5g | carbs: 46.5g | fiber: 1.5g |
sodium: 645mg

Grits with Shrimp

Prep time: 5 minutes | Cook time: 15 minutes | Serves 8

Ingredients:
tablespoon oil
cups quick grits
12 ounces (340 g) Parmesan cheese, shredded
2 cups heavy cream
24 ounces (680 g) tail-on shrimp
2 tablespoons Old Bay seasoning
A pinch of ground black pepper
4 cups water

Directions:
Add a tablespoon of oil to the Instant Pot. Select the Sauté function for cooking.
Add the shrimp to the oil and drizzle old bay seasoning over it.
Cook the shrimp for 3-4 minutes while stirring then set them aside.
Now add the water, cream, and quick grits to the pot. Select the Manual function for 3 minutes at High Pressure.
After the beep, do a Quick release then remove the lid.
Add the shredded cheese to the grits then stir well.
Take a serving bowl, first pour in the creamy grits mixture then top it with shrimp.
Sprinkle black pepper on top then serve hot.

Per Serving:
calories: 528 | fat: 38.6g | protein: 30.7g | carbs: 15.2g | fiber: 0.7g | sodium: 1249mg

Salmon Baked in Foil

Prep time: 5 minutes | Cook time: 25 minutes | Serves 4

Ingredients:
cups cherry tomatoes
tablespoons extra-virgin olive oil
3 tablespoons lemon juice
3 tablespoons almond butter
1 teaspoon oregano
½ teaspoon salt
4 (5-ounce / 142-g) salmon fillets

Directions:
Preheat the oven to 400°F (205°C).
Cut the tomatoes in half and put them in a bowl.
Add the olive oil, lemon juice, butter, oregano, and salt to the tomatoes
and gently toss to combine.
Cut 4 pieces of foil, about 12-by-12 inches each.
Place the salmon fillets in the middle of each piece of foil.
Divide the tomato mixture evenly over the 4 pieces of salmon. Bring
the ends of the foil together and seal to form a closed pocket.
Place the 4 pockets on a baking sheet. Bake in the preheated oven for
25 minutes.
Remove from the oven and serve on a plate.

Per Serving:
calories: 410 | fat: 32.0g | protein: 30.0g | carbs: 4.0g | fiber: 1.0g |
sodium: 370mg

Instant Pot Poached Salmon

Prep time: 10 minutes | Cook time: 3 minutes | Serves 4

Ingredients:
1 lemon, sliced ¼ inch thick
4 (6-ounce / 170-g) skinless salmon fillets, 1½ inches thick
½ teaspoon salt
¼ teaspoon pepper
½ cup water

Directions:
Layer the lemon slices in the bottom of the Instant Pot.
Season the salmon with salt and pepper, then arrange the salmon
(skinside down) on top of the lemon slices. Pour in the water.
Secure the lid. Select the Manual mode and set the cooking time for 3
minutes at High Pressure.
Once cooking is complete, do a quick pressure release. Carefully open
the lid.
Serve warm.

Per Serving:
calories: 350 | fat: 23.0g | protein: 35.0g | carbs: 0g | fiber: 0g |
sodium: 390mg

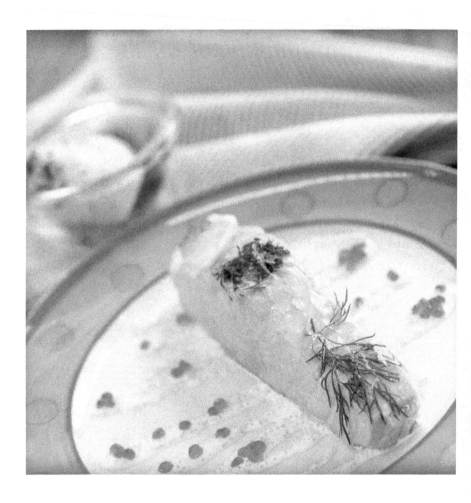

Balsamic-Honey Glazed Salmon

Prep time: 2 minutes | Cook time: 8 minutes | Serves 4

Ingredients:
½ cup balsamic vinegar
1 tablespoon honey
4 (8-ounce / 227-g) salmon fillets
Sea salt and freshly ground pepper, to taste
1 tablespoon olive oil

Directions:
Heat a skillet over medium-high heat. Combine the vinegar and honey in a small bowl.
Season the salmon fillets with the sea salt and freshly ground pepper; brush with the honey-balsamic glaze.
Add olive oil to the skillet, and sear the salmon fillets, cooking for 3 to 4 minutes on each side until lightly browned and medium rare in the center.
Let sit for 5 minutes before serving.

Per Serving:
calories: 454 | fat: 17.3g | protein: 65.3g | carbs: 9.7g | fiber: 0g | sodium: 246mg

Seared Salmon with Lemon Cream Sauce

Prep time: 10 minutes | Cook time: 20 minutes | Serves 4

Ingredients:
4 (5-ounce / 142-g) salmon fillets
Sea salt and freshly ground black pepper, to taste
1 tablespoon extra-virgin olive oil
½ cup low-sodium vegetable broth
Juice and zest of 1 lemon
1 teaspoon chopped fresh thyme
½ cup fat-free sour cream
1 teaspoon honey
1 tablespoon chopped fresh chives

Directions:
Preheat the oven to 400°F (205°C).
Season the salmon lightly on both sides with salt and pepper.
Place a large ovenproof skillet over medium-high heat and add the
olive oil. Sear the salmon fillets on both sides until golden, about 3
minutes per side. Transfer the salmon to a baking dish and bake in the
preheated oven until just cooked through, about 10 minutes.
Meanwhile, whisk together the vegetable broth, lemon juice and zest,
and thyme in a small saucepan over medium-high heat until the liquid
reduces by about one-quarter, about 5 minutes. Whisk in the sour
cream and honey. Stir in the chives and serve the sauce over the
salmon.

Per Serving:
calories: 310 | fat: 18.0g | protein: 29.0g | carbs: 6.0g | fiber: 0g |
sodium: 129mg

Tuna and Zucchini Patties

Prep time: 10 minutes | Cook time: 12 minutes | Serves 4

Ingredients:
3 slices whole-wheat sandwich bread, toasted
2 (5-ounce / 142-g) cans tuna in olive oil, drained
1 cup shredded zucchini
1 large egg, lightly beaten
¼ cup diced red bell pepper
1 tablespoon dried oregano
1 teaspoon lemon zest
¼ teaspoon freshly ground black pepper
¼ teaspoon kosher or sea salt
1 tablespoon extra-virgin olive oil
Salad greens or 4 whole-wheat rolls, for serving (optional)

Directions:
Crumble the toast into bread crumbs with your fingers (or use a knife to cut into ¼-inch cubes) until you have 1 cup of loosely packed crumbs. Pour the crumbs into a large bowl. Add the tuna, zucchini, beaten egg, bell pepper, oregano, lemon zest, black pepper, and salt. Mix well with a fork. With your hands, form the mixture into four (½-cup-size) patties. Place them on a plate, and press each patty flat to about ¾-inch thick.

In a large skillet over medium-high heat, heat the oil until it's very hot, about 2 minutes.

Add the patties to the hot oil, then reduce the heat down to medium. Cook the patties for 5 minutes, flip with a spatula, and cook for an additional 5 minutes. Serve the patties on salad greens or whole-wheat rolls, if desired.

Per Serving:
calories: 757 | fat: 72.0g | protein: 5.0g | carbs: 26.0g | fiber: 4.0g | sodium: 418mg

---

Baked Fish with Pistachio Crust

Prep time: 10 minutes | Cook time: 15 to 20 minutes | Serves 4

Ingredients:
½ cup extra-virgin olive oil, divided
1 pound (454 g) flaky white fish (such as cod, haddock, or halibut), skin removed
½ cup shelled finely chopped pistachios
½ cup ground flaxseed
Zest and juice of 1 lemon, divided
1 teaspoon ground cumin
1 teaspoon ground allspice
½ teaspoon salt
¼ teaspoon freshly ground black pepper

Directions:
Preheat the oven to 400°F (205°C).
Line a baking sheet with parchment paper or aluminum foil and drizzle 2 tablespoons of olive oil over the sheet, spreading to evenly coat the bottom.
Cut the fish into 4 equal pieces and place on the prepared baking sheet. In a small bowl, combine the pistachios, flaxseed, lemon zest, cumin, allspice, salt, and pepper. Drizzle in ¼ cup of olive oil and stir well. Divide the nut mixture evenly on top of the fish pieces. Drizzle the lemon juice and remaining 2 tablespoons of olive oil over the fish and bake until cooked through, 15 to 20 minutes, depending on the thickness of the fish.
Cool for 5 minutes before serving.

Per Serving:
calories: 509 | fat: 41.0g | protein: 26.0g | carbs: 9.0g | fiber: 6.0g | sodium: 331mg

Dill Baked Sea Bass

Prep time: 10 minutes | Cook time: 10 to 15 minutes | Serves 6

Ingredients:
¼ cup olive oil
2 pounds (907 g) sea bass
Sea salt and freshly ground pepper, to taste
1 garlic clove, minced
¼ cup dry white wine
3 teaspoons fresh dill
2 teaspoons fresh thyme

Directions:
Preheat the oven to 425°F (220°C).
Brush the bottom of a roasting pan with the olive oil. Place the fish in the pan and brush the fish with oil.
Season the fish with sea salt and freshly ground pepper. Combine the remaining ingredients and pour over the fish.
Bake in the preheated oven for 10 to 15 minutes, depending on the size of the fish.
Serve hot.

Per Serving:
calories: 224 | fat: 12.1g | protein: 28.1g | carbs: 0.9g | fiber: 0.3g | sodium: 104mg

Tomato Tuna Melts

Prep time: 5 minutes | Cook time: 3 to 4 minutes | Serves 2

Ingredients:
(5-ounce / 142-g) can chunk light tuna packed in water, drained
tablespoons plain Greek yogurt
2 tablespoons finely chopped celery
tablespoon finely chopped red onion
teaspoons freshly squeezed lemon juice
Pinch cayenne pepper
1 large tomato, cut into ¾-inch-thick rounds
½ cup shredded Cheddar cheese

Directions:
Preheat the broiler to High.
Stir together the tuna, yogurt, celery, red onion, lemon juice, and cayenne pepper in a medium bowl.
Place the tomato rounds on a baking sheet. Top each with some tuna salad and Cheddar cheese.
Broil for 3 to 4 minutes until the cheese is melted and bubbly. Cool for 5 minutes before serving.

Per Serving:
calories: 244 | fat: 10.0g | protein: 30.1g | carbs: 6.9g | fiber: 1.0g | sodium: 445mg

Mackerel and Green Bean Salad

Prep time: 10 minutes | Cook time: 10 minutes | Serves 2

Ingredients:
2 cups green beans
tablespoon avocado oil
mackerel fillets
4 cups mixed salad greens
2 hard-boiled eggs, sliced
avocado, sliced
tablespoons lemon juice
2 tablespoons olive oil
1 teaspoon Dijon mustard
Salt and black pepper, to taste

Directions:
Cook the green beans in a medium saucepan of boiling water for about
3 minutes until crisp-tender. Drain and set aside.
Melt the avocado oil in a pan over medium heat. Add the mackerel
fillets and cook each side for 4 minutes.
Divide the greens between two salad bowls. Top with the mackerel,
sliced egg, and avocado slices.
In another bowl, whisk together the lemon juice, olive oil, mustard,
salt, and pepper, and drizzle over the salad. Add the cooked green
beans and toss to combine, then serve.

Per Serving:
calories: 737 | fat: 57.3g | protein: 34.2g | carbs: 22.1g | fiber: 13.4g |
sodium: 398mg

Shrimp and Pea Paella

Prep time: 20 minutes | Cook time: 60 minutes | Serves 2

Ingredients:
2 tablespoons olive oil
1 garlic clove, minced
½ large onion, minced
1 cup diced tomato
½ cup short-grain rice
½ teaspoon sweet paprika
½ cup dry white wine
1¼ cups low-sodium chicken stock
8 ounces (227 g) large raw shrimp
1 cup frozen peas
¼ cup jarred roasted red peppers, cut into strips
Salt, to taste

Directions:
Heat the olive oil in a large skillet over medium-high heat.
Add the garlic and onion and sauté for 3 minutes, or until the onion is
softened. Add the tomato, rice, and paprika and stir for 3 minutes to
toast the rice. Add the wine and chicken stock and stir to combine.
Bring the mixture to a boil. Cover and reduce the heat to medium-low,
and simmer for 45 minutes, or until the rice is just about tender and
most of the liquid has been absorbed. Add the shrimp, peas, and
roasted red peppers. Cover and cook for an additional 5 minutes.
Season with salt to taste and serve.

Per Serving:
calories: 646 | fat: 27.1g | protein: 42.0g | carbs: 59.7g | fiber: 7.0g |
sodium: 687mg

Garlic Shrimp with Arugula Pesto

Prep time: 20 minutes | Cook time: 5 minutes | Serves 2

Ingredients:
3 cups lightly packed arugula
½ cup lightly packed basil leaves
¼ cup walnuts
3 tablespoons olive oil
3 medium garlic cloves
2 tablespoons grated Parmesan cheese
1 tablespoon freshly squeezed lemon juice
Salt and freshly ground black pepper, to taste
1 (10-ounce / 283-g) package zucchini noodles
8 ounces (227 g) cooked, shelled shrimp
2 Roma tomatoes, diced

Directions:
Process the arugula, basil, walnuts, olive oil, garlic, Parmesan cheese, and lemon juice in a food processor until smooth, scraping down the sides as needed. Season with salt and pepper to taste.
Heat a skillet over medium heat. Add the pesto, zucchini noodles, and cooked shrimp. Toss to combine the sauce over the noodles and shrimp, and cook until heated through.
Taste and season with more salt and pepper as needed. Serve topped with the diced tomatoes.

Per Serving:
calories: 435 | fat: 30.2g | protein: 33.0g | carbs: 15.1g | fiber: 5.0g | sodium: 413mg

Teriyaki Salmon

Prep time: 10 minutes | Cook time: 8 minutes | Serves 4

Ingredients:
4 (8-ounce / 227-g) thick salmon fillets.
cup soy sauce
cups water
½ cup mirin
2 tablespoons sesame oil
4 teaspoons sesame seeds
2 cloves garlic, minced
2 tablespoons freshly grated ginger
4 tablespoons brown sugar
1 tablespoon corn starch
4 green onions, minced

Directions:
Add the soy sauce, sesame oil, sesame seeds, mirin, ginger, water, garlic, green onions, and brown sugar to a small bowl. Mix them well.
In a shallow dish place the salmon fillets and pour half of the prepared mixture over the fillets. Let it marinate for 30 minutes in a refrigerator. Pour 1 cup of water into the insert of your Instant pot and place trivet inside it. Arrange the marinated salmon fillets over the trivet and secure the lid. Select the Manual settings with High Pressure and 8 minutes cooking time. Meanwhile, take a skillet and add the remaining marinade mixture in it. Let it cook for 2 minutes, then add the corn starch mixed with water. Stir well and cook for 1 minute. Check the pressure cooker, do a Quick release if it is done. Transfer the fillets to a serving platter and pour the sesame mixture over it.
Garnish with chopped green chilies then serve hot.

Per Serving: calories: 622 | fat: 28.6g | protein: 51.3g | carbs: 29.6g | fiber: 2.0g | sodium: 1086mg

Coconut Tangy Cod Curry

Prep time: 5 minutes | Cook time: 3 minutes | Serves 6

Ingredients:
(28-ounce / 794-g) can coconut milk
Juice of 2 lemons
tablespoons red curry paste
2 teaspoons fish sauce
2 teaspoons honey
4 teaspoons Sriracha
4 cloves garlic, minced
2 teaspoons ground turmeric
2 teaspoons ground ginger
1 teaspoon sea salt
teaspoon white pepper
pounds (907 g) codfish, cut into 1-inch cubes
½ cup chopped fresh cilantro, for garnish
4 lime wedges, for garnish

Directions:
Add all the ingredients, except the cod cubes and garnish, to a large
bowl and whisk them well.
Arrange the cod cube at the base of the Instant Pot and pour the
coconut milk mixture over it.
Secure the lid and hit the Manual key, select High Pressure with 3
minutes cooking time.
After the beep, do a Quick release then remove the lid.
Garnish with fresh cilantro and lemon wedges then serve.

Per Serving:
calories: 396 | fat: 29.1g | protein: 26.6g | carbs: 11.4g | fiber: 2.0g |
sodium: 1024mg

Shrimps with Broccoli

Prep time: 5 minutes | Cook time: 10 minutes | Serves 2

Ingredients:
2 teaspoons vegetable oil
2 tablespoons corn starch
1 cup broccoli florets
¼ cup chicken broth
8 ounces (227 g) large shrimp, peeled and deveined
¼ cup soy sauce
¼ cup water
¼ cup sliced carrots
3 tablespoons rice vinegar
2 teaspoons sesame oil
1 tablespoon chili garlic sauce
Coriander leaves to garnish
Boiled rice or noodles, for serving

Directions:
Add 1 tablespoon of corn starch and shrimp to a bowl. Mix them well then set it aside.
In a small bowl, mix the remaining corn starch, chicken broth, carrots, chili garlic sauce, rice vinegar and soy sauce together. Keep the mixture aside.
Select the Sauté function on your Instant pot, add the sesame oil and broccoli florets to the pot and sauté for 5 minutes.
Add the water to the broccoli, cover the lid and cook for 5 minutes.
Stir in shrimp and vegetable oil to the broccoli, sauté it for 5 minutes.
Garnish with coriander leaves on top.
Serve with rice or noodles.

Per Serving:
calories: 300 | fat: 16.5g | protein: 19.6g | carbs: 17.1g | fiber: 2.2g | sodium: 1241mg

Shrimp and Spaghetti Squash Bowls

Prep time: 5 minutes | Cook time: 25 minutes | Serves 4

Ingredients:
½ cup dry white wine
¼ teaspoon crushed red pepper flakes
1 large shallot, finely chopped
1 pound (454 g) jumbo shrimp, peeled and deveined
(28-ounce / 794-g) can crushed tomatoes
cloves garlic, minced
2½ pounds (1.1 kg) spaghetti squash
1 teaspoon olive oil
Salt and pepper, to taste
Parsley leaves (garnish)

Directions:
At first, sprinkle some salt and pepper over the shrimp and keep them in a refrigerator until further use. Hit the Sauté function on your Instant Pot, then add the olive oil and red pepper flakes into it. Sauté for 1 minute. Add the shallot and cook for 3 minutes. Then add the garlic, cook for 1 minute. Add the dry wine, tomatoes, and whole spaghetti squash in the pot. Select Manual settings with medium pressure for 20 minutes. After the beep, do a Natural release. Remove the lid and the spaghetti squash. Cut squash in half, remove its seed and stab with a fork to form spaghetti strands out of it. Keep them aside. Select the Sauté function on your instant pot again, stir in shrimp. Mix well the shrimp with sauce.
To serve, top the spaghetti squash with shrimp and sauce. Garnish it with parsley.

Per Serving:
calories: 222 | fat: 4.4g | protein: 19.3g | carbs: 30.1g | fiber: 8.5g | sodium: 974mg

Shrimp and Potato Curry

Prep time: 5 minutes | Cook time: 9 minutes | Serves 8

Ingredients:
2 tablespoons olive oil
1½ medium onions, chopped
1½ teaspoons ground cumin
2 teaspoons red chili powder
teaspoons ground turmeric
medium white rose potatoes, diced
6 medium tomatoes, chopped
2 pounds (907 g) medium shrimp, peeled and deveined
1½ tablespoons fresh lemon juice
Salt, to taste
½ cup fresh cilantro, chopped

Directions:
Select the Sauté function on your Instant Pot. Add the oil and onions
then cook for 2 minutes.
Add the tomatoes, potatoes, cilantro, lemon juice and all the spices into
the pot and secure the lid.
Select the Manual function at medium pressure for 5 minutes.
Do a natural release then remove the lid. Stir shrimp into the pot.
Secure the lid again then set the Manual function with High Pressure
for 2 minutes.
After the beep, use Natural release and let it stand for 10 minutes.
Remove the lid and serve hot.

Per Serving:
calories: 197 | fat: 5.0g | protein: 18.1g | carbs: 20.3g | fiber: 3.9g |
sodium: 700mg

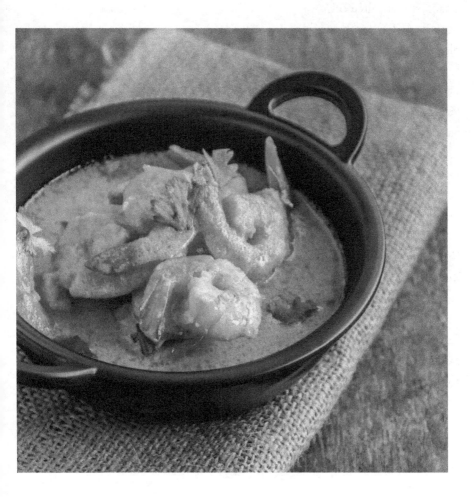

Sardines and Plum Tomato Curry

Prep time: 10 minutes | Cook time: 8 hours 2 minutes | Serves 4

Ingredients:
1 tablespoon olive oil
pound (454 g) fresh sardines, cubed
plum tomatoes, chopped finely
½ large onion, sliced
1 garlic clove, minced
½ cup tomato purée
Salt and ground black pepper, to taste

Directions:
Select the Sauté function on your Instant pot then add the oil and sardines to it.
Let it sauté for 2 minutes then add all the remaining ingredients.
Cover the lid and select Slow Cook function for 8 hours.
Remove the lid and stir the cooked curry.
Serve warm.

Per Serving:
calories: 292 | fat: 16.5g | protein: 28.9g | carbs: 6.0g | fiber: 1.3g | sodium: 398mg

Scallop Teriyaki

Prep time: 5 minutes | Cook time: 5 minutes | Serves 6

Ingredients:
2 pounds (907 g) jumbo sea scallops
2 tablespoons olive oil
6 tablespoons pure maple syrup
1 cup coconut aminos
1 teaspoon ground ginger
1 teaspoon garlic powder
1 teaspoon sea salt

Directions:
Add the olive oil to the Instant pot and heat it on the Sauté settings of your pot.
Add the scallops to the pot and cook for a minute from each side.
Stir in all the remaining ingredients in the pot and mix them well.
Secure the lid and select the Steam function to cook for 3 minutes.
After the beep, do a Quick release then remove the lid.
Serve hot.

Per Serving:
calories: 228 | fat: 5.3g | protein: 23.4g | carbs: 21.4g | fiber: 0.5g | sodium: 3664mg

Shrimp and Tomato Creole

Prep time: 20 minutes | Cook time: 7 hours 10 minutes | Serves 4

Ingredients:
1 pound (454 g) shrimp (peeled and deveined)
1 tablespoon olive oil
1 (28-ounce / 794-g) can crush whole tomatoes
1 cup celery stalk (sliced)
¾ cup chopped white onion
½ cup green bell pepper (chopped)
1 (8-ounce / 227-g) can tomato sauce
½ teaspoon minced garlic
¼ teaspoon ground black pepper
1 tablespoon Worcestershire sauce
4 drops hot pepper sauce
Salt, to taste
White rice for serving

Directions:
Put the oil to the Instant Pot along with all the ingredients except the shrimp. Secure the cooker lid and keep the pressure handle valve turned to the venting position. Select the Slow Cook function on your cooker and set it on medium heat. Let the mixture cook for 6 hours. Remove the lid afterwards and add the shrimp to the pot. Stir and let the shrimp cook for another 1 hour on Slow Cook function. Keep the lid covered with pressure release handle in the venting position.
To serve, pour the juicy shrimp creole over steaming white rice.

Per Serving:
calories: 231 | fat: 4.8g | protein: 27.6g | carbs: 23.8g | fiber: 6.1g | sodium: 646m

Fruits and Desserts

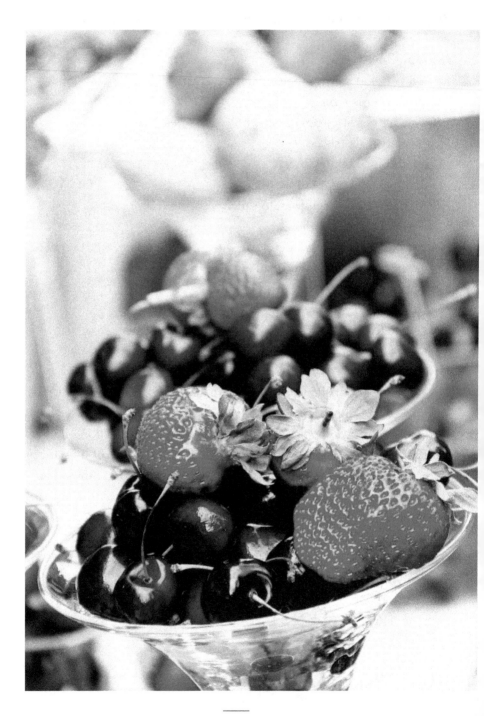

Mango and Coconut Frozen Pie

Prep time: 1 hour 10 minutes | Cook time: 0 minutes | Serves 8

Crust:
cup cashews
½ cup rolled oats 1 cup soft pitted dates
Filling:
large mangoes, peeled and chopped
½ cup unsweetened shredded coconut
1 cup unsweetened coconut milk
½ cup water

Directions:
Combine the ingredients for the crust in a food processor. Pulse to combine well.
Pour the mixture in an 8-inch springform pan, then press to coat the bottom. Set aside.
Combine the ingredients for the filling in the food processor, then pulse to purée until smooth.
Pour the filling over the crust, then use a spatula to spread the filling evenly. Put the pan in the freeze for 30 minutes.
Remove the pan from the freezer and allow to sit for 15 minutes under room temperature before serving.

Per Serving: (1 slice) calories: 426 | fat: 28.2g | protein: 8.1g | carbs: 14.9g | fiber: 6.0g | sodium: 174mg

Mini Nuts and Fruits Crumble

Prep time: 15 minutes | Cook time: 15 minutes | Serves 6

Ingredients:
¼ cup coarsely chopped hazelnuts
1 cup coarsely chopped walnuts
1 teaspoon ground cinnamon
Sea salt, to taste
1 tablespoon melted coconut oil Filling:
6 fresh figs, quartered
2 nectarines, pitted and sliced
cup fresh blueberries
teaspoons lemon zest
½ cup raw honey
1 teaspoon vanilla extract

Directions:
Combine the ingredients for the topping in a bowl. Stir to mix well. Set aside until ready to use.
Preheat the oven to 375°F (190°C).
Combine the ingredients for the fillings in a bowl. Stir to mix well.
Divide the filling in six ramekins, then divide and top with nut topping.
Bake in the preheated oven for 15 minutes or until the topping is lightly browned and the filling is frothy.
Serve immediately.

Per Serving:
calories: 336 | fat: 18.8g | protein: 6.3g | carbs: 41.9g | fiber: 6.0g | sodium: 31mg

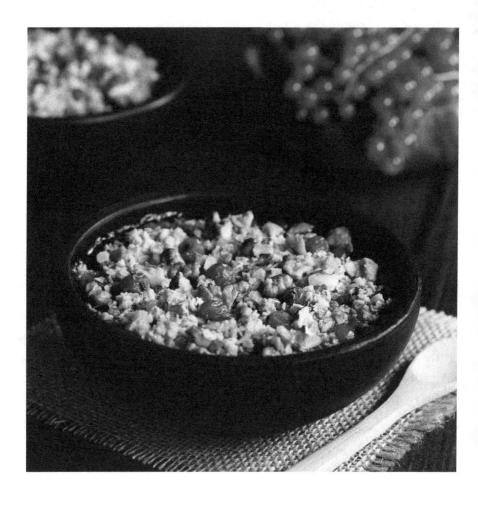

Rice Pudding with Roasted Orange

Prep time: 10 minutes | Cook time: 19 to 20 minutes | Serves 6

Ingredients:

2 medium oranges

2 teaspoons extra-virgin olive oil

⅛ teaspoon kosher salt

2 large eggs

2 cups unsweetened almond milk

1 cup orange juice

1 cup uncooked instant brown rice

¼ cup honey

½ teaspoon ground cinnamon

1 teaspoon vanilla extract

Cooking spray

Directions:

Preheat the oven to 450°F (235°C). Spritz a large, rimmed baking sheet with cooking spray. Set aside.

Slice the unpeeled oranges into ¼-inch rounds. Brush with the oil and sprinkle with salt. Place the slices on the baking sheet and roast for 4 minutes. Flip the slices and roast for 4 more minutes, or until they begin to brown. Remove from the oven and set aside.

Crack the eggs into a medium bowl. In a medium saucepan, whisk together the milk, orange juice, rice, honey and cinnamon. Bring to a boil over medium-high heat, stirring constantly. Reduce the heat to mediumlow and simmer for 10 minutes, stirring occasionally.

Using a measuring cup, scoop out ½ cup of the hot rice mixture and whisk it into the eggs. While constantly stirring the mixture in the pan, slowly pour the egg mixture back into the saucepan. Cook on low heat for 1 to 2 minutes, or until thickened, stirring constantly. Remove from the heat and stir in the vanilla.

Let the pudding stand for a few minutes for the rice to soften. The rice will be cooked but slightly chewy. For softer rice, let stand for another half hour.

Top with the roasted oranges. Serve warm or at room temperature.

Per Serving:

calories: 204 | fat: 6.0g | protein: 5.0g | carbs: 34.0g | fiber: 1.0g | sodium: 148mg

Cherry Walnut Brownies

Prep time: 10 minutes | Cook time: 20 minutes | Serves 9

Ingredients:
2 large eggs
½ cup 2% plain Greek yogurt
½ cup sugar
⅓ cup honey
¼ cup extra-virgin olive oil
1 teaspoon vanilla extract
½ cup whole-wheat pastry flour
⅓ cup unsweetened dark chocolate cocoa powder
¼ teaspoon baking powder
¼ teaspoon salt
⅓ cup chopped walnuts
9 fresh cherries, stemmed and pitted
Cooking spray

Directions:
Preheat the oven to 375°F (190°C) and set the rack in the middle of the oven. Spritz a square baking pan with cooking spray. In a large bowl, whisk together the eggs, yogurt, sugar, honey, oil and vanilla.
In a medium bowl, stir together the flour, cocoa powder, baking powder and salt. Add the flour mixture to the egg mixture and whisk until all the dry ingredients are incorporated. Fold in the walnuts.
Pour the batter into the prepared pan. Push the cherries into the batter, three to a row in three rows, so one will be at the center of each brownie once you cut them into squares. Bake the brownies for 20 minutes, or until just set. Remove from the oven and place on a rack to cool for 5 minutes. Cut into nine squares and serve.

Per Serving: calories: 154 | fat: 6.0g | protein: 3.0g | carbs: 24.0g | fiber: 2.0g | sodium: 125mg

Citrus Cranberry and Quinoa Energy Bites

Prep time: 25 minutes | Cook time: 0 minutes | Makes 12 bites

Ingredients:
2 tablespoons almond butter
2 tablespoons maple syrup
¾ cup cooked quinoa
1 tablespoon dried cranberries
1 tablespoon chia seeds
¼ cup ground almonds
¼ cup sesame seeds, toasted
Zest of 1 orange
½ teaspoon vanilla extract

Directions:
Line a baking sheet with parchment paper.
Combine the butter and maple syrup in a bowl. Stir to mix well.
Fold in the remaining ingredients and stir until the mixture holds together and smooth.
Divide the mixture into 12 equal parts, then shape each part into a ball.
Arrange the balls on the baking sheet, then refrigerate for at least 15 minutes.
Serve chilled.

Per Serving: (1 bite)
calories: 110 | fat: 10.8g | protein: 3.1g | carbs: 4.9g | fiber: 3.0g | sodium: 211mg

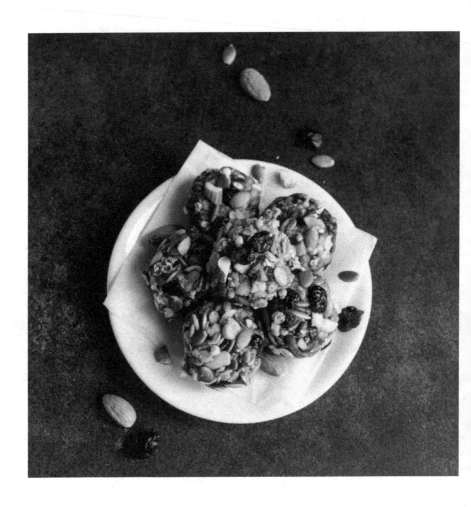

Lemony Blackberry Granita

Prep time: 10 minutes | Cook time: 0 minutes | Serves 4

Ingredients:
1 pound (454 g) fresh blackberries
1 teaspoon chopped fresh thyme
¼ cup freshly squeezed lemon juice
½ cup raw honey
½ cup water

Directions:
Put all the ingredients in a food processor, then pulse to purée.
Pour the mixture through a sieve into a baking dish. Discard the seeds remain in the sieve.
Put the baking dish in the freezer for 2 hours. Remove the dish from the refrigerator and stir to break any frozen parts.
Return the dish back to the freezer for an hour, then stir to break any frozen parts again.
Return the dish to the freezer for 4 hours until the granita is completely frozen.
Remove it from the freezer and mash to serve.

Per Serving:
calories: 183 | fat: 1.1g | protein: 2.2g | carbs: 45.9g | fiber: 6.0g | sodium: 6mg

Lemony Tea and Chia Pudding

Prep time: 30 minutes | Cook time: 0 minutes | Serves 3 to 4

Ingredients:
2 teaspoons matcha green tea powder (optional)
2 tablespoons ground chia seeds
to 2 dates
cups unsweetened coconut milk
Zest and juice of 1 lime

Directions:
Put all the ingredients in a food processor and pulse until creamy and smooth.
Pour the mixture in a bowl, then wrap in plastic. Store in the refrigerator for at least 20 minutes, then serve chilled.

Per Serving:
calories: 225 | fat: 20.1g | protein: 3.2g | carbs: 5.9g | fiber: 5.0g | sodium: 314mg

Honey Baked Cinnamon Apples

Prep time: 5 minutes | Cook time: 20 minutes | Serves 2

Ingredients:
1 teaspoon extra-virgin olive oil
4 firm apples, peeled, cored, and sliced
½ teaspoon salt
1½ teaspoons ground cinnamon, divided 2 tablespoons unsweetened almond milk
2 tablespoons honey

Directions:
Preheat the oven to 375°F (190°C). Coat a small casserole dish with the olive oil.
Toss the apple slices with the salt and ½ teaspoon of the cinnamon in a medium bowl. Spread the apples in the prepared casserole dish and bake in the preheated oven for 20 minutes.
Meanwhile, in a small saucepan, heat the milk, honey, and remaining 1 teaspoon of cinnamon over medium heat, stirring frequently.
When it reaches a simmer, remove the pan from the heat and cover to keep warm.
Divide the apple slices between 2 plates and pour the sauce over the apples. Serve warm.

Per Serving:
calories: 310 | fat: 3.4g | protein: 1.7g | carbs: 68.5g | fiber: 12.6g | sodium: 593mg

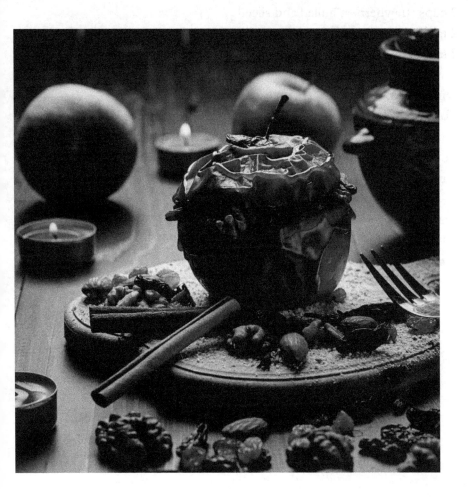

Strawberries with Balsamic Vinegar

Prep time: 5 minutes | Cook time: 0 minutes | Serves 2

Ingredients:
2 cups strawberries, hulled and sliced
2 tablespoons sugar
2 tablespoons balsamic vinegar

Directions:
Place the sliced strawberries in a bowl, sprinkle with the sugar, and drizzle lightly with the balsamic vinegar.
Toss to combine well and allow to sit for about 10 minutes before serving.

Per Serving:
calories: 92 | fat: 0.4g | protein: 1.0g | carbs: 21.7g | fiber: 2.9g | sodium: 5mg

Banana, Cranberry, and Oat Bars

Prep time: 15 minutes | Cook time: 40 minutes | Makes 16 bars

Ingredients:
2 tablespoon extra-virgin olive oil
2 medium ripe bananas, mashed
½ cup almond butter
½ cup maple syrup
⅓ cup dried cranberries
1½ cups old-fashioned rolled oats
¼ cup oat flour
¼ cup ground flaxseed
¼ teaspoon ground cloves
½ cup shredded coconut
½ teaspoon ground cinnamon
1 teaspoon vanilla extract

Directions:
Preheat the oven to 400°F (205°C). Line a 8-inch square pan with parchment paper, then grease with olive oil.
Combine the mashed bananas, almond butter, and maple syrup in a bowl. Stir to mix well.
Mix in the remaining ingredients and stir to mix well until thick and sticky.
Spread the mixture evenly on the square pan with a spatula, then bake in the preheated oven for 40 minutes or until a toothpick inserted in the center comes out clean.
Remove them from the oven and slice into 16 bars to serve.

Per Serving:
calories: 145 | fat: 7.2g | protein: 3.1g | carbs: 18.9g | fiber: 2.0g | sodium: 3m

Chocolate, Almond, and Cherry Clusters

Prep time: 15 minutes | Cook time: 3 minutes | Makes 10 clusters

Ingredients:
1 cup dark chocolate (60% cocoa or higher), chopped
1 tablespoon coconut oil
½ cup dried cherries
1 cup roasted salted almonds

Directions:
Line a baking sheet with parchment paper.
Melt the chocolate and coconut oil in a saucepan for 3 minutes. Stir constantly.
Turn off the heat and mix in the cherries and almonds.
Drop the mixture on the baking sheet with a spoon. Place the sheet in the refrigerator and chill for at least 1 hour or until firm.
Serve chilled.

Per Serving:
calories: 197 | fat: 13.2g | protein: 4.1g | carbs: 17.8g | fiber: 4.0g | sodium: 57mg

Chocolate and Avocado Mousse

Prep time: 40 minutes | Cook time: 5 minutes | Serves 4 to 6

Ingredients:
8 ounces (227 g) dark chocolate (60% cocoa or higher), chopped
¼ cup unsweetened coconut milk
2 tablespoons coconut oil
2 ripe avocados, deseeded
¼ cup raw honey
Sea salt, to taste

Directions:
Put the chocolate in a saucepan. Pour in the coconut milk and add the coconut oil.
Cook for 3 minutes or until the chocolate and coconut oil melt. Stir constantly.
Put the avocado in a food processor, then drizzle with honey and melted chocolate. Pulse to combine until smooth.
Pour the mixture in a serving bowl, then sprinkle with salt. Refrigerate to chill for 30 minutes and serve.

Per Serving:
calories: 654 | fat: 46.8g | protein: 7.2g | carbs: 55.9g | fiber: 9.0g | sodium: 112mg

Apple Compote

Prep time: 15 minutes | Cook time: 10 minutes | Serves 4

Ingredients:
6 apples, peeled, cored, and chopped
¼ cup raw honey
1 teaspoon ground cinnamon
¼ cup apple juice
Sea salt, to taste

Directions:
Put all the ingredients in a stockpot. Stir to mix well, then cook over medium-high heat for 10 minutes or until the apples are glazed by honey and lightly saucy. Stir constantly.
Serve immediately.

Per Serving:
calories: 246 | fat: 0.9g | protein: 1.2g | carbs: 66.3g | fiber: 9.0g | sodium: 62mg

Peanut Butter and Chocolate Balls

Prep time: 45 minutes | Cook time: 0 minutes | Serves 15 balls

Ingredients:
¾ cup creamy peanut butter
¼ cup unsweetened cocoa powder
2 tablespoons softened almond butter
½ teaspoon vanilla extract
1¾ cups maple syrup

Directions:
Line a baking sheet with parchment paper.
Combine all the ingredients in a bowl. Stir to mix well.
Divide the mixture into 15 parts and shape each part into a 1-inch ball.
Arrange the balls on the baking sheet and refrigerate for at least 30 minutes, then serve chilled.

Per Serving:(1 ball)
calories: 146 | fat: 8.1g | protein: 4.2g | carbs: 16.9g | fiber: 1.0g | sodium: 70mg

Grilled Stone Fruit with Honey

Prep time: 8 minutes | Cook time: 6 minutes | Serves 2

Ingredients:
3 apricots, halved and pitted
2 plums, halved and pitted
2 peaches, halved and pitted ½ cup low-fat ricotta cheese
2 tablespoons honey
Cooking spray

Directions:
Preheat the grill to medium heat. Spray the grill grates with cooking spray.
Arrange the fruit, cut side down, on the grill, and cook for 2 to 3 minutes per side, or until lightly charred and softened.
Serve warm with a sprinkle of cheese and a drizzle of honey.

Per Serving:
calories: 298 | fat: 7.8g | protein: 11.9g | carbs: 45.2g | fiber: 4.3g | sodium: 259mg

Mascarpone Baked Pears

Prep time: 10 minutes | Cook time: 20 minutes | Serves 2

Ingredients:

2 ripe pears, peeled
1 tablespoon plus 2 teaspoons honey, divided
1 teaspoon vanilla, divided
¼ teaspoon ground coriander
¼ teaspoon ginger
¼ cup minced walnuts
¼ cup mascarpone cheese
Pinch salt
Cooking spray

Directions:

Preheat the oven to 350°F (180°C). Spray a small baking dish with cooking spray.

Slice the pears in half lengthwise. Using a spoon, scoop out the core from each piece. Put the pears, cut side up, in the baking dish.

Whisk together 1 tablespoon of honey, ½ teaspoon of vanilla, ginger, and coriander in a small bowl. Pour this mixture evenly over the pear halves.

Scatter the walnuts over the pear halves.

Bake in the preheated oven for 20 minutes, or until the pears are golden and you're able to pierce them easily with a knife.

Meanwhile, combine the mascarpone cheese with the remaining 2 teaspoons of honey, ½ teaspoon of vanilla, and a pinch of salt. Stir to combine well.

Divide the mascarpone among the warm pear halves and serve.

Per Serving:

calories: 308 | fat: 16.0g | protein: 4.1g | carbs: 42.7g | fiber: 6.0g | sodium: 88mg

Coconut Blueberries with Brown Rice

Prep time: 55 minutes | Cook time: 10 minutes | Serves 4

Ingredients:
cup fresh blueberries
cups unsweetened coconut milk
teaspoon ground ginger
¼ cup maple syrup
Sea salt, to taste
cups cooked brown rice

Directions:
Put all the ingredients, except for the brown rice, in a pot. Stir to combine well.
Cook over medium-high heat for 7 minutes or until the blueberries are tender.
Pour in the brown rice and cook for 3 more minute or until the rice is soft. Stir constantly.
Serve immediately.

Per Serving:
calories: 470 | fat: 24.8g | protein: 6.2g | carbs: 60.1g | fiber: 5.0g | sodium: 75mg

Blueberry and Oat Crisp

Prep time: 15 minutes | Cook time: 20 minutes | Serves 4

Ingredients:
2 tablespoons coconut oil, melted, plus more for greasing
4 cups fresh blueberries
Juice of ½ lemon
2 teaspoons lemon zest
¼ cup maple syrup
1 cup gluten-free rolled oats
½ cup chopped pecans
½ teaspoon ground cinnamon
Sea salt, to taste

Directions:
Preheat the oven to 350°F (180°C). Grease a baking sheet with coconut oil.
Combine the blueberries, lemon juice and zest, and maple syrup in a bowl. Stir to mix well, then spread the mixture on the baking sheet.
Combine the remaining ingredients in a small bowl. Stir to mix well. Pour the mixture over the blueberries mixture.
Bake in the preheated oven for 20 minutes or until the oats are golden brown.
Serve immediately with spoons.

Per Serving:
calories: 496 | fat: 32.9g | protein: 5.1g | carbs: 50.8g | fiber: 7.0g | sodium: 41mg

Frozen Mango Raspberry Delight

Prep time: 5 minutes | Cook time: 0 minutes | Serves 2

Ingredients:
3 cups frozen raspberries
1 mango, peeled and pitted
1 peach, peeled and pitted
1 teaspoon honey

Directions:
Place all the ingredients into a blender and purée, adding some water as needed.
Put in the freezer for 10 minutes to firm up if desired. Serve chilled or at room temperature.

Per Serving:
calories: 276 | fat: 2.1g | protein: 4.5g | carbs: 60.3g | fiber: 17.5g | sodium: 4mg

Mixed Berry Crisp

Prep time: 15 minutes | Cook time: 30 minutes | Serves 2

Ingredients:
1½ cups frozen mixed berries, thawed
1 tablespoon coconut sugar 1 tablespoon almond butter
¼ cup oats
¼ cup pecans

Directions:
Preheat the oven to 350°F (180°C).
Divide the mixed berries between 2 ramekins
Place the coconut sugar, almond butter, oats, and pecans in a food processor, and pulse a few times, until the mixture resembles damp sand.
Divide the crumble topping over the mixed berries.
Put the ramekins on a sheet pan and bake for 30 minutes, or until the top is golden and the berries are bubbling.
Serve warm.

Per Serving:
calories: 268 | fat: 17.0g | protein: 4.1g | carbs: 26.8g | fiber: 6.0g | sodium: 44mg

Mint Banana Chocolate Sorbet

Prep time: 4 hours 5 minutes | Cook time: 0 minutes | Serves 1

Ingredients:
1 frozen banana
tablespoon almond butter
tablespoons minced fresh mint
2 to 3 tablespoons dark chocolate chips (60% cocoa or higher)
2 to 3 tablespoons goji (optional)

Directions:
Put the banana, butter, and mint in a food processor. Pulse to purée until creamy and smooth.
Add the chocolate and goji, then pulse for several more times to combine well.
Pour the mixture in a bowl or a ramekin, then freeze for at least 4 hours before serving chilled.

Per Serving:
calories: 213 | fat: 9.8g | protein: 3.1g | carbs: 2.9g | fiber: 4.0g | sodium: 155mg

Glazed Pears with Hazelnuts

Prep time: 10 minutes | Cook time: 20 minutes | Serves 4

Ingredients:
4 pears, peeled, cored, and quartered lengthwise
1 cup apple juice
1 tablespoon grated fresh ginger
½ cup pure maple syrup
¼ cup chopped hazelnuts

Directions:
Put the pears in a pot, then pour in the apple juice. Bring to a boil over medium-high heat, then reduce the heat to medium-low. Stir constantly.
Cover and simmer for an additional 15 minutes or until the pears are tender.
Meanwhile, combine the ginger and maple syrup in a saucepan. Bring to a boil over medium-high heat. Stir frequently. Turn off the heat and transfer the syrup to a small bowl and let sit until ready to use.
Transfer the pears in a large serving bowl with a slotted spoon, then top the pears with syrup.
Spread the hazelnuts over the pears and serve immediately.

Per Serving:
calories: 287 | fat: 3.1g | protein: 2.2g | carbs: 66.9g | fiber: 7.0g | sodium: 8mg

Sweet Spiced Pumpkin Pudding

Prep time: 2 hours 10 minutes | Cook time: 0 minutes | Serves 6

Ingredients:
cup pure pumpkin purée
cups unsweetened coconut milk
teaspoon ground cinnamon
¼ teaspoon ground nutmeg
½ teaspoon ground ginger
Pinch cloves
¼ cup pure maple syrup
tablespoons chopped pecans, for garnish

Directions:
Combine all the ingredients, except for the chopped pecans, in a large bowl. Stir to mix well.

Wrap the bowl in plastic and refrigerate for at least 2 hours.

Remove the bowl from the refrigerator and discard the plastic. Spread the pudding with pecans and serve chilled.

Per Serving:
calories: 249 | fat: 21.1g | protein: 2.8g | carbs: 17.2g | fiber: 3.0g | sodium: 46mg

Spiced Sweet Pecans

Prep time: 4 minutes | Cook time: 17 minutes | Serves 4

Ingredients:
1 cup pecan halves
3 tablespoons almond butter
1 teaspoon ground cinnamon
½ teaspoon ground nutmeg
¼ cup raw honey
¼ teaspoon sea salt

Directions:
Preheat the oven to 350°F (180°C). Line a baking sheet with parchment paper.
Combine all the ingredients in a bowl. Stir to mix well, then spread the mixture in the single layer on the baking sheet with a spatula.
Bake in the preheated oven for 16 minutes or until the pecan halves are well browned.
Serve immediately.

Per Serving:
calories: 324 | fat: 29.8g | protein: 3.2g | carbs: 13.9g | fiber: 4.0g | sodium: 180mg

Greek Yogurt Affogato with Pistachios

Prep time: 5 minutes | Cook time: 0 minutes | Serves 4

Ingredients:
24 ounces (680 g) vanilla Greek yogurt
2 teaspoons sugar
4 shots hot espresso
4 tablespoons chopped unsalted pistachios
4 tablespoons dark chocolate chips

Directions:
Spoon the yogurt into four bowls or tall glasses.
Mix ½ teaspoon of sugar into each of the espresso shots.
Pour one shot of the hot espresso over each bowl of yogurt.
Top each bowl with 1 tablespoon of the pistachios and 1 tablespoon of the chocolate chips and serve.

Per Serving:
calories: 190 | fat: 6.0g | protein: 20.0g | carbs: 14.0g | fiber: 1.0g | sodium: 99mg

Fruit and Nut Chocolate Bark

Prep time: 15 minutes | Cook time: 2 minutes | Serves 2

Ingredients:
tablespoons chopped nuts
ounces (85 g) dark chocolate chips
¼ cup chopped dried fruit (blueberries, apricots, figs, prunes, or any combination of those)

Directions:
Line a sheet pan with parchment paper and set aside.
Add the nuts to a skillet over medium-high heat and toast for 60 seconds, or just fragrant. Set aside to cool.
Put the chocolate chips in a microwave-safe glass bowl and microwave on High for 1 minute.
Stir the chocolate and allow any unmelted chips to warm and melt. If desired, heat for an additional 20 to 30 seconds.
Transfer the chocolate to the prepared sheet pan. Scatter the dried fruit and toasted nuts over the chocolate evenly and gently pat in so they stick.
Place the sheet pan in the refrigerator for at least 1 hour to let the chocolate harden.
When ready, break into pieces and serve.

Per Serving:
calories: 285 | fat: 16.1g | protein: 4.0g | carbs: 38.7g | fiber: 2.0g | sodium: 2mg

Pecan and Carrot Cake

Prep time: 15 minutes | Cook time: 45 minutes | Serves 12

Ingredients:

½ cup coconut oil, at room temperature, plus more for greasing the baking dish

2 teaspoons pure vanilla extract

¼ cup pure maple syrup

6 eggs

½ cup coconut flour

1 teaspoon baking powder

1 teaspoon baking soda

½ teaspoon ground nutmeg

1 teaspoon ground cinnamon

⅛ teaspoon sea salt

½ cup chopped pecans

3 cups finely grated carrots

Directions:

Preheat the oven to 350°F (180°C). Grease a 13-by-9-inch baking dish with coconut oil. Combine the vanilla extract, maple syrup, and ½ cup of coconut oil in a large bowl. Stir to mix well. Break the eggs in the bowl and whisk to combine well. Set aside. Combine the coconut flour, baking powder, baking soda, nutmeg, cinnamon, and salt in a separate bowl. Stir to mix well. Make a well in the center of the flour mixture, then pour the egg mixture into the well. Stir to combine well. Add the pecans and carrots to the bowl and toss to mix well. Pour the mixture in the single layer on the baking dish. Bake in the preheated oven for 45 minutes or until puffed and the cake spring back when lightly press with your fingers. Remove the cake from the oven. Allow to cool for at least 15 minutes, then serve.

Per Serving: calories: 255 | fat: 21.2g | protein: 5.1g | carbs: 12.8g | fiber: 2.0g | sodium: 202mg

Raspberry Yogurt Basted Cantaloupe

Prep time: 15 minutes | Cook time: 0 minutes | Serves 6

Ingredients:
2 cups fresh raspberries, mashed
1 cup plain coconut yogurt
½ teaspoon vanilla extract
1 cantaloupe, peeled and sliced
½ cup toasted coconut flakes

Directions:
Combine the mashed raspberries with yogurt and vanilla extract in a small bowl. Stir to mix well.
Place the cantaloupe slices on a platter, then top with raspberry mixture and spread with toasted coconut.
Serve immediately.

Per Serving:
calories: 75 | fat: 4.1g | protein: 1.2g | carbs: 10.9g | fiber: 6.0g | sodium: 36mg

Crispy Sesame Cookies

Prep time: 5 minutes | Cook time: 8 to 10 minutes | Serves 14 to 16

Ingredients:
1 cup hulled sesame seeds
1 cup sugar
8 tablespoons almond butter
2 large eggs
1¼ cups flour

Directions:
Preheat the oven to 350°F (180°C).
Toast the sesame seeds on a baking sheet for 3 minutes. Set aside and let cool.
Using a mixer, whisk together the sugar and butter. Add the eggs one at a time until well blended. Add the flour and toasted sesame seeds and mix until well blended.
Drop spoonfuls of cookie dough onto a baking sheet and form them into round balls, about 1-inch in diameter, similar to a walnut.
Put in the oven and bake for 5 to 7 minutes, or until golden brown.
Let the cookies cool for 5 minutes before serving.

Per Serving:
calories: 218 | fat: 12.0g | protein: 4.0g | carbs: 25.0g | fiber: 2.0g | sodium: 58mg

Crunchy Almond Cookies

Prep time: 5 minutes | Cook time: 5 to 7 minutes | Serves 4 to 6

Ingredients:
½ cup sugar
8 tablespoons almond butter
1 large egg
1½ cups all-purpose flour
1 cup ground almonds

Directions:
Preheat the oven to 375°F (190°C). Line a baking sheet with parchment paper.
Using a mixer, whisk together the sugar and butter. Add the egg and mix until combined. Alternately add the flour and ground almonds, ½ cup at a time, while the mixer is on slow.
Drop 1 tablespoon of the dough on the prepared baking sheet, keeping the cookies at least 2 inches apart.
Put the baking sheet in the oven and bake for about 5 to 7 minutes, or until the cookies start to turn brown around the edges.
Let cool for 5 minutes before serving.

Per Serving:
calories: 604 | fat: 36.0g | protein: 11.0g | carbs: 63.0g | fiber: 4.0g | sodium: 181mg

Apple and Berries Ambrosia

Prep time: 15 minutes | Cook time: 0 minutes | Serves 4

Ingredients:
2 cups unsweetened coconut milk, chilled
2 tablespoons raw honey
apple, peeled, cored, and chopped
cups fresh raspberries
2 cups fresh blueberries

Directions:
Spoon the chilled milk in a large bowl, then mix in the honey. Stir to mix well.
Then mix in the remaining ingredients. Stir to coat the fruits well and serve immediately.

Per Serving:
calories: 386 | fat: 21.1g | protein: 4.2g | carbs: 45.9g | fiber: 11.0g | sodium: 16mg

Berry and Rhubarb Cobbler

Prep time: 15 minutes | Cook time: 35 minutes | Serves 8

Cobbler:
cup fresh raspberries
cups fresh blueberries
1 cup sliced (½-inch) rhubarb pieces
tablespoon arrowroot powder
¼ cup unsweetened apple juice
tablespoons melted coconut oil
¼ cup raw honey Topping:
1 cup almond flour
1 tablespoon arrowroot powder
½ cup shredded coconut
¼ cup raw honey
½ cup coconut oil

Make the Cobbler:
Preheat the oven to 350°F (180°C). Grease a baking dish with melted coconut oil. Combine the ingredients for the cobbler in a large bowl. Stir to mix well. Spread the mixture in the single layer on the baking dish. Set aside. Make the Topping Combine the almond flour, arrowroot powder, and coconut in a bowl. Stir to mix well. Fold in the honey and coconut oil. Stir with a fork until the mixture crumbled. Spread the topping over the cobbler, then bake in the preheated oven for 35 minutes or until frothy and golden brown. Serve immediately.

Per Serving:
calories: 305 | fat: 22.1g | protein: 3.2g | carbs: 29.8g | fiber: 4.0g | sodium: 3mg

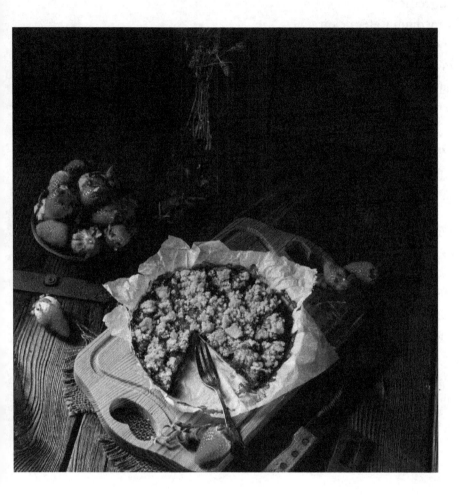

Watermelon and Blueberry Salad

Prep time: 5 minutes | Cook time: 0 minutes | Serves 6 to 8

Ingredients:
1 medium watermelon
cup fresh blueberries
⅓ cup honey
tablespoons lemon juice
2 tablespoons finely chopped fresh mint leaves

Directions:
Cut the watermelon into 1-inch cubes. Put them in a bowl.
Evenly distribute the blueberries over the watermelon.
In a separate bowl, whisk together the honey, lemon juice and mint.
Drizzle the mint dressing over the watermelon and blueberries.
Serve cold.

Per Serving:
calories: 238 | fat: 1.0g | protein: 4.0g | carbs: 61.0g | fiber: 3.0g |
sodium: 11mg

Grilled Peaches with Whipped Ricotta

Prep time: 5 minutes | Cook time: 14 to 22 minutes | Serves 4

Ingredients:
4 peaches, halved and pitted
2 teaspoons extra-virgin olive oil
¾ cup whole-milk Ricotta cheese
1 tablespoon honey
¼ teaspoon freshly grated nutmeg
4 sprigs mint
Cooking spray

Directions:
Spritz a grill pan with cooking spray. Heat the grill pan to medium heat. Place a large, empty bowl in the refrigerator to chill.

Brush the peaches all over with the oil. Place half of the peaches, cut-side down, on the grill pan and cook for 3 to 5 minutes, or until grill marks appear.

Using tongs, turn the peaches over. Cover the grill pan with aluminum foil and cook for 4 to 6 minutes, or until the peaches are easily pierced with a sharp knife. Set aside to cool. Repeat with the remaining peaches.

Remove the bowl from the refrigerator and add the Ricotta. Using an electric beater, beat the Ricotta on high for 2 minutes. Add the honey and nutmeg and beat for 1 more minute.

Divide the cooled peaches among 4 serving bowls. Top with the Ricotta mixture and a sprig of mint and serve.

Per Serving:
calories: 176 | fat: 8.0g | protein: 8.0g | carbs: 20.0g | fiber: 3.0g | sodium: 63mg

Walnut and Date Balls

Prep time: 5 minutes | Cook time: 8 to 10 minutes | Serves 6 to 8

Ingredients:
1 cup walnuts
1 cup unsweetened shredded coconut
14 medjool dates, pitted
8 tablespoons almond butter

Directions:
Preheat the oven to 350°F (180°C).
Put the walnuts on a baking sheet and toast in the oven for 5 minutes.
Put the shredded coconut on a clean baking sheet. Toast for about 3 to
5 minutes, or until it turns golden brown. Once done, remove it from
the oven and put it in a shallow bowl. In a food processor, process the
toasted walnuts until they have a medium chop. Transfer the chopped
walnuts into a medium bowl. Add the dates and butter to the food
processor and blend until the dates become a thick paste. Pour the
chopped walnuts into the food processor with the dates and pulse just
until the mixture is combined, about 5 to 7 pulses. Remove the mixture
from the food processor and scrape it into a large bowl. To make the
balls, spoon 1 to 2 tablespoons of the date mixture into the palm of
your hand and roll around between your hands until you form a ball.
Put the ball on a clean, lined baking sheet. Repeat until all the mixture
is formed into balls. Roll each ball in the toasted coconut until the
outside of the ball is coated. Put the ball back on the baking sheet and
repeat. Put all the balls into the refrigerator for 20 minutes before
serving. Store any leftovers in the refrigerator in an airtight container.

Per Serving:
calories: 489 | fat: 35.0g | protein: 5.0g | carbs: 48.0g | fiber: 7.0g |
sodium: 114mg

Orange Mug Cakes

Prep time: 10 minutes | Cook time: 3 minutes | Serves 2

Ingredients:
6 tablespoons flour
2 tablespoons sugar
1 teaspoon orange zest
½ teaspoon baking powder
Pinch salt
egg
tablespoons olive oil
2 tablespoons unsweetened almond milk
2 tablespoons freshly squeezed orange juice
½ teaspoon orange extract ½ teaspoon vanilla extract

Directions:
Combine the flour, sugar, orange zest, baking powder, and salt in a small bowl.
In another bowl, whisk together the egg, olive oil, milk, orange juice, orange extract, and vanilla extract.
Add the dry ingredients to the wet ingredients and stir to incorporate. The batter will be thick.
Divide the mixture into two small mugs. Microwave each mug separately. The small ones should take about 60 seconds, and one large mug should take about 90 seconds, but microwaves can vary.
Cool for 5 minutes before serving.

Per Serving:
calories: 303 | fat: 16.9g | protein: 6.0g | carbs: 32.5g | fiber: 1.0g | sodium: 118mg

Cozy Superfood Hot Chocolate

Prep time: 5 minutes | Cook time: 8 minutes | Serves 2

Ingredients:

2 cups unsweetened almond milk
1 tablespoon avocado oil
tablespoon collagen protein powder
teaspoons coconut sugar
2 tablespoons cocoa powder
1 teaspoon ground cinnamon
1 teaspoon ground ginger
1 teaspoon vanilla extract
½ teaspoon ground turmeric
Dash salt
Dash cayenne pepper (optional)

Directions:

In a small saucepan over medium heat, warm the almond milk and avocado oil for about 7 minutes, stirring frequently.
Fold in the protein powder, which will only properly dissolve in a heated liquid.
Stir in the coconut sugar and cocoa powder until melted and dissolved.
Carefully transfer the warm liquid into a blender, along with the cinnamon, ginger, vanilla, turmeric, salt, and cayenne pepper (if desired). Blend for 15 seconds until frothy.
Serve immediately.

Per Serving:

calories: 217 | fat: 11.0g | protein: 11.2g | carbs: 14.8g | fiber: 6.0g | sodium: 202mg

Sauces, Dips, and Dressings

Homemade Blackened Seasoning

Prep time: 10 minutes | Cook time: 0 minutes | Makes about ½ cup

Ingredients:
2 tablespoons smoked paprika
2 tablespoons garlic powder 2 tablespoons onion powder
1 tablespoon sweet paprika
1 teaspoon dried dill
1 teaspoon freshly ground black pepper
½ teaspoon ground mustard
¼ teaspoon celery seeds

Directions:
Add all the ingredients to a small bowl and mix well.
Serve immediately, or transfer to an airtight container and store in a cool, dry and dark place for up to 3 months.

Per Serving: (1 tablespoon)
calories: 22 | fat: 0.9g | protein: 1.0g | carbs: 4.7g | fiber: 1.0g | sodium: 2mg

Not Old Bay Seasoning

Prep time: 10 minutes | Cook time: 0 minutes | Makes about ½ cup

Ingredients:
3 tablespoons sweet paprika

tablespoon mustard seeds

tablespoons celery seeds

2 teaspoons freshly ground black pepper

1½ teaspoons cayenne pepper

1 teaspoon red pepper flakes

½ teaspoon ground ginger

½ teaspoon ground nutmeg

½ teaspoon ground cinnamon

¼ teaspoon ground cloves

Directions:
Mix together all the ingredients in an airtight container until well combined.

You can store it in a cool, dry, and dark place for up to 3 months.

Per Serving: (1 tablespoon)

calories: 26 | fat: 1.9g | protein: 1.1g | carbs: 3.6g | fiber: 2.1g | sodium: 3mg

Ginger Teriyaki Sauce

Prep time: 5 minutes | Cook time: 0 minutes | Serves 2

Ingredients:
¼ cup pineapple juice
¼ cup low-sodium soy sauce
2 tablespoons packed coconut sugar
1 tablespoon grated fresh ginger
1 tablespoon arrowroot powder or cornstarch
1 teaspoon garlic powder

Directions:
Whisk the pineapple juice, soy sauce, coconut sugar, ginger, arrowroot powder, and garlic powder together in a small bowl.
Store in an airtight container in the fridge for up to 5 days.

Per Serving:
calories: 37 | fat: 0.1g | protein: 1.1g | carbs: 12.0g | fiber: 0g | sodium: 881mg

Aioli

Prep time: 5 minutes | Cook time: 0 minutes | Makes ½ cup

Ingredients:
½ cup plain Greek yogurt
2 teaspoons Dijon mustard
½ teaspoon hot sauce
¼ teaspoon raw honey
Pinch salt

Directions:
In a small bowl, whisk together the yogurt, mustard, hot sauce, honey, and salt.
Serve immediately or refrigerate in an airtight container for up to 3 days.

Per Serving:
calories: 47 | fat: 2.5g | protein: 2.1g | carbs: 3.5g | fiber: 0g | sodium: 231mg

Cheesy Pea Pesto

Prep time: 5 minutes | Cook time: 0 minutes | Serves 4

Ingredients:
½ cup fresh green peas
½ cup grated Parmesan cheese
¼ cup extra-virgin olive oil
¼ cup pine nuts
¼ cup fresh basil leaves
2 garlic cloves, minced
¼ teaspoon sea salt

Directions:
Add all the ingredients to a food processor or blender and pulse until the nuts are chopped finely.
Transfer to an airtight container and refrigerate for up to 2 days. You can also store it in ice cube trays in the freezer for up to 6 months.

Per Serving:
calories: 247 | fat: 22.8g | protein: 7.1g | carbs: 4.8g | fiber: 1.0g | sodium: 337mg

Ranch-Style Cauliflower Dressing

Prep time: 10 minutes | Cook time: 0 minutes | Serves 8

Ingredients:

2 cups frozen cauliflower, thawed

½ cup unsweetened plain almond milk

2 tablespoons apple cider vinegar

2 tablespoons extra-virgin olive oil

garlic clove, peeled

teaspoons finely chopped fresh parsley

2 teaspoons finely chopped scallions (both white and green parts)

1 teaspoon finely chopped fresh dill

½ teaspoon onion powder

½ teaspoon Dijon mustard

½ teaspoon salt

¼ teaspoon freshly ground black pepper

Directions:

Place all the ingredients in a blender and pulse until creamy and smooth.

Serve immediately, or transfer to an airtight container to refrigerate for up to 3 days.

Per Serving: (2 tablespoons)

calories: 41 | fat: 3.6g | protein: 1.0g | carbs: 1.9g | fiber: 1.1g | sodium: 148mg

Asian-Inspired Vinaigrette

Prep time: 5 minutes | Cook time: 0 minutes | Serves 2

Ingredients:

¼ cup extra-virgin olive oil

3 tablespoons apple cider vinegar

1 garlic clove, minced

1 tablespoon peeled and grated fresh ginger

1 tablespoon chopped fresh cilantro

1 tablespoon freshly squeezed lime juice

½ teaspoon sriracha

Directions:

Add all the ingredients in a small bowl and stir to mix well.

Serve immediately, or store covered in the refrigerator and shake before using.

Per Serving:

calories: 251 | fat: 26.8g | protein: 0g | carbs: 1.8g | fiber: 0.7g | sodium: 3mg

Garlic Lemon-Tahini Dressing

Prep time: 5 minutes | Cook time: 0 minutes | Serves 8 to 10

Ingredients:

½ cup tahini

¼ cup extra-virgin olive oil

¼ cup freshly squeezed lemon juice

garlic clove, finely minced

teaspoons salt

Directions:

In a glass mason jar with a lid, combine the tahini, olive oil, lemon juice, garlic, and salt. Cover and shake well until combined and creamy. Store in the refrigerator for up to 2 weeks.

Per Serving:

calories: 121 | fat: 12.0g | protein: 2.0g | carbs: 3.0g | fiber: 1.0g | sodium: 479mg

Creamy Grapefruit and Tarragon Dressing

Prep time: 5 minutes | Cook time: 0 minutes | Serves 4 to 6

Ingredients:
½ cup avocado oil mayonnaise
2 tablespoons Dijon mustard
1 teaspoon dried tarragon or 1 tablespoon chopped fresh tarragon
½ teaspoon salt
Zest and juice of ½ grapefruit
¼ teaspoon freshly ground black pepper
1 to 2 tablespoons water (optional)

Directions:
In a large mason jar with a lid, combine the mayonnaise, Dijon, tarragon, grapefruit zest and juice, salt, and pepper and whisk well with a fork until smooth and creamy. If a thinner dressing is preferred, thin out with water.
Serve immediately or refrigerate until ready to serve.

Per Serving:
calories: 86 | fat: 7.0g | protein: 1.0g | carbs: 6.0g | fiber: 0g | sodium: 390mg

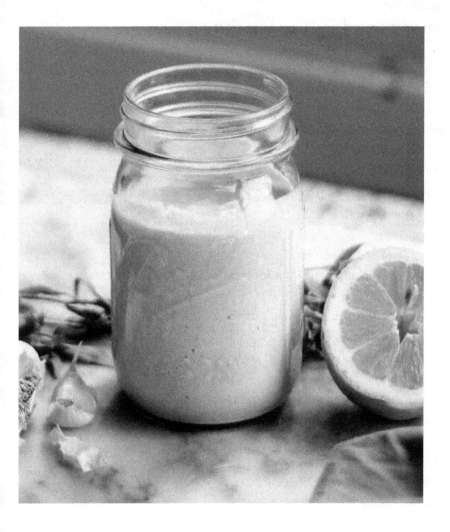

Peri-Peri Sauce

Prep time: 10 minutes | Cook time: 5 minutes | Serves 4

Ingredients:
1 tomato, chopped
1 red onion, chopped
1 red bell pepper, deseeded and chopped
1 red chile, deseeded and chopped
4 garlic cloves, minced
2 tablespoons extra-virgin olive oil
Juice of 1 lemon
1 tablespoon dried oregano
1 tablespoon smoked paprika
1 teaspoon sea salt

Directions:
Process all the ingredients in a food processor or a blender until smooth.
Transfer the mixture to a small saucepan over medium-high heat and bring to a boil, stirring often.
Reduce the heat to medium and allow to simmer for 5 minutes until heated through.
You can store the sauce in an airtight container in the refrigerator for up to 5 days.

Per Serving:
calories: 98 | fat: 6.5g | protein: 1.0g | carbs: 7.8g | fiber: 3.0g | sodium: 295mg

Lemon-Tahini Sauce

Prep time: 10 minutes | Cook time: 0 minutes | Makes 1 cup

Ingredients:
½ cup tahini
1 garlic clove, minced
Juice and zest of 1 lemon
½ teaspoon salt, plus more as needed
½ cup warm water, plus more as needed

Directions:
Combine the tahini and garlic in a small bowl.
Add the lemon juice and zest and salt to the bowl and stir to mix well.
Fold in the warm water and whisk until well combined and creamy.
Feel free to add more warm water if you like a thinner consistency.
Taste and add more salt as needed.
Store the sauce in a sealed container in the refrigerator for up to 5 days.

Per Serving: (¼ cup)
calories: 179 | fat: 15.5g | protein: 5.1g | carbs: 6.8g | fiber: 3.0g |
sodium: 324mg

Peanut Sauce with Honey

Prep time: 5 minutes | Cook time: 0 minutes | Serves 4

Ingredients:
¼ cup peanut butter
1 tablespoon peeled and grated fresh ginger
1 tablespoon honey
1 tablespoon low-sodium soy sauce
1 garlic clove, minced
Juice of 1 lime
Pinch red pepper flakes

Directions:
Whisk together all the ingredients in a small bowl until well incorporated.
Transfer to an airtight container and refrigerate for up to 5 days.

Per Serving:
calories: 117 | fat: 7.6g | protein: 4.1g | carbs: 8.8g | fiber: 1.0g | sodium: 136mg

Pineapple Salsa

Prep time: 10 minutes | Cook time: 0 minutes | Serves 6 to 8

Ingredients:
1 pound (454 g) fresh or thawed frozen pineapple, finely diced, juices reserved
1 white or red onion, finely diced
1 bunch cilantro or mint, leaves only, chopped
1 jalapeño, minced (optional)
Salt, to taste

Directions:
Stir together the pineapple with its juice, onion, cilantro, and jalapeño (if desired) in a medium bowl. Season with salt to taste and serve.
The salsa can be refrigerated in an airtight container for up to 2 days.

Per Serving:
calories: 55 | fat: 0.1g | protein: 0.9g | carbs: 12.7g | fiber: 1.8g | sodium: 20mg

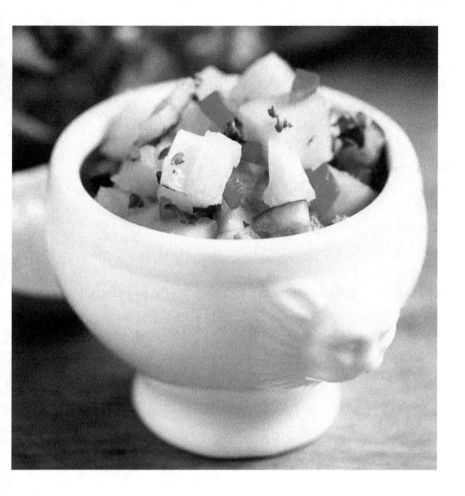

Vinaigrette

Prep time: 5 minutes | Cook time: 0 minutes | Makes 1 cup

Ingredients:
½ cup extra-virgin olive oil
¼ cup red wine vinegar
1 tablespoon Dijon mustard
1 teaspoon dried rosemary
½ teaspoon salt
½ teaspoon freshly ground black pepper

Directions:
In a cup or a mansion jar with a lid, combine the olive oil, vinegar, mustard, rosemary, salt, and pepper and shake until well combined. Serve chilled or at room temperature.

Per Serving:
calories: 124 | fat: 14.0g | protein: 0g | carbs: 1.0g | fiber: 0g | sodium: 170mg

Hot Pepper Sauce

Prep time: 10 minutes | Cook time: 20 minutes | Makes 4 cups

Ingredients:
2 red hot fresh chiles, deseeded
2 dried chiles
2 garlic cloves, peeled
½ small yellow onion, roughly chopped
2 cups water
2 cups white vinegar

Directions:
Place all the ingredients except the vinegar in a medium saucepan over medium heat. Allow to simmer for 20 minutes until softened.
Transfer the mixture to a food processor or blender. Stir in the vinegar and pulse until very smooth.
Serve immediately or transfer to a sealed container and refrigerate for up to 3 months.

Per Serving: (2 tablespoons)
calories: 20 | fat: 1.2g | protein: 0.6g | carbs: 4.4g | fiber: 0.6g | sodium: 12mg

Cilantro-Tomato Salsa

Prep time: 10 minutes | Cook time: 0 minutes | Serves 6

Ingredients:
2 or 3 medium, ripe tomatoes, diced
1 serrano pepper, seeded and minced
½ red onion, minced
¼ cup minced fresh cilantro
Juice of 1 lime
¼ teaspoon salt, plus more as needed

Directions:
Place the tomatoes, serrano pepper, onion, cilantro, lime juice, and salt in a small bowl and mix well.
Taste and add additional salt, if needed.
Store in an airtight container in the refrigerator for up to 3 days.

Per Serving: (¼ cup)
calories: 17 | fat: 0g | protein: 1.0g | carbs: 3.9g | fiber: 1.0g | sodium: 83mg

Lentil-Tahini Dip

Prep time: 10 minutes | Cook time: 15 minutes | Makes 3 cups

Ingredients:
1 cup dried green or brown lentils, rinsed
2½ cups water, divided
⅓ cup tahini
1 garlic clove
½ teaspoon salt, plus more as needed

Directions:
Add the lentils and 2 cups of water to a medium saucepan and bring to a boil over high heat.

Once it starts to boil, reduce the heat to low, and then cook for 14 minutes, stirring occasionally, or the lentils become tender but still hold their shape. You can drain any excess liquid.

Transfer the lentils to a food processor, along with the remaining water, tahini, garlic, and salt and process until smooth and creamy. Taste and adjust the seasoning if needed. Serve immediately.

Per Serving: (¼ cup)
calories: 100 | fat: 3.9g | protein: 5.1g | carbs: 10.7g | fiber: 6.0g | sodium: 106mg

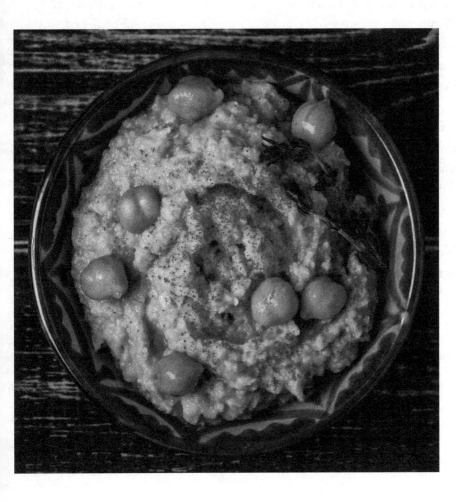

Lemon-Dill Cashew Dip

Prep time: 10 minutes | Cook time: 0 minutes | Makes 1 cup

Ingredients:

¾ cup cashews, soaked in water for at least 4 hours and drained well

¼ cup water

Juice and zest of 1 lemon

2 tablespoons chopped fresh dill

¼ teaspoon salt, plus more as needed

Directions:

Put the cashews, water, lemon juice and zest in a blender and blend until smooth.

Add the dill and salt to the blender and blend again.

Taste and adjust the seasoning, if needed.

Transfer to an airtight container and refrigerate for at least 1 hour to blend the flavors.

Serve chilled.

Per Serving: (1 tablespoon)

calories: 37 | fat: 2.9g | protein: 1.1g | carbs: 1.9g | fiber: 0g | sodium: 36mg

Basil Pesto

Prep time: 5 minutes | Cook time: 0 minutes | Makes 1 cup

Ingredients:
cups packed fresh basil leaves
garlic cloves, peeled
½ cup freshly grated Parmesan cheese
½ cup extra-virgin olive oil
⅓ cup pine nuts
Kosher salt and freshly ground black pepper, to taste

Directions:
Place all the ingredients, except for the salt and pepper, in a food processor. Pulse a few times until smoothly pur é ed. Season with salt and pepper to taste.
Store in an airtight container in the fridge for up to 2 weeks.

Per Serving:
calories: 100 | fat: 10.2g | protein: 2.2g | carbs: 1.2g | fiber: 0g | sodium: 72mg

Orange-Garlic Dressing

Prep time: 5 minutes | Cook time: 0 minutes | Serves 2

Ingredients:
¼ cup extra-virgin olive oil
orange, zested
tablespoons freshly squeezed orange juice
¾ teaspoon za'atar seasoning
1 teaspoon garlic powder
½ teaspoon salt
¼ teaspoon Dijon mustard
Freshly ground black pepper, to taste

Directions:
Whisk together all ingredients in a bowl until well combined.
Serve immediately or refrigerate until ready to serve.

Per Serving:
calories: 287 | fat: 26.7g | protein: 1.2g | carbs: 12.0g | fiber: 2.1g |
sodium: 592mg

Italian Dressing

Prep time: 5 minutes | Cook time: 0 minutes | Serves 12

Ingredients:
½ cup extra-virgin olive oil
¼ cup red wine vinegar
1 teaspoon dried Italian seasoning
1 teaspoon Dijon mustard
¼ teaspoon salt
¼ teaspoon freshly ground black pepper
1 garlic clove, minced

Directions:
Place all the ingredients in a mason jar and cover. Shake vigorously for 1 minute until completely mixed.
Store in the refrigerator for up to 1 week.

Per Serving: (1 tablespoon)
calories: 80 | fat: 8.6g | protein: 0g | carbs: 0g | fiber: 0g | sodium: 51mg

Parsley Vinaigrette

Prep time: 5 minutes | Cook time: 0 minutes | Makes about ½ cup

Ingredients:

½ cup lightly packed fresh parsley, finely chopped

⅓ cup extra-virgin olive oil

3 tablespoons red wine vinegar

1 garlic clove, minced

¼ teaspoon salt, plus additional as needed

Directions:

Place all the ingredients in a mason jar and cover. Shake vigorously for 1 minute until completely mixed.

Taste and add additional salt as needed.

Serve immediately or serve chilled.

Per Serving: (1 tablespoon)

calories: 92 | fat: 10.9g | protein: 0g | carbs: 0g | fiber: 0g | sodium: 75mg

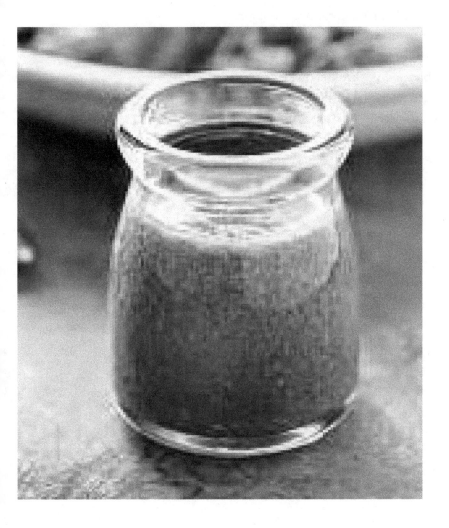

Tzatziki

Prep time: 15 minutes | Cook time: 0 minutes | Serves 4 to 6

Ingredients:

½ English cucumber, finely chopped

1 teaspoon salt, divided

1 cup plain Greek yogurt

8 tablespoons olive oil, divided

1 garlic clove, finely minced

1 to 2 tablespoons chopped fresh dill

1 teaspoon red wine vinegar

½ teaspoon freshly ground black pepper

Directions:

In a food processor, pulse the cucumber until puréed. Place the cucumber on several layers of paper towels lining the bottom of a colander and sprinkle with ½ teaspoon of salt. Allow to drain for 10 to 15 minutes. Using your hands, squeeze out any remaining liquid.

In a medium bowl, whisk together the cucumber, yogurt, 6 tablespoons of olive oil, garlic, dill, vinegar, remaining ½ teaspoon of salt, and pepper until very smooth.

Drizzle with the remaining 2 tablespoons of olive oil. Serve immediately or refrigerate until ready to serve.

Per Serving:

calories: 286 | fat: 29.0g | protein: 3.0g | carbs: 5.0g | fiber: 0g | sodium: 615mg

Guacamole

Prep time: 10 minutes | Cook time: 0 minutes | Serves 6

Ingredients:
2 large avocados
¼ white onion, finely diced
small, firm tomato, finely diced
¼ cup finely chopped fresh cilantro
tablespoons freshly squeezed lime juice
¼ teaspoon salt
Freshly ground black pepper, to taste

Directions:
Slice the avocados in half and remove the pits. Using a large spoon to scoop out the flesh and add to a medium bowl.
Mash the avocado flesh with the back of a fork, or until a uniform consistency is achieved. Add the onion, tomato, cilantro, lime juice, salt, and pepper to the bowl and stir to combine.
Serve immediately, or transfer to an airtight container and refrigerate until chilled.

Per Serving: (¼ cup)
calories: 81 | fat: 6.8g | protein: 1.1g | carbs: 5.7g | fiber: 3.0g | sodium: 83mg

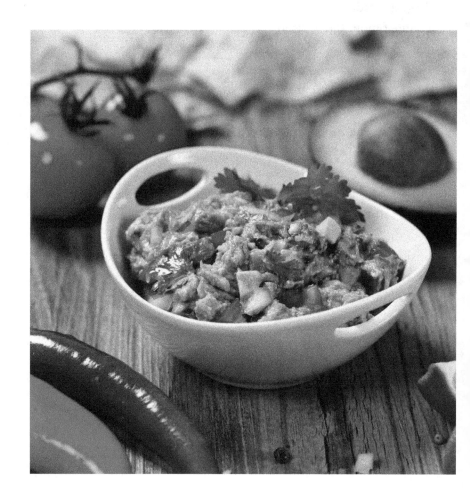

Creamy Cucumber Dip

Prep time: 10 minutes | Cook time: 0 minutes | Serves 6

Ingredients:
1 medium cucumber, peeled and grated
¼ teaspoon salt
cup plain Greek yogurt
garlic cloves, minced
1 tablespoon extra-virgin olive oil
1 tablespoon freshly squeezed lemon juice
¼ teaspoon freshly ground black pepper

Directions:
Place the grated cucumber in a colander set over a bowl and season with salt. Allow the cucumber to stand for 10 minutes. Using your hands, squeeze out as much liquid from the cucumber as possible. Transfer the grated cucumber to a medium bowl.
Add the yogurt, garlic, olive oil, lemon juice, and pepper to the bowl and stir until well blended.
Cover the bowl with plastic wrap and refrigerate for at least 2 hours to blend the flavors.
Serve chilled.

Per Serving: (¼ cup)
calories: 47 | fat: 2.8g | protein: 4.2g | carbs: 2.7g | fiber: 0g | sodium: 103mg

Creamy Cider Yogurt Dressing

Prep time: 5 minutes | Cook time: 0 minutes | Serves 2

Ingredients:
1 cup plain, unsweetened, full-fat Greek yogurt
½ cup extra-virgin olive oil
½ lemon, juiced
1 tablespoon chopped fresh oregano
1 tablespoon apple cider vinegar
½ teaspoon dried parsley
½ teaspoon kosher salt
¼ teaspoon garlic powder
¼ teaspoon freshly ground black pepper

Directions:
In a large bowl, whisk all ingredients to combine.
Serve chilled or at room temperature.

Per Serving:
calories: 407 | fat: 40.7g | protein: 8.3g | carbs: 3.8g | fiber: 0.5g |
sodium: 382mg

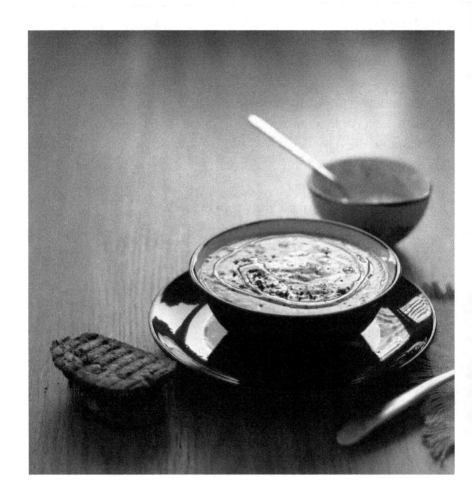

Harissa Sauce

Prep time: 10 minutes | Cook time: 20 minutes | Makes 3 to 4 cups

Ingredients:
1 large red bell pepper, deseeded, cored, and cut into chunks
1 yellow onion, cut into thick rings
4 garlic cloves, peeled
cup vegetable broth
tablespoons tomato paste
1 tablespoon tamari
1 teaspoon ground cumin
1 tablespoon Hungarian paprika

Directions:
Preheat the oven to 450°F (235°C). Line a baking sheet with parchment paper.
Place the bell pepper on the prepared baking sheet, flesh-side up, and space out the onion and garlic around the pepper.
Roast in the preheated oven for 20 minutes. Transfer to a blender.
Add the vegetable broth, tomato paste, tamari, cumin, and paprika.
Purée until smooth. Served chilled or warm.

Per Serving: (¼ cup)
calories: 15 | fat: 1.0g | protein: 1.0g | carbs: 3.0g | fiber: 1.0g | sodium: 201mg

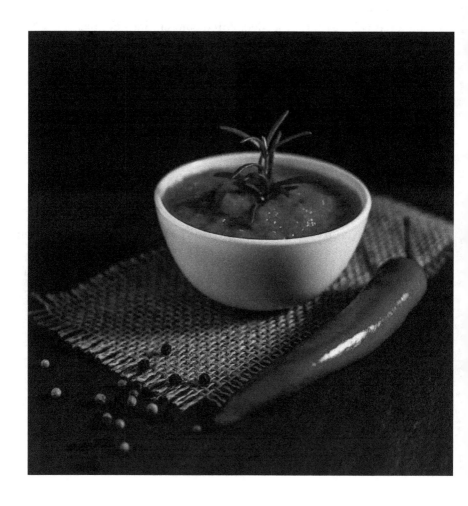

Basic French Vinaigrette

Prep time: 5 minutes | Cook time: 0 minutes | Serves 2

Ingredients:
3 tablespoons apple cider vinegar
2 tablespoons minced shallot (or 1 tablespoon minced red onion)
1 tablespoon balsamic vinegar
½ teaspoon dried thyme
1 teaspoon Dijon mustard
¼ cup olive oil
Salt and black pepper, to taste

Directions:
Stir together the apple cider vinegar, shallot, and balsamic vinegar in a medium jar with a tight-fitting lid. Allow to sit for 5 minutes.
Stir in the mustard and thyme. Whisk in the olive oil in a slow, steady stream and season to taste with salt and pepper.
Store in an airtight container in the fridge for up to 5 days.

Per Serving:
calories: 256 | fat: 27.1g | protein: 0.3g | carbs: 3.4g | fiber: 0.4g | sodium: 207mg

CPSIA information can be obtained
at www.ICGtesting.com
Printed in the USA
LVHW081957100521
686587LV00025B/102